Monoclonal Antibodies
for Cancer Detection and Therapy

Contributors

N. C. Armitage
Ruth Arnon
Bernard Aubert
Florent Aubry
J. Aubry
K. D. Bagshawe
R. W. Baldwin
L. Barrelet
Jean Pierre Bazin
R. H. J. Begent
J. Berthe
A. Bischof-Delaloye
H. E. Blythman
A. R. Bradwell
K. E. Britton
F. Buchegger
Joy M. Burchell
X. Canat
P. Carayon
S. Carrel
D. Carriere
P. Casellas
J. F. Chatal
C. Curtet
B. Delaloye
J. M. Derocq
Robert Di Paola
J. Y. Douillard
D. Dussossoy
P. W. Dykes
M. J. Embleton
D. S. Fairweather
A. A. Fauser
M. C. Garnett
N. C. Gorin
M. Granowska
J.-Ph. Grob
O. Gros

P. Gros
J. D. Hardcastle
Ingegerd Hellström
Karl Erik Hellström
Esther Hurwitz
F. K. Jansen
S. Junqua
J. T. Kemshead
M. Kremer
G. Laurent
J. C. Laurent
B. Le Mevel
J. B. Le Pecq
M. C. Liance
Jean Lumbroso
Jean-Pierre Mach
C. Maurel
Chris Myers
Stanley E. Order
Claude Parmentier
A. C. Perkins
Jean Daniel Piekarski
M. V. Pimm
P. Poncelet
B. Remandet
Marcel Ricard
G. Richer
Philippe Rougier
G. F. Rowland
Jean Claude Saccavini
J. Shepherd
R. G. Simmonds
Joyce Taylor-Papadimitriou
Maurice Tubiana
T. Tursz
H. Vidal
V. von Fliedner
J. Wiels
P. Wils

Monoclonal Antibodies for Cancer Detection and Therapy

Edited by

R. W. BALDWIN

Cancer Research Campaign Laboratories
University of Nottingham
Nottingham, United Kingdom

VERA S. BYERS

Xoma Corporation
Berkeley, California

1985

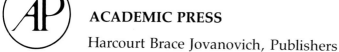

ACADEMIC PRESS

Harcourt Brace Jovanovich, Publishers

London   Orlando   San Diego   New York
Austin   Montreal   Sydney   Tokyo   Toronto

ACADEMIC PRESS INC. (LONDON) LTD.
24–28 Oval Road
LONDON NW1 7DX

United States Edition published by
ACADEMIC PRESS, INC.
Orlando, Florida 32887

British Library Cataloguing in Publication Data

Monoclonal antibodies for cancer detection and
    therapy.
    1. Cancer–Diagnosis   2. Cancer–Treatment
    3. Antibodies, Monoclonal
    I. Baldwin, R. W.   II. Byers, Vera S.
    616.99'4   RC271.A6/

Library of Congress Cataloging in Publication Data
Main entry under title:

Monoclonal antibodies for cancer detection and therapy.

    Includes index.
    1. Cancer.   2. Antibodies, Monoclonal–Diagnostic
use.   3. Antibodies, Monoclonal–Therapeutic use.
I. Baldwin, R. W. (Robert William), Date.
II. Byers, Vera S.   [DNLM: 1. Antibodies, Monoclonal
–diagnostic use.   2. Antibodies, Monoclonal–
therapeutic use.   3. Neoplasms–diagnosis.   4. Neoplasms–
therapy. QZ 266 M751]
RC262.M665   1985   616.99'4   85-6207
ISBN 0–12–077020–2 (alk. paper)
ISBN 0–12–077021–0 (paperback)

PRINTED IN THE UNITED STATES OF AMERICA

85 86 87 88   9 8 7 6 5 4 3 2 1

Contents

Contributors

Numbers in parentheses indicate the pages on which the authors' contributions begin.

N. C. Armitage (129), Department of Surgery, University Hospital, Queen's Medical Centre, Nottingham NG7 2UH, United Kingdom

Ruth Arnon (365), Department of Chemical Immunology, The Weizmann Institute of Science, Rehovot 76100, Israel

Bernard Aubert (87), Institut Gustave-Roussy, and Unité de Recherches de Radiobiologie Clinique, INSERM U66, 94805 Villejuif, France

Florent Aubry (87), Institut Gustave-Roussy, and Unité de Recherches de Radiobiologie Clinique, INSERM U66, 94805 Villejuif, France

J. Aubry (159), Unité 211 INSERM, 44035 Nantes, France

K. D. Bagshawe (181), Cancer Research Campaign Laboratories, Department of Medical Oncology, Charing Cross Hospital, London W6 8RF, United Kingdom

R. W. Baldwin (97, 129), Cancer Research Campaign Laboratories, University of Nottingham, Nottingham NG7 2RD, United Kingdom

L. Barrelet (53), Ludwig Institute for Cancer Research, 1066 Epalinges, Lausanne, Switzerland, and Policlinique Médicale Universitaire and Division of Nuclear Medicine, 1011 Lausanne, Switzerland

Jean Pierre Bazin (87), Institut Gustave-Roussy, and Unité de Recherches de Radiobiologie Clinique, INSERM U66, 94805 Villejuif, France

R. H. J. Begent (181), Cancer Research Campaign Laboratories, Department of Medical Oncology, Charing Cross Hospital, London W6 8RF, United Kingdom

J. Berthe (223), Department of Toxicology, Centre de Recherches Clin. Midy, Groupe Sanofi, 34082 Montpellier, France

A. Bischof-Delaloye (53), Ludwig Institute for Cancer Research, 1066 Epalinges, Lausanne, Switzerland, and Policlinique Médicale Universitaire and Division of Nuclear Medicine, 1011 Lausanne, Switzerland

H. E. Blythman (223), Immunotoxin Project, Centre de Recherches Clin. Midy, Groupe Sanofi, 34082 Montpellier, France

A. R. Bradwell (65), Immunodiagnostic Research Laboratory, Department of Immunology, Medical School, University of Birmingham, Birmingham B15 2TH, United Kingdom

K. E. Britton (201), Department of Nuclear Medicine, St. Bartholomew's Hospital, London EC1A 7BE, United Kingdom

F. Buchegger (53), Ludwig Institute for Cancer Research, 1066 Epalinges, Lausanne, Switzerland

Joy M. Burchell (1), Imperial Cancer Research Fund Laboratories, London WC2A 3PX, United Kingdom

X. Canat (223), Immunotoxin Project, Centre de Recherches Clin. Midy, Groupe Sanofi, 34082 Montpellier, France

P. Carayon (223), Immunotoxin Project, Centre de Recherches Clin. Midy, Groupe Sanofi, 34082 Montpellier, France

S. Carrel (53), Ludwig Institute for Cancer Research, 1066 Epalinges, Lausanne, Switzerland

D. Carriere (223), Department of Toxicology, Centre de Recherches Clin. Midy, Groupe Sanofi, 34082 Montpellier, France

P. Casellas (223), Immunotoxin Project, Centre de Recherches Clin. Midy, Groupe Sanofi, 34082 Montpellier, France

J. F. Chatal (159), Unité 211 INSERM, 44035 Nantes, France, and Centre René Gauducheau, 44035 Nantes, France

C. Curtet (159), Unité 211 INSERM, 44035 Nantes, France, and Centre René Gauducheau, 44035 Nantes, France

B. Delaloye (53), Ludwig Institute for Cancer Research, 1066 Epalinges, Lausanne, Switzerland, and Policlinique Médicale Universitaire and Division of Nuclear Medicine, 1011 Lausanne, Switzerland

J. M. Derocq (223), Immunotoxin Project, Centre de Recherches Clin. Midy, Groupe Sanofi, 34082 Montpellier, France

Robert Di Paola (87), Institut Gustave-Roussy, and Unité de Recherches de Radiobiologie Clinique, INSERM U66, 94805 Villejuif, France

J. Y. Douillard (159), Unité 211 INSERM, 44035 Nantes, France, and Centre René Gauducheau, 44035 Nantes, France

D. Dussossoy (223), Immunotoxin Project, Centre de Recherches Clin. Midy, Groupe Sanofi, 34082 Montpellier, France

P. W. Dykes (65), Immunodiagnostic Research Laboratory, Department of Immunology, Medical School, University of Birmingham, Birmingham B15 2TH, United Kingdom

M. J. Embleton (317), Cancer Research Campaign Laboratories, University of Nottingham, Nottingham NG7 2RD, United Kingdom

D. S. Fairweather[1] (65), Immunodiagnostic Research Laboratory, Department of Immunology, Medical School, University of Birmingham, Birmingham B15 2TH, United Kingdom

A. A. Fauser (223), Med. Univ. Klinik, Freiburg, Federal Republic of Germany

M. C. Garnett (317), Cancer Research Campaign Laboratories, University of Nottingham, Nottingham NG7 2RD, United Kingdom

N. C. Gorin (223), Hôpital St. Antoine, Paris 75012, France

M. Granowska (201), Department of Nuclear Medicine, St. Bartholomew's Hospital, London EC1A 7BE, United Kingdom

J. -Ph. Grob (53), Ludwig Institute for Cancer Research, 1066 Epalinges, Lausanne, Switzerland

O. Gros (223), Immunotoxin Project, Centre de Recherches Clin. Midy, Groupe Sanofi, 34082 Montpellier, France

P. Gros (223), Immunotoxin Project, Centre de Recherches Clin. Midy, Groupe Sanofi, 34082 Montpellier, France

J. D. Hardcastle (129), Department of Surgery, University Hospital, Queen's Medical Centre, Nottingham NG7 2UH, United Kingdom

Ingegerd Hellström (17), ONCOGEN, Seattle, Washington 98121 U.S.A., and Departments of Pathology and Microbiology/Immunology, University of Washington, Seattle, Washington 98195 U.S.A.

Karl Erik Hellström (17), ONCOGEN, Seattle, Washington 98121 U.S.A., and Departments of Pathology and Microbiology/Immunology, University of Washington, Seattle, Washington 98195 U.S.A.

Esther Hurwitz (365), Department of Chemical Immunology, The Weizmann Institute of Science, Rehovot 76100, Israel

F. K. Jansen (223), Immunotoxin Project, Centre de Recherches Clin. Midy, Groupe Sanofi, 34082 Montpellier, France

S. Junqua (269), Laboratoire de Physico-Chimie Macromoléculaire, Institut Gustave-Roussy, 94805 Villejuif, France

J. T. Kemshead (281), Imperial Cancer Research Fund Laboratories, Oncology Laboratory, Institute of Child Health, London WC1, United Kindom

M. Kremer (159), Unité 211 INSERM, 44035 Nantes, France, and Centre René Gauducheau, 44035 Nantes, France

G. Laurent (223), Immunotoxin Project, Centre de Recherches Clin. Midy, Groupe Sanofi, 34082 Montpellier, France

[1]Present address: Department of Geriatric Medicine, University Hospital of South Manchester, Manchester M20 8LR, United Kingdom.

J. C. Laurent (223), Immunotoxin Project, Centre de Recherches Clin.
  Midy, Groupe Sanofi, 34082 Montpellier, France
B. Le Mevel (159), Unité 211 INSERM, 44035 Nantes, France, and Centre
  René Gauducheau, 44035 Nantes, France
J. B. Le Pecq (269), Laboratoire de Physico-Chimie Macromoléculaire,
  Institut Gustave-Roussy, 94805 Villejuif, France
M. C. Liance (223), Immunotoxin Project, Centre de Recherches Clin.
  Midy, Groupe Sanofi, 34082 Montpellier, France
Jean Lumbroso (87), Institut Gustave-Roussy, and Unité de Recherches
  de Radiobiologie Clinique, INSERM U66, 94805 Villejuif, France
Jean-Pierre Mach (53, 87), Ludwig Institute for Cancer Research, 1066
  Epalinges, Lausanne, Switzerland
C. Maurel (159), Unité 211 INSERM, 44035 Nantes, France
Chris Myers[2] (249), Membrane Immunology Laboratory, Imperial Cancer
  Research Fund, London, WC2A 3PX, United Kindom
Stanley E. Order (303), Radiation Oncology, The Johns Hopkins Hospital
  Oncology Center, Baltimore Maryland 21205, U.S.A.
Claude Parmentier (87), Institut Gustave-Roussy, and Unité de Re-
  cherches de Radiobiologie Clinique, INSERM U66, 94805 Villejuif,
  France
A. C. Perkins (129), Department of Medical Physics, University Hospital,
  Queen's Medical Centre, Nottingham NG7 2UH, United Kingdom
Jean Daniel Piekarski (87), Institut Gustave-Roussy, and Unité de Re-
  cherches de Radiobiologie Clinique, INSERM U66, 94805 Villejuif,
  France
M. V. Pimm (97, 129), Cancer Research Campaign Laboratories, Uni-
  versity of Nottingham, Nottingham NG7 2RD, United Kingdom
P. Poncelet (223), Immunotoxin Project, Centre de Recherches Clin.
  Midy, Groupe Sanofi, 34082 Montpellier, France
B. Remandet (223), Department of Toxicology, Centre de Recherches
  Clin. Midy, Groupe Sanofi, 34082 Montpellier, France
Marcel Ricard (87), Institut Gustave-Roussy, and Unité de Recherches
  de Radiobiologie Clinique, INSERM U66, 94805 Villejuif, France
G. Richer (223), Immunotoxin Project, Centre de Recherches Clin. Midy,
  Groupe Sanofi, 34082 Montpellier, France
Philippe Rougier (87), Institut Gustave-Roussy, and Unité de Recherches
  de Radiobiologie Clinique, INSERM U66, 94805 Villejuif, France
G. F. Rowland[3] (345), Lilly Research Centre Ltd., Eli Lilly and Co., Win-
  dlesham, Surrey GU20 6PH, United Kingdom

[2]Present address: Department of Microbiology, University of Texas Health Science Center
at Dallas, Dallas, Texas 75235, U.S.A.
[3]Present address: Department of Biochemistry, University of Stellenbosch, Stellenbosch,
South Africa, 7600.

Jean Claude Saccavini (87, 159), Office des Rayonnements Ionisants, 91190 Gif-sur-Yvette, France

J. Shepherd (201), Department of Nuclear Medicine and Department of Gynaecological Surgery, St. Bartholomew's Hospital, London EC1A 7BE, United Kingdom

R. G. Simmonds (345), Lilly Research Centre Ltd., Eli Lilly and Co., Windlesham, Surrey GU20 6PH, United Kingdom

Joyce Taylor-Papadimitriou (1), Imperial Cancer Research Fund Laboratories, London WC2A 3PX, United Kingdom

Maurice Tubiana (87), Institut Gustave-Roussy, and Unité de Recherches de Radiobiologie Clinique, INSERM U66, 94805 Villejuif, France

T. Tursz (269), Laboratoire d'Immuno-Biologie des Tumeurs, Institut Gustave-Roussy, 94805 Villejuif, France

H. Vidal (223), Immunotoxin Project, Centre de Recherches Clin. Midy, Groupe Sanofi, 34082 Montpellier, France

V. von Fliedner (53), Ludwig Institute for Cancer Research, 1066 Epalinges, Lausanne, Switzerland

J. Wiels (269), Laboratoire d'Immuno-Biologie des Tumeurs, Institut Gustave-Roussy, 94805 Villejuif, France

P. Wils (269), Laboratoire de Physico-Chimie Macromoléculaire, Institut Gustave-Roussy, 94805 Villejuif, France

Preface

The notion that antibodies recognising antigens associated with tumours may be used for targeting diagnostic and/or therapeutic agents has been under investigation for many years. These approaches have gained fresh impetus with the developments in hybridoma technology, since it is now feasible to produce unlimited amounts of monoclonal antibodies which recognise antigenic determinants associated with human malignant cells. Originally it was anticipated that fusion of spleen cells, from donors (typically mice or rats) immunized with human tumour cells or subcellular fractions, with cultured myeloma cells of the appropriate species would readily yield monoclonal antibodies reacting specifically with a particular tumour. In most instances, however, hybridomas produce antibodies showing restricted, but not necessarily tumour-specific, reactivities. This is exemplified by the extensive studies on malignant melanoma, where melanoma-specific antibodies have still to be described. Also monoclonal antibodies against breast cancer and osteogenic sarcoma react with a range of tumours. Methods for producing monoclonal antibodies with improved tumour specificity continue to be researched, and this includes the development of human monoclonal antibodies following 'immortalizing' human B lymphocytes by various means. Even so, the reviews presented in this book demonstrate very clearly that, notwithstanding the limitation of the monoclonal antibodies currently available, their applications for cancer detection and therapy represent a potential major advance in the management of cancer patients. Particularly impressive are the advances being made in the application of radiolabelled monoclonal antibodies for tumour detection using gamma camera imaging procedures. This is clearly illustrated in three independent trials on colorectal cancer patients, whilst studies in ovarian cancer and malignant melanoma attest to the potential of immunoscintigraphy. The overall impression gained from these trials is that immunoscintigraphy 'works' and further refinements in technique will aid in the overall evaluation of the clinical application of the technique in comparison with other diagnostic methods. These include the use of antibody fragments [Fab and F(ab')$_2$] as well as radiolabelling of antibodies with a range of radionuclides, especially ^{111}In. This radionuclide is more suitable than ^{131}I for gamma camera imaging, and its use in a number of trials has made possible tumour imaging without the use of blood pool subtraction techniques, which can introduce artefacts. ^{111}In-Labelled antibodies are also more suitable for emission tomography, which provides the opportunity to obtain three-dimensional images of antibody distribution. The improvements in immunoscintigraphic technology described in the book indicate that a critical assessment of the potential of these procedures for tumour detection will soon be forthcoming.

A second major advance is the application of monoclonal antibodies for therapy. Here the situation is potentially exciting, although one senses that more basic developments are required before a critical evaluation of antibody-mediated therapy is possible. The therapeutic potential of unmodified monoclonal antibodies *in vivo* is still far from clear, apart from the one lymphoma patient treated with a mouse anti-idiotypic monoclonal antibody. There are, however, well-documented applications *in vitro*, where monoclonal antibodies are being used to eliminate unwanted cell populations from bone marrow cells used for reconstitution of patients following high-dose chemotherapy and radiotherapy. This approach is exemplified by the use of a monoclonal antibody reacting with neuroblastoma cells coupled to polystyrene beads containing a magnetic material for eliminating neuroblastoma cells from bone marrow preparations.

A major objective of many investigations reviewed in the book is to develop methods for targeting therapeutic agents, which include radioactive isotopes and cytotoxic agents. Administration of monoclonal antibodies carrying therapeutic levels of radioisotope is being attempted and, for example, has been used to treat patients with malignant pleural and pericardiac effusions in ovarian cancer. The alternative approach of monoclonal antibody targeting of cytotoxic agents is being actively explored using either 'conventional' chemotherapeutic agents or highly cytotoxic molecules, such as plant toxins. These investigations are described in considerable detail with respect to methods of antibody coupling to cytotoxic agents. These studies validate the concept of using monoclonal antibodies for targeting cytotoxic agents, but further refinements in the design of these immunocytotoxic agents are clearly desirable. In the meanwhile, therapeutic potential of a range of immunocytotoxics can be evaluated against a range of human tumour xenografts, so providing the basis for establishing clinical trials.

R. W. Baldwin
Vera S. Byers

CHAPTER 1

Monoclonal Antibodies to Breast Cancer and Their Application

Joy M. Burchell and Joyce Taylor-Papadimitriou

Imperial Cancer Research Fund Laboratories
London, United Kingdom

I. INTRODUCTION

One out of eleven women in Great Britain and the United States will develop breast cancer during her lifetime and it accounts for 27% of all cancers that develop in women (Leis, 1981). Since tumours which are diagnosed before they have become invasive have a better prognosis, there is considerable interest in developing reagents which would be effective in early diagnosis. Moreover, since those women who do show lymph node involvement form a heterogeneous group, there is also a need for prognostic indicators which would aid in the management of the disease. Thus, in addition to their potential as drug targeting agents, monoclonal antibodies to breast tumour antigens may be powerful tools for the detection and subclassification of breast cancers.

Although a large number of monoclonals directed to breast tumour antigens have been developed (see Table I) nearly all are tumour associated rather than tumour specific and, where a high specificity for tu-

1

TABLE I

MONOCLONAL ANTIBODIES TO BREAST CANCER

Antibody	Immunogen	Antigenic determinant	Reference
10-302 (and others)	BT20 cells	10-302 present in 126-kDa protein	Soule and Edgington, 1982
MBr1	MCF-7 cells	Carbohydrate	Menard et al., 1983; Canevari et al., 1983
MBr2	MCF-7 cells		Menard et al., 1983
MBr3			
F36/22	MCF-7 cells and SK-Br-3 cells		Papsidero et al., 1983
H7/105			
H59	ZR-75-1	30K	Yuan et al., 1982
24-17-1	MCF-7 cells	95K	Thompson et al., 1983
24-17-2		100K	
B series of monoclonals including B6.2, B72.3	Membrane fraction of breast tumour metastases to the liver	B72.3 present on 220–400-kDa protein. B6.2–90K	Colcher et al., 1981; Nuti et al., 1982
M18	Human milk fat globule	I(MA) blood group determinant	Foster et al., 1982; Gooi et al., 1983; Foster and Neville, 1984
M39			Foster et al., 1982
M8	Human milk fat globule		
HMFG-1	Human milk fat globule	Carbohydrate antigen on large molecular weight molecule (>400K)	Taylor-Papadimitriou et al., 1981; Burchell et al., 1983
HMFG-2			
MAM series	Human milk fat globule	Some recognise a large molecular weight component	Hilkens et al., 1984
Mc3	Human milk fat globule	46K	Ceriani et al., 1982
Human monoclonal antibodies	—	—	Schlom et al., 1980

mours is claimed (Colcher *et al.*, 1981; Nuti *et al.*, 1982), some primary tumours show no reaction and metastases from positive primary tumours may become negative. The available antibodies to breast cancer can be divided into four groups: (1) Those that have been derived by immunizing the mouse with whole tumour cells, either in the form of cell lines derived from breast cancers or tumour cells taken directly from the patient; (2) antibodies that have been derived by using membrane-enriched fractions of breast tumour cells; (3) human monoclonal antibodies generated by the fusion of lymphocytes, obtained from lymph nodes of mastectomy patients, with mouse myeloma cells; and (4) antibodies which have been derived by using human milk fat globule as the antigen which is an easily accessible source of plasma membrane from terminally differentiated breast epithelial cells (Table I). Although the latter components have been raised against normal components of the differentiated membrane, they have been useful for *in vivo* imaging of breast carcinomas (Epenetos *et al.*, 1982a; Rainsbury *et al.*, 1983) and the HMFG-2 monoclonal antibody has been especially useful in the imaging of ovarian carcinomas (Epenetos *et al.*, 1982a; Granowska *et al.*, 1983; Pateisky *et al.*, 1983).

II. NATURE OF THE ANTIGENIC DETERMINANTS

Attempts to raise monoclonals which might be useful for drug targeting have focussed on membrane antigens, since an interaction with the cell membrane is a necessary prerequisite for specific delivery of highly toxic substances like ricin. However, antibodies to intracellular components, such as the intermediate filament proteins, and to extracellular matrix components found in the vicinity of the tumour are being used in tumour diagnosis and localisation (Gatter *et al.*, 1982). The cytokeratins which form the intermediate filaments of epithelial cells are members of a large family of proteins. Since these proteins are only found in epithelial (and mesothelial) cells (Sun and Green, 1978; Franke *et al.*, 1978), they can be very effective diagnostic tools discriminating between carcinomas and lymphomas (Gatter *et al.*, 1982). They also have potential for discriminating between carcinomas from different tissues and for identifying the target cells within a tissue (Taylor-Papadimitriou *et al.*, 1983). Anti-keratin antibodies are also beginning to be used for tumour localisation where presumably they can only be effective where there is extensive necrosis. Their advantage lies in the fact they are expressed consistently on epithelial cells and are not lost in the change to malignancy (Osborn and Weber, 1982).

The antibodies listed in Table I are all directed to components of the cell membrane and many of them react with carbohydrate antigens (Gooi et al., 1983; Canevari et al., 1983; Burchell et al., 1983; Foster and Neville, 1984). The fact that so many of the antibodies showing some specificity for tumour cell membranes are directed to oligosaccharide determinants is interesting in view of the fact that alterations in carbohydrate residues have been observed in differentiation (Kapadia et al., 1981; Feizi, 1981; Boland et al., 1982) and in malignancy (Springer et al., 1975; Feizi et al., 1979; Javadpour, 1983). In general, these antigenic determinants have been better characterised than the polypeptide antigens recognised by monoclonal antibodies which are usually only identified by the molecular weight of the protein.

The monoclonal antibodies HMFG-1 and HMFG-2 react with oligo-saccharide determinants present on a large molecular weight component (>400K) of human milk fat globule. This protein has been described as a mucin-like molecule, containing at least 50% carbohydrate (Shimizu and Yamauchi, 1982), and appears to be highly immunogenic as M8, M18, M39 and the MAM-6 series of monoclonal antibodies may also be directed towards determinants carried on this protein. HMFG-1 has a greater number of binding sites on this mucin-like molecule than HMFG-2 and reacts strongly with lactating breast but only weakly with resting breast, while the HMFG-2 determinant is more strongly expressed on carcinoma cells and can be carried on a range of molecular weight proteins (80–300K). Thus, the HMFG-1 monoclonal may recognise an oligosac-charide determinant present on a large, complex carbohydrate side chain which is more representative of normal differentiation, while the HMFG-2 antibody may recognise an antigen present on a simpler carbohydrate side chain which may represent an abortive attempt at correct glyco-sylation by the malignant cell.

From lectin-blocking experiments it has been shown that sialic acid may form part of the HMFG-2 determinant (Burchell et al., 1983) and the M18 determinant present on the luminal plasma membranes of ep-ithelial cells in the normal breast has been shown to be masked by sialic acid in some types of mammary carcinoma (Foster and Neville, 1984). This is of interest as it has been shown that sialylation of cellular gly-coproteins is increased in a variety of tumours (Yogeeswaran and Salk, 1981) and sialylation of particular carbohydrate residues on tumour cells may facilitate their metastatic spread (Altevogt et al., 1983).

The tumour-associated monoclonal antibodies that react with carbo-hydrate residues may be reflecting changes in the pattern of activity of

glycosyltransferases associated with the malignant change. These antibodies may prove to be very useful for tumour imaging, as a single oligosaccharide sequence can be repeated many times on the same molecule, thus increasing the number of sites available for antibody binding.

The large number of antibodies reacting with carbohydrate determinants is indicative of the highly immunogenic nature of certain oligo-
saccharide sequences in the mouse (Brockhaus *et al.*, 1982). One approach
to obtaining a monoclonal antibody which is tumour specific may be to
change the species of the spleen donor and so perhaps reveal a new
profile of immunogenic determinants. In this context, it is interesting to
note that most investigators have used BALB/c mice, and the rather
unique monoclonal B6.2 was obtained using the C57 black strain.

A. Specificity of the Monoclonal Antibody

Since the antibodies which have been developed so far are not tumour
specific, at least as judged by their reaction with tissue sections, they
are clearly not appropriate vehicles for the targeting of toxins. They may,
however, be suitable for targeting of some cytotoxic drugs, and are being
used quite effectively for *in vivo* imaging of carcinomas where some cross-
reactivity can be tolerated if it is not adjacent to the area to be scanned.
In fact, antibodies may show a more restricted reaction *in vivo* compared
to their spectrum of reactivity as judged by immunohistological staining
of tissue sections. For example, the HMFG-2 antibody has been successfully used in the imaging of ovarian carcinoma although this antibody
reacts with a component present on normal ovarian tubules in tissue
sections. In the normal ovary, antigens found lining the tubules are not
exposed to the bloodstream and only in the malignant change when the
normal architecture of the tissue is disrupted is the antibody afforded
access to its antigen. Another factor which may restrict access of the
antibody to normal cells is that epithelial cells commonly secrete mucins
which form a barrier over the cells and prevent access of the antibody
to the cell membrane.

B. Affinity

In order to obtain efficient tumour imaging and drug targeting, it is
important to use an antibody which shows high-affinity binding to its
antigen. It is important to remember that a monoclonal antibody is di-

rected to a specific epitope, and when this is oligosaccharide in nature, it may be expressed on several molecules which can vary in molecular weight and in their affinity for the antibody. We have, therefore, measured the rate of dissociation of purified iodinated HMFG-1 and HMFG-2 from normal breast epithelial cells and from cell lines derived from metastatic breast cancers. It has been shown (Froese *et al.*, 1978; Mason and Williams, 1980; Burchell *et al.*, 1983) that differences in the antibody's affinity are due mainly to differences in the rates of dissociation from the antigen. Thus, by measuring the rate of dissociation, an idea of relative affinities can be obtained. As seen in Fig. 1A and 1B, both antibodies bind to normal breast epithelial cells with relatively high affinity but each antibody shows differing affinities in its binding to breast cancer cell lines. Thus, HMFG-1 binds with low affinity to T47D cells but shows relatively high-affinity binding on ZR-75-1 and MCF-7 cells. This may well be important in deciding on the time to image patients as the period of time that an antibody will remain bound to a tumour may differ with the individual.

The affinity of an antibody may also play a part in deciding whether subtraction techniques should be employed in *in vivo* imaging. The advantage of using ^{131}I is that it has a half-life of 13 days; thus, scanning may be carried out a few days after the administration of the antibody by which time non-specific radioactivity should have been cleared from the blood pool. This requires a very high-affinity antibody that remains bound to the antigen for a number of days and for the antigen to be carried on a molecule with a long metabolic half-life.

III. APPLICATIONS OF THE MONOCLONAL ANTIBODIES

A. Tumour Targeting

Colcher *et al.*, (1983; Schlom *et al.*, 1983) described the successful localisation of the ^{125}I-labelled monoclonal antibody B6.2 to human mammary tumours transplanted into athymic mice. Using intact IgG, tumour : tissue ratios of 10 : 1 were achieved in the liver, spleen and kidneys but lower tumour : blood ratios were obtained. No localisation was seen when normal mouse immunoglobulin was used and iodinated B6.2 did not localize to a human melanoma transplanted into the mice. Higher tumour : tissue ratios were observed when using F(ab')₂ fragments of B6.2 to localize mammary tumours, but the use of Fab fragments resulted in large amounts of label in the kidney and bladder.

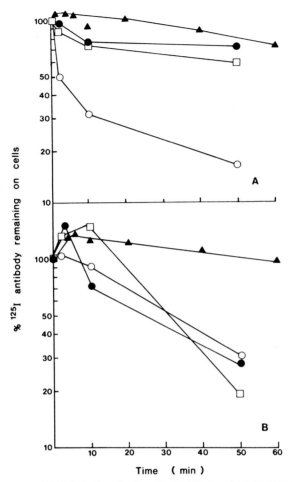

Fig. 1. Dissociation of ^{125}I-labelled antibodies (A) HMFG-1 and (B) HMFG-2, after binding to □—□ MCF-7, ●—● ZR-75-1, ○—○ T47D, ▲—▲ normal breast epithelial cells from human milk. Cells were incubated for 40 min with ^{125}I-labelled antibody, then 1000 times excess of cold antibody was added and radioactivity associated with the cells was measured at times indicated.

The M8 antibody raised at the Ludwig Institute (Foster *et al.*, 1982) has been used to locate metastatic breast carcinomas (Rainsbury *et al.*, 1983). All 10 patients with skeletal metastases, as confirmed by X-rays and MDP scans, showed positive scans with the indium-labelled monoclonal antibody which also localized to the primary tumour, although soft tissue metastases were not detectable on the antibody scans of any of the patients. In this study, Rainsbury *et al.* were able to visualize some bone metastases that conventional techniques did not detect (and vice versa). Thus, the combination of antibody imaging with X-rays and MDP scans may increase the number of bone metastases that are identified.

Trials using the HMFG-2 monoclonal antibody to image local skin metastases in patients with breast carcinoma are now underway at Guy's Hospital in London. Preliminary studies with ^{123}I-labelled HMFG-2 have been unsuccessful and this may be due to the limited blood supply associated with this type of secondary tumour because of its extreme necrotic nature.

One of the most successful applications of a monoclonal antibody directed towards a breast differentiation antigen has been in the localization of tumours, not from the breast, but of ovarian origin (Epenetos *et al.*, 1982a; Granowska *et al.*, 1983; Pateisky *et al.*, 1983). Although this is discussed in detail in a separate chapter, it is interesting to note that in one study the HMFG-2 antibody, labelled with ^{123}I has been used to successfully locate 20 out of 22 ovarian tumours and their metastasis as confirmed by surgery (Granowska *et al.*, 1983). Benign lesions are, however, also localized with the antibody, thus limiting its application to ascertaining the extent and spread of a tumour rather than in preliminary diagnosis. The success obtained with the HMFG-2 antibody in this study can be attributed to a number of factors which include: (1) It is a relatively high-affinity antibody and there are a large number of antigenic sites on the tumour cells; (2) the antibody does not react with normal tissue *in vivo* to a sufficient extent to be detected by imaging; and (3) the ovaries are situated away from the central blood pool thus making images easier to interpret.

B. Monoclonal Antibodies in Therapy

Some success in the inhibition of tumour growth after the administration of a monoclonal antibody has been reported in animals and humans (Herlyn *et al.*, 1980; Miller *et al.*, 1982). Recently, Capone *et al.*, (1983) showed that the passive administration of the monoclonal antibody F36/22 (which reacts with an antigen on differentiated mammary epithelium which is also highly expressed on breast and ovarian carcinomas) to nude mice bearing human mammary carcinomas resulted in the rapid reduction of the tumour to 25% of the pre-treatment volume. This reduction was only seen when intact immunoglobulin was used, which suggests the cytolytic effect is due to events mediated through the Fc portion of the antibody.

Although specific antibodies are not available which allow therapeutic

doses of radiation linked to antibodies to be given intravenously, Epenetos *et al.*, (1984) described the use of HMFG-2 to administer large doses
of radiation into restricted environments, i.e., intrapleurally, intraperi-
cardially or intraperitoneally. They report that the antibody delivers 250–
500 times the radiation dose to its target tumour compared with other
organs, thus allowing repeated treatment in the same patient.

C. Problems Involved in Tumour Targeting

1. Drug Targeting and Antibody Specificity

Until tumour-specific antibodies are available, the targeting of toxins
in human subjects remains a theoretical possibility, although the targeting
of drugs already used in cancer therapy may be possible using the existing
tumour-associated monoclonal antibodies. The successful targeting of
existing drugs could be of considerable benefit to the patient since many
have extremely hazardous side effects. For example, adriamycin, often
used alone or in combination with other drugs in the treatment of breast
cancer, can cause nausea, frequent vomiting, hair loss and has a specific
action on the myocardium (Arcamone, 1981). Pimm *et al.*, (1982) showed
that in an animal model system, adriamycin, conjugated to a monoclonal
antibody, significantly retarded the growth of a rat mammary carcinoma
at a twenty-fifth of the effective dose of the free drug. Unfortunately,
one of the problems that exists in targeting drugs in the human subject
is the very small absolute amounts of antibody which reach the target
tumour (Epenetos *et al.*, 1985a).

2. Location

The location of the breast, close to the central blood pool, is a disadvantage when imaging primary or local recurrences because of the
high non-specific radioactivity associated with the circulatory system.
F(ab′)$_2$ fragments of immunoglobulins may clear from the bloodstream
faster than intact immunoglobulins; investigations by Colcher *et al.* (1983),
using antibodies to image human mammary tumours transplanted into
athymic mice, have shown the F(ab′)$_2$ fragments clear from the blood
two to three times faster than intact IgG and high tumour : tissue ratios
were obtained.

The clear imaging of distant breast metastases may be easier to achieve
but massive liver uptake (one of the common sites of breast metastases)
of [111]I-labelled M8 antibody has been observed (Rainsbury *et al.*, 1983).

Using this antibody, unsubtracted images failed to show any soft tissue metastases although it was successful in imaging bone metastases.

3. Accessibility of Antigen

If antibodies are to be administered intravenously, then the tumour to be imaged must have an adequate blood supply to allow access of the antibody to the antigen; the success of imaging skeletal metastases has been in part attributed to the rich local medullary blood supply in this site (Rainsbury et al., 1983). One possibility which would allow greater accessibility of antibody to antigen is to alter the route of administration which may also reduce the non-specific radioactivity attributed to the blood pool. It has been demonstrated, using polyclonal antiserum to carcinoembryonic antigen (CEA) that administration of labelled antibody to the lymphatic system via subcutaneous injections in the finger webs can result in the specific concentration of antibody in the lymph node metastases from breast carcinomas (DeLand et al., 1979). On the other hand, Epenetos et al., (1985c) described non-specific uptake of antibody when ^{123}I-labelled HMFG-2 was administered intralymphatically to patients with cervical cancer. Assessment of axillary lymph node involvement is still the best prognostic indicator in breast cancer; if radiolabelled monoclonal antibodies could be used to estimate the nodal involvement within the internal mammary chain, the prognostic value of nodal involvement may be improved.

Imperial Cancer Research Fund group at Guy's Hospital, London, is now carrying out a study using ^{131}I-labelled HMFG-2 injected intrapleurally to determine if the antibody will localize to malignant cells invading the pleural cavity. By investigating the kinetics involved in the appearance of labelled antibody in the blood, knowledge as to how easily antibody passes the blood tumour barrier will be obtained.

D. Use as Prognostic and Diagnostic Indicators

As yet, only a few monoclonal antibodies have been applied to tumour targeting in the human subject, and in breast cancer patients the success has been rather limited; however, other clinical applications are being pursued and some show considerable promise. Most tumours show marked heterogeneity in their staining patterns with monoclonal antibodies, both within a single tumour and among tumours (Colcher et al.,

1981; Rasmussen *et al.*, 1982) and it may be possible to exploit this heterogeneity both in the classification of tumour types (Kufe *et al.*, 1983) and in the prognosis of the disease. It has been reported that high levels of extracellular staining of breast carcinomas with HMFG-1 is associated with an extended disease-free interval (Wilkinson *et al.*, 1984). This may reflect the data of Chang and Taylor-Papadimitriou, who reported that normal mammary epithelial cells expressing the secreted high molecular weight molecule recognised by HMFG-1 have a decreased growth potential (Chang and Taylor-Papadimitriou, 1983); these data provided evidence for the theory discussed earlier that the expression of the HMFG-1 antigen is representative of the normal, terminally differentiated cell.

To obtain accurate staging of breast cancer it is desirable to identify all metastatic deposits—the sensitivity and ease of identification may be greatly increased by the use of monoclonal antibodies for the detection of micrometastases in histological sections. The tumour-associated, epithelial-specific antibodies, for example, those directed to the human milk fat globule, may be used in this context although the expression of these antigens can be modulated by the environment. As indicated earlier, the intermediate filaments of epithelial cells, the cytokeratins, are totally conserved in tumours and metastatic cells of epithelial origins. Thus, anti-keratin antibodies are ideal for detecting metastases in tissues such as bone marrow and lymph nodes where epithelial cells are not normally found.

In serous effusions, the identification of malignant epithelial cells from activated mesothelial cells can often present a problem to the cytologist; monoclonal antibodies that distinguish between the two cell types would be extremely useful. The antibodies HMFG-2 (Epenetos *et al.*, 1982b) and Cal (Woods *et al.*, 1982) have been used in this context. Although some activated mesothelial cells may exhibit a weak reaction with antibodies of this type depending on fixation conditions (Ghosh *et al.*, 1983), they are proving to be useful for identification of carcinoma cells in effusions. Anti-keratin antibodies have not been used for this purpose since a very specific antibody is required which reacts with the keratins found in carcinomas but not with the mesothelial keratins.

A reliable breast tumour marker that may be used in prognosis and diagnosis and identified in the serum has long been sought, but as yet no successful marker has been identified. Monoclonal antibodies have the potential to specifically identify circulating tumour-associated antigens; molecules reacting with monoclonal antibodies directed towards the human milk fat globule have been identified in the serum of some breast cancer patients (Ceriani *et al.*, 1982; Burchell *et al.*, 1984). In advanced breast cancer patients, 53% of serum showed elevated levels of the HMFG-2 antigen compared to 16% of healthy control women, and 30% of the cancer patients showed high levels of the HMFG-1 antigen with only 6% of controls showing elevated levels. Although it is doubtful whether these antibodies could be used in diagnosis, in patients where high levels of the antigen are detected they may be useful to monitor the course of the disease. As there appears to be a correlation between high levels of the HMFG-2 antigen and early death, this antibody may be potentially useful as a prognostic indicator (Burchell *et al.*, 1984).

IV. CONCLUSIONS

The search for a totally specific monoclonal antibody to breast cancer has, as yet, been unfruitful but, perhaps surprisingly, the tumour-associated monoclonal antibodies have been used successfully in a number of clinical situations. *In vivo* topographical barriers exist that prevent access of antibody to normal tissue; thus, an antibody may show higher specificity *in vivo* than *in vitro*. This may create a dilemma for the scientist and clinician in deciding at what stage an antibody should be used in the clinic for non-invasive techniques like *in vivo* imaging. Immunological staining of sections may overestimate the cross-reactivity of the antibody *in vivo* as, in this situation, the monoclonal is afforded access to all parts of the tissue; studies using human tumours transplanted into animals may underestimate the cross-reactivity as the tumour is isolated from other human material.

Even with a highly specific antibody showing a consistently high affinity for antigen, special problems remain in the *in vivo* imaging of primary breast tumours and their local metastases because of their proximity to the blood pool. Further work using antibody fragments and other radiolabels will be necessary to overcome these problems. In the field of drug targeting, however, it could be that breast tumours may be feasible targets since, in this case, specificity does not have to be so limited as to be restricted to the tumour. An antibody reacting with a tissue-specific antigen would suffice and the elimination of the normal mammary epithelial cell would be a much less drastic way to eradicate the disease than mastectomy.

REFERENCES

Altevogt, P., Fogel, M., Cheingsong-Popov, R., Dennis, J., Robinson, P., and Schirrmacher, V. (1983). *Cancer Res.* **43**, 5138–5144.

Arcamone, E. (1981). "Doxorubicin: Antreancer Antibiotics," pp. 25–32. Academic Press, New York.

Boland, C. R., Montgomery, C. K., and Kim, Y. S. (1982). *Proc. Natl. Acad. Sci. U.S.A.* **79**, 2051–2055.

Brockhaus, M., Magnani, J. L., Herlyn, M., Blaszczyt, M., Steplewski, Koprowski, H., and Ginsberg, V. (1982). *Arch. Biochem. Biophys.* **217**, 647–651.

Burchell, J., Durbin, H., and Taylor-Papadimitriou, J. (1983). *J. Immunol.* **131**, 508–513.

Burchell, J., Wang, D. and Taylor-Papadimitriou, J. (1984). *Int. J. Cancer* **34**, 763–768.

Canevari, S., Fossati, G., Bulsari, A., Sonnino, S., and Colnaghi, M. (1983). *Cancer Res.* **43**, 1301–1305.

Capone, P. M., Papsidero, L. D., Croghan, G. A., and Ming Chu, T. (1983). *Proc. Natl. Acad. Sci. U.S.A.* **80**, 7328–7332.

Ceriani, R. L., Sasaki, M., Sussman, M., Wara, W. M., and Blank, E. W. (1982). *Proc. Natl. Acad. Sci. U.S.A.* **79**, 5420–5424.

Chang, S. E., and Taylor-Papadimitriou, J. (1983). *Cell Differ.* **12**, 143–154.

Colcher, D., Horan Hand, P., Nuti, M., and Schlom, J. (1981). *Proc. Natl. Acad. Sci. U.S.A.* **78**, 3199–3203.

Colcher, D., Zalutsky, M., Kaplan, W., Kufe, D., Austin, F., and Schlom, J. (1983). *Cancer Res.* **43**, 736–742.

DeLand, F. M., Kim, E. E., Corgan, R. L., Casper, S., Primus, F. J., Spremulli, E., Estes, N., and Goldenberg, D. M. (1979). *J. Nucl. Med.* **20**, 1243–1250.

Epenetos, A. A., Britton, K. E., Mather, S., Shepherd, J., Granowska, M., Taylor-Papadimitriou, J., Nimmon, C. C., Durbin, H., Hawkins, L. R., Malpas, J. S., and Bodmer, W. F. (1982a). *Lancet* **2**, 999–1004.

Epenetos, A. A., Canti, G., Taylor-Papadimitriou, J., Curling, M., and Bodmer, W. F. (1982b). *Lancet* **2**, 1004–1006.

Epenetos, A. A., Courtenay-Luck, N., Halnan, K. E., Hooker, G., Hughes, J. M. B., Krausz, T., Lambert, J., Lavender, J. P., MacGregor, W. G., McKenzie, C. J., Munro, A., Myers, M. J., Orr, J. S., Pearse, E. E., Snook, D., Webb, B., Burchell, J., Durbin, H., Kemshead, J., and Taylor-Papadimitriou, J. (1984). *Lancet* **1**, 1441–1443.

Epenetos, A. A., Snook, D., Halnan, K., Lambert, J., Field, S. B., MacGregor, W., Wood, C., Orr, J. S., Durbin, H., Taylor-Papadimitriou, J., Bodmer, W. F., and Johnson, P. (1985a). *Cancer Res.* (in press).

Epenetos, A. A., Gibson, R., Halnan, K. E., Henderson, B., Lambert, J., Lavender, J. P., McKenzie, C. J., MacGregor, W. G., Munro, A., Orr, J. S., Snook, D., Bodmer, W. F., Durbin, H., Kemshead, J., and Taylor-Papadimitriou, J. (1985b). *Br. J. Cancer* **51**, 805–808.

Feizi, T. (1981). *Trends Biochem. Sci.* **6**, 333–335.

Feizi, T., Picard, J., Kapadia, A., and Slavin, G. (1979). *Protides Biol. Fluids* **27**, 221–224.

Foster, C. S., and Neville, A. M. (1984). *Hum. Pathol.* **15**, 1–12.

Foster, C. S., Edwards, P.A.W., Dinsedale, E. A., and Neville, A. M. (1982). *Virchows Arch. A-Pathol. Anat. Histol.* **394**, 279–293.

Franke, W. W., Weber, K., Osborn, M., Schmid, E., and Freundenstein, C. (1978). *Exp. Cell Res.* **116**, 429–445.

Froese, A. (1968). Immunochemistry **5**, 253–264.

Gatter, K. C., Abdulaziz, Z., Beverley, P., Corvalan, J. R., Ford, C., Lane, E. B., Mota, M., Nash, J. R. G., Pulford, K., Stein, M., Taylor-Papadimitriou, J., Woodhouse, C., and Mason, D. Y. (1982). *J. Clin. Pathol.* **35**, 1253–1267.

Ghosh, A. K., Spriggs, A. I., Taylor-Papadimitriou, J., and Mason, D. Y. (1983). *J. Clin. Pathol.* **36**, 1154–1164.

Gooi, M. C., Uermura, K. I., Edwards, P. A. W., Foster, C. S., Pickering, N., and Feizi, T. (1983). *Carbohydr. Res.* **20**, 293.

Granowska, M., Shepherd, J., Britton, K. E., Waird, B., Mather, S., Taylor-Papadimitriou, J., Epenetos, A. A., Carroll, M. J., Nimmon, C. C., Hawkins, L. A., and Bodmer, W. F. (1983). *Proc. Annu. Meet. Soc. Nucl. Med.* **24**, No. 5.

Herlyn, E. M., Stepleswki, Z., Herlyn, M. F., and Koprowski, H. (1980). *Cancer Res.* **40**, 717–721.

Hilkens, J., Buijs, F., Hilgers, J., Hageman, Ph., Calafat, J., Sonnenberg, A. and Van der Volk, M. (1984). *Int. J. Cancer* **34**, 197–206.

Javadpour, N. (1983). *Urology* **21**, 1–7.

Kapadia, A., Feizi, T., and Evans, M. J. (1981). *Exp. Cell Res.* **131**, 185–195.

Kufe, D., Inghirami, G., Abe, M., Hayes, D., Justi-Wheeler, H. and Schlom, J. (1984). *Hybridoma* **3**, 223–232.

Leis, M. P. (1981). *Breast Cancer Res. Treat.* **1**, 5–15.

Mason, D. W., and Williams, A. F. (1980). *Biochem. J.* **187**, 1–20.

Menard, S., Tagliabue, E., Canevari, S., Fossati, G., and Colnaghi, M. (1983). *Cancer Res.* **43**, 1295–1300.

Miller, R. A., Maloney, D. G., Warnke, R., and Levy, R. (1982). *N. Engl. J. Med.* **306**, 517–522.

Nuti, M., Teramoto, J. A., Mariani-Constantini, R., Horan Hand, P., Colcher, D., and Schlom, J. (1982). *Int. J. Cancer* **29**, 539–545.

Osborn, M., and Weber, K. (1982). *Cell* **31**, 303–306.

Papsidero, L. D., Croghan, G. A., O'Connell, M. J., Valenzuela, L. A., Nemoto, T., and Ming Chu, T. (1983). *Cancer Res.* **43**, 1741–1747.

Pateisky, N., Philipp, K., Skodler, W. D., Spona, J., and Taylor-Papadimitriou, J. (1983). *Cancer Detect. Prev.* **6**(6), 625 (abstr.).

Pimm, M. V., Jones, J. A., Price, M. R., Middle, J. G., Embleton, M. J., and Baldwin, R. W. (1982). *Cancer Immunol. Immunother.* **12**, 125–134.

Rainsbury, R. M., Westwood, J. M., Coombs, R. C., Neville, A. M., Orr, R. J., Kalirui, T. S., McCready, V. R., and Gazet, J. C. (1983). *Lancet* **2**, 934–938.

Rasmussen, B. B., Hilkens, J., Hilgers, J., Nielsen, H. H., Thorpe, S. M., and Rose, C. (1982). *Breast Cancer Res. Treat.* **2**, 401–405.

Schlom, J., Wunderlich, D., and Teramoto, Y. A. (1980). *Proc. Natl. Acad. Sci. U.S.A.* **77**, 6841–6845.

Schlom, J., Colcher, D., Horan Hand, P., Wunderlich, D., Nuti, M., and Teramoto, J. A. (1983). *In* "Understanding Breast Cancer" (M. Rich, J. C. Hager, and P. Furmanski, eds.), pp. 169–213. Dekker, New York.

Shimizu, M., and Yamauchi, K. (1982). *J. Biochem. (Tokyo)* **91**, 515–518.

Soule, M. R., and Edgington, T. S. (1982). *Breast Cancer Res. Treat.* **2**, 294 (abstr.).

Springer, G. E., Desai, P. R., and Banatwala, I. (1975). *J. Natl. Cancer Inst. (U.S.)* **54**, 335–339.

Sun, T.-T., and Green, H. (1978). *J. Biol. Chem.* **253**, 2053–2060.

Taylor-Papadimitriou, J., Peterson, J. A., Arklie, J., Burchell, J., Ceriani, R. L., and Bodmer, W. F. (1981). *Int. J. Cancer* **28**, 17–21.

Taylor-Papadimitriou, J., Lane, E. B., and Chang, S. E. (1983). *In* "Understanding Breast Cancer" (M. A. Rich, J. C. Hager, and P. Furmanski, eds.), pp. 215–245. Dekker, New York.

Thompson, C. H., Jones, S. L., Whitehead, R. M., and McKenzie, I.F.C. (1983). *JNCI, J. Natl. Cancer Inst.* **70,** 409–419.

Wilkinson, M. J. S., Howell, A., Harris, H., Taylor-Papadimitriou J., Swindell, R., and Sellwood, R. A. (1984). *Int. J. Cancer* **33,** 299–304.

Woods, J. C., Spriggs, A. L., Harris, H., and McGee, J. O. (1982), *Lancet* **2,** 512–514.

Yogeeswaran, G., and Salk, P. L. (1981). *Science* **212,** 1514–1516.

Yuan, D., Hendler, F. J., and Vitetta, E. S. (1982). *JNCI, J. Natl. Cancer Inst.* **68,** 719–728.

CHAPTER **2**

Monoclonal Anti-melanoma Antibodies and Their Possible Clinical Use

Karl Erik Hellström and Ingegerd Hellström

ONCOGEN
Seattle, Washington, U.S.A.
and Departments of Pathology and Microbiology/Immunology
University of Washington
Seattle, Washington, U.S.A.

I. INTRODUCTION

Tumor immunologists have been interested in malignant melanoma for many years. There are several reasons for this. Melanomas regress

MONOCLONAL ANTIBODIES FOR CANCER
DETECTION AND THERAPY

occasionally (Everson and Cole, 1966), as would be the case if some patients react immunologically to their tumors. They grow well in culture, which facilitates the use of various *in vitro* assays to measure cell-mediated and humoral immune responses to melanoma-associated antigens. Their prognosis is very poor, unless the tumors are diagnosed early and removed, which is an incitement to seek knowledge that can lead to new therapeutic modalities.

Some of the first evidence that there are cell surface antigens which are preferentially associated with melanomas came from the demonstration that lymphocytes from patients with melanoma displayed cell-mediated anti-tumor immunity since they could specifically inhibit (or kill) plated melanoma cells (Hellström *et al.*, 1968, 1971). This observation was confirmed and extended by studies with leukocyte migration inhibition (McCoy *et al.*, 1975) and leukocyte adherence inhibition (Halliday *et al.*, 1975) techniques. Nevertheless, there was substantial controversy about the initial findings (Herberman and Oldham, 1975; Baldwin, 1975), particularly in view of uncertainties as to whether they reflected T cell reactivity (Wybran *et al.*, 1974), antibody-dependent cellular cytotoxicity (Hellström *et al.*, 1971; Kodera and Bean, 1975; Hersey *et al.*, 1976, 1983) or activities of natural killer (NK) cells (Takasugi and Mickey, 1976); this has been discussed in view of more recent information (Hellström and Hellström, 1983). It is noteworthy that cloned T cells from patients with melanoma have been shown to selectively kill allogeneic melanoma cells *in vitro* (de Vries and Spits, 1984). Although the latter finding is surprising by being in apparent contradiction to the expected genetic restriction of T cell-mediated cytotoxicity (Zinkernagel and Doherty, 1974), it is in agreement with the early claim that T cells are responsible for some of the lymphocyte-mediated cytotoxic reactions to antigens shared by different melanomas (Wybran *et al.*, 1974).

Serological assays have many advantages over tests for cell-mediated immunity when attempting to define the specificity and molecular nature of antigens (Old, 1981). Such assays have consequently been applied to search for antibodies in the sera of patients with melanoma, and they have given strong indication that some melanoma patients form antibodies to their tumors. Some of these antibodies are directed to antigens that are shared by different melanomas (Morton *et al.*, 1968; Cornain *et al.*, 1975), while others define antigens that appear to be unique to each tumor (Lewis *et al.*, 1969). The most extensive of the serological studies were by Shiku *et al.* (1976), who tested patient sera for antibodies to autochthonous melanoma cells and employed adsorption techniques to establish their specificity. The data confirmed the existence of antibodies to antigens that are unique to a given melanoma ("Class I") as well as of antigens shared by many melanomas ("Class II"). In addition ("Class

III''), antigens were demonstrated which were common to many cultured normal and neoplastic cells (Shiku et al., 1977).

In view of the evidence that there are melanoma-associated antigens that can be recognized by patients with such tumors, it is not surprising that melanomas were among the neoplasms that were first investigated by the monoclonal antibody technique (Kohler and Milstein, 1975). Koprowski et al. (1978), Yeh et al. (1979), Carrel et al. (1980), Woodbury et al. (1980), and Dippold et al. (1980) were among the first to establish antibody-forming cell hybrids (hybridomas) by immunizing mice with human melanomas and they obtained many monoclonal antibodies with specificity for such tumors. Although some antibodies did not live up to their promise of tumor specificity, there are, as a result of the initial studies and subsequent investigations, several antigens that have been defined by monoclonal antibodies and are preferentially expressed in melanoma. In-depth studies of these antigens may be informative about key events during the neoplastic transformation, and some antigens offer promise as both diagnostic markers and therapeutic targets. Those antigens that are expressed at the cell surface are, at least to us, the most interesting ones, since they may be targets for diagnostic and therapeutic procedures based on antibody localization to tumor.

In this chapter we discuss cell surface antigens of human melanoma as defined by monoclonal antibodies. Rather than attempting to provide an overall literature survey, we shall concentrate on three antigens (p97, a GD3 ganglioside, a proteoglycan) which have two features in common: They have general interest in that they are among the antigens most specific for melanoma so far detected, and we have worked with them ourselves. Several other contributors to this volume are responsible for much of our present understanding of the immunology of melanoma. Their chapters are, therefore, likely to deal with aspects beyond those which we discuss. We are not, in this review, considering intracellular antigens, such as S100 (Cochran et al., 1982).

II. MELANOMA-ASSOCIATED CELL SURFACE ANTIGENS

A. Establishment and Screening of Hybridomas

Essentially all monoclonal antibodies to human melanoma antigens that are presently available have been obtained by immunizing mice (in vivo) with human melanomas and hybridizing their spleen cells with cells from drug-marked mouse myelomas, such as NS-1 (Kohler and Milstein, 1975) or SP2/O (Galfre *et al.*, 1977). Although human hybridomas have been isolated which make antibodies binding to melanoma cells (Cote *et al.*, 1983; C. Berglund, personal communication), those antibodies appear to be less specific for melanoma than the better of the monoclonal mouse antibodies. The same appears, so far, to hold true for antibodies made by EBV-transformed lymphocytes from patients with melanoma. A possible exception to this is a recent group of antibodies which was obtained by hybridizing lymphocytes from regional lymph nodes of melanoma patients with mouse myeloma cells (M. Mitchell, personal communication). Several human monoclonal antibodies were obtained by this approach and were found to bind to intra-cellular antigens expressed in melanomas but not in normal nevi; some antigen expression was also detected in kidney tubuli and in sebaceous glands. Since the antigens were not detectable at the cell surface, they are beyond the scope of this chapter.

It is important to note that whenever one establishes hybridomas, one will, at best, get what one searches for. Thus, if one needs antibodies for diagnosis of tumor in formalin-fixed, paraffin-embedded sections, the early screening of antibodies against such sections is called for; if one searches for antibodies to tumor antigen in serum (Koprowski *et al.*, 1981; Bast *et al.*, 1983), this should be reflected in the immunization and the screening procedures used; and if one wants antibodies that are cytotoxic or growth inhibitory to tumor cells (Vollmers and Birchmeyer, 1983a,b) or give antibody-dependent cellular cytotoxicity (ADCC) (Hellström *et al.*, 1981a; Steplewski *et al.*, 1979; Schultz *et al.*, 1983), or activate human complement (I. Hellström *et al.*, 1985a) that should, likewise, be reflected in the screening. We also like to emphasize that it is relatively easy to make additional monoclonal antibodies to an antigen that has already been identified (e.g., antibodies with different isotype and/or biological characteristics or with higher affinity). One can, for example, use the purified antigen for screening in binding assays (Nudelman *et al.*, 1982), one can screen with radioimmunoprecipitation techniques and take advantage of one's knowledge of the antigen's molecular weight (Brown *et al.*, 1980), and one can screen with a two-site immunoradiometric assay (Brown *et al.*, 1981b) using an available antibody to one determinant of the antigen and selecting for an antibody to another determinant of the same antigen. Since antibodies that bind protein A from *Staphylococcus aureus* are practical to work with, it is often time-saving to first select those hybridomas that form antibodies that bind to protein A (Brown *et al.*, 1980). Likewise, time may be saved by the early elimination of hybridomas that make antibodies of low stability.

Almost all of the existing monoclonal anti-melanoma antibodies identify antigens that are shared by many melanomas (Hellström et al., 1968; Morton et al., 1968; Shiku et al., 1976) rather than antigens that are unique to just one or a few such tumors (Lewis et al., 1969; Shiku et al., 1976). The only exception to this appeared to be an antigen, called 3.1, to which three different monoclonal antibodies were made (Yeh et al., 1979). When binding assays were used to test cell lines, antigen 3.1 was preferentially expressed by the immunizing melanoma, and thus appeared to be very similar to the unique Class I antigens (Shiku et al., 1976) as these had been studied by also using cultivated cells. However, antigen 3.1 was detected in several normal tissues when biopsy material was subsequently studied (Brown et al., 1981a), a finding that illustrates the need to always confirm observations on cell lines by testing tissues. In view of the fact that monoclonal mouse antibodies to clone-specific antigens of human leukemias can be made relatively easily (Miller et al., 1981), the disppointing lack of in vivo specificity for antigen 3.1 should not be taken as evidence that monoclonal mouse antibodies cannot be made to true Class I antigens.

B. Antigen Specificity

The question of antigen specificity (for tumor versus normal tissues and for tumor type) is, of course, a key question in any study of tumor antigens. For melanoma antigens, as defined by monoclonal antibodies, it must, at least so far, be answered in relative rather than absolute terms. That is, although the expression of some melanoma antigens is 20- to 1000-fold greater in melanomas than in normal tissues, there are no absolute, qualitative differences (Brown et al., 1981b; K. E. Hellström et al., 1985). Consequently, specificity is best defined in quantitative terms, for example, as the number of antibody-binding sites per cell. The history of our own work on p97, one of the more specific melanoma antigens thus far identified, illustrates the question of antigen specificity rather well. In initial studies with radioimmunoprecipitation and indirect binding assays on cell lines, p97 appeared to be entirely confined to tumor (Woodbury et al., 1980). However, when more sensitive assays were applied, a significant, albeit small, amount of antigen was found also in normal tissues (Brown et al., 1981b). Studies on other antigens in melanomas (and in different tumors) have since led to similar conclusions.

Two-site immunoradiometric assays (Brown et al., 1981b) are useful for the quantitative definition of antigen expression. They are based on the use of monoclonal antibodies to two different determinants of the same antigen molecule, so that an antigen must bind to two different antibodies in order to be recognized. The background is thereby low and, for certain antigens, the sensitivity sufficient to demonstrate only a few (10 or less) molecules per cell (Plowman et al., 1983; J. P. Brown, unpublished findings).

The detection of melanoma-associated antigens in tissue sections by immunohistology using, for example, the peroxidase–antiperoxidase technique (Sternberger, 1979) or avidin–biotin technology has also contributed a great deal to our understanding of antigen specificity (Garrigues et al., 1982). The immunohistological approach is not quantitative but has the advantage of selectively identifying which cells in a sample express the antigen of interest. This is important, since melanomas are mixtures of different types of cells, including many stroma cells, and also since most melanomas, at least if they are large, contain live areas and areas of necrosis: An immunochemical test could give erroneous results when the samples consist primarily of normal stroma or are derived from necrotic areas.

Although the initial hope for truly melanoma-specific antigens has not (yet) been realized, the degree of specificity of several of the melanoma-associated antigens so far identified is sufficient for most practical purposes. It can be as great as is the difference between transformed and nontransformed cells in the expression of some known oncogene products (Slamon et al., 1984; Schimke, 1984), and it is greater than the differences between normal and neoplastic cells in sensitivity to inhibition by interferon or to killing by NK cells (Herberman, 1980) or chemotherapeutic drugs.

Another question that deserves consideration is that of antibody specificity for tumor *type*. The early studies with lymphocytes and sera from cancer patients established the concept of tumor-type specific antigens, i.e., of antigens that are primarily confined to tumors of one histological type, for example, to melanomas (Hellström and Hellström, 1969). Studies with monoclonal antibodies have confirmed the existence of such antigens (Koprowski and Steplewski, 1981; Dippold et al., 1980; Woodbury et al., 1980; Bumol et al., 1982; Hellström and Hellstöm, 1983). However, the degree of tumor-type specificity is less absolute than it appeared to be in the early studies. This is amply illustrated with respect to the expression of melanoma-associated antigens. For example, p97 is not only strongly expressed by most melanomas but is present in some carcinomas of the bladder, salivary gland, and breast and in a few other carcinomas as well (Woodbury et al., 1981; Brown et al., 1981b; K. E. Hellström et al., 1984b). Although the lack of absolute tumor-type specificity detracts from the use of an antibody to distinguish diagnostically between different tumors (see further below), a positive aspect of this finding is that antibodies to melanoma antigens may be useful for the *in vivo* diagnosis, and therapy, also of certain tumors other than melanoma.

C. Three Melanoma Antigens of Particular Interest

According to published reports, there are at least some 10 different cell surface antigens which are expressed more strongly by melanoma cells than by various other cells (Koprowski *et al.*, 1978, 1981; Yeh *et al.*, 1979; Woodbury *et al.*, 1980; Dippold *et al.*, 1980; Carrel *et al.*, 1980; Loop *et al.*, 1981; Steplewski *et al.*, 1981; Imai *et al.*, 1982; Reisfeld *et al.*, 1982; Bumol and Reisfeld, 1982; Houghton *et al.*, 1982; Liao *et al.*, 1982; Johnson *et al.*, 1984). The total number of such "melanoma-associated" antigens depends on how stringent one's criteria for specificity are.

As indicated in the Introduction, we consider three antigens to be of particular interest, i.e., p97 (Woodbury *et al.*, 1980, 1981), a proteoglycan (Bumol and Reisfeld, 1982; Imai *et al.*, 1982; Hellström *et al.*, 1983a), and a GD3 ganglioside (Dippold *et al.*, 1980; Yeh *et al.*, 1982; Pukel *et al.*, 1982; Nudelman *et al.*, 1982). Two of them, p97 and the proteoglycan, are proteins, and one, the sialoganglioside, is a glycolipid. In this chapter we shall, for the sake of brevity, refer to these three antigens as "the major melanoma antigens," but are fully aware that the list of major antigens is likely to be extended in the future.

All three major antigens are oncofetal or differentiation antigens, a trait which they have in common with most other antigens detected in human tumors by monoclonal antibodies (K. E. Hellström *et al.*, 1982a) and, for that matter, with most human tumor antigens defined by other assays as well, e.g., by microcytotoxicity testing of patient lymphocytes (Hellström and Brown, 1979). They can be demonstrated in biopsies of melanomas and, less frequently and in smaller amounts, in biopsies of some other tumors, and they are present in nevi but not in resting skin melanocytes. Hematopoietic stem cells have very little, if any, of these antigens, since they are not killed, nor functionally interfered with, by *in vitro* exposure to antibodies to any of the three antigens (B. Torok-Storb, personal communication).

It should be noted that monoclonal antibodies to the three major antigens have been made in many laboratories and by using different cell lines as immunogens, different mouse stains and protocols for immunization, and different techniques for screening. This suggests that the number of antigens that can be detected by monoclonal mouse antibodies as strongly associated with human melanoma is rather limited. One may argue, however, that other and perhaps more melanoma-specific antigens could be identified by using another species for immunization (rats, for example), by immunizing *in vitro* (which might decrease the impact of suppressor cell-mediated immunoregulatory mechanisms), or by concentrating on human monoclonal antibodies; it has, for example, been difficult to obtain monoclonal mouse antibodies to many HLA specificities, most of the antibodies defining common "framework" determinants, and one must realize that the same might be the case for many mouse antibodies to human tumor antigens. One may also argue that the reason why relatively few melanoma-associated antigens have been demonstrated is that the selection methods used have eliminated those hybridomas which make antibodies to antigens that are expressed in relatively small amounts at the cell surface, and this may include hypothetical antigens of very high (or absolute) tumor specificity. If the latter would be the case, however, one still must realize that antigens that are expressed only at low concentrations may be unsuitable for many diagnostic and therapeutic purposes.

An important question is whether any of the antigens so far defined by monoclonal mouse antibodies induce immune responses in patients with melanoma and are related to the Class II melanoma antigens referred to in the Introduction. At this time we know very little about this. If the number of melanoma-associated cell surface antigens is quite limited, one would expect some of the antigens recognized by the immune system of patients to be the same as those recognized by the mouse. However, attempts to detect immune responses in patients to antigens defined by monoclonal mouse antibodies have generally failed.

One approach to investigate whether patients can respond immunologically to an antigen that is defined by a mouse antibody is to study whether they have any lymphocyte clones that can recognize the given antigen. Anti-idiotypic antibodies (see below) can be employed for this in conjunction with cell-sorting techniques and can be induced by using the respective monoclonal antibodies as immunogens (Nepom *et al.*, 1984). If any melanoma-specific lymphocytes can be identified by this approach, they can be subsequently characterized with respect to phenotype and function and used to establish lymphocyte clones which, depending on the nature of the idiotype-positive lymphocytes isolated, could be used to obtain human monoclonal antibodies, or as T cell lines with helper, suppressor, or cytolytic activities.

The three major melanoma antigens are now discussed under separate headings.

1. p97

Antigen p97 was one of the first melanoma-associated antigens defined by monoclonal antibodies (Hellström *et al.*, 1980). It is a phosphorylated sialoglycoprotein with a molecular weight (MW) that is slightly less than that of rabbit phosphorylase b (97,400) on sodium dodecyl sulfate–poly-acrylamide gel electrophoresis (SDS–PAGE) (Woodbury *et al.*, 1980, 1981); the same antigen (Brown *et al.*, 1981c) was described as gp95 by Dippold *et al.* (1980). Antigen p97 is present in most melanomas, although its expression varies between different such tumors with the positive ones having 50,000–500,000 molecules per cell and a small group of ("negative") melanomas expressing less than 20,000 molecules per cell. It is also expressed, although in smaller amounts (less than 50,000 molecules per cell) in certain carcinomas, e.g., in some salivary gland tumors and bladder carcinomas. The antigen is present, although in trace levels only (less than 8,000 molecules per cell), in various adult human tissues (Brown *et al.*, 1981b) and, in relatively high amounts, in fetal intestine (Woodbury *et al.*, 1981); it is not significantly expressed in any cells of the blood.

Five different epitopes of p97 have been identified (Brown *et al.*, 1981b), and some 20 different monoclonal antibodies to p97 have been made, which differ in epitope specificity, isotype, etc. (Brown *et al.*, 1981c; Dippold *et al.*, 1980). Three of the five epitopes have been detected on a 40-kDa fragment, which can be cleaved off from p97 by using papain (Brown *et al.*, 1981c).

A partial amino acid sequencing of its N-terminal end has shown that p97 is structurally related to transferrin (Brown *et al.*, 1982), a known growth factor. Although antibodies to native p97 do not bind transferrin, antibodies to denatured p97 do. Like transferrin, p97 binds iron (Brown *et al.*, 1982). The N-terminus of p97, which is situated on the 40-kDa fragment, is extracellular, while the C-terminus appears to be cytoplasmic (J. P. Brown, unpublished findings).

Antigen p97 is coded for by a gene on chromosome 3 (Plowman *et al.*, 1983). This is the chromosome to which the genes for both transferrin (McAlpine and Bootsma, 1982) and the transferrin receptor (Enns *et al.*, 1981; Goodfellow *et al.*, 1982) have been assigned. In view of this, and since it has been surmised that p97 and the transferrin receptor (Sutherland *et al.*, 1981; Trowbridge and Omary, 1981) are identical (Sutherland

Antigen p97 is coded for by a gene on chromosome 3 (Plowman *et al.*, 1983). This is the chromosome to which the genes for both transferrin (McAlpine and Bootsma, 1982) and the transferrin receptor (Enns *et al.*, 1981; Goodfellow *et al.*, 1982) have been assigned. In view of this, and since it has been surmised that p97 and the transferrin receptor (Sutherland *et al.*, 1981; Trowbridge and Omary, 1981) are identical (Sutherland *et al.*, 1981), we must point out, first, that these are two distinct markers that are expressed on different cell populations (lymphoblasts, for example, express very little p97 but large amounts of the transferrin receptor) and that the distinctiveness of the two molecules has been formally proven by sequential immunoprecipitation analysis (Brown *et al.*, 1982; J. P. Brown, unpublished findings).

A structural homology has been reported between an oncogene, Blym, and transferrin (Goubin *et al.*, 1983), suggesting that there is likely to be homology also between p97 and Blym. Recent studies have established cDNA clones (Brown *et al.*, 1985) and genomic clones (G. D. Plowman, T. Rose, and J. P. Brown, unpublished findings) coding for p97, and it should, therefore, become possible to prove experimentally, or disprove, the assumed relationship between p97 and Blym. Using the cloned p97 gene, it should also be feasible to test whether p97 can transform indicator cells *in vitro* and thereby, itself, behave as an oncogene, and, of course, to investigate the functional role of p97 in melanomas and in the normal embryo, as well as the regulation of antigen expression in various types of cells. Furthermore, the cloned gene can be used to transfect (human) p97 into mouse tumor cells and to search for a mouse homologue to p97 (G.D. Plowman, T. Rose, and J.P. Brown, unpublished findings). This way, animal models can be developed of great potential use for studies on passive and active immunity to (human) tumor-associated differentiation antigens.

It is interesting that two of the tumor cell surface antigens which have been studied the most, p97 and the transferrin receptor (Trowbridge and Omary, 1981; Sutherland *et al.*, 1981), are coded for by genes on the same chromosome and that they are both able to bind iron (directly for p97 and via transferrin for the transferrin receptor), an ability that may confer selective advantage to cells.

2. GD3

The second of the major melanoma antigens is a GD3 sialoganglioside which is strongly expressed by most melanomas and only weakly, if at all, by normal adult tissues (Dippold *et al.*, 1980; Yeh *et al.*, 1982). As for p97, the degree of antigen expression varies between different melanomas (Yeh *et al.*, 1982). It is present in human embryos, particularly in brain and kidney (K. Hudkins and I. Hellström, unpublished observations). Some carcinomas, including some salivary gland tumors, sarcomas, breast carcinomas and transitional cell bladder tumors, also express the melanoma-associated GD3 antigen, although generally in lower amounts than most melanomas (I. Hellström, unpublished observations).

In our own laboratory, we first obtained an IgM antibody, 4.2, which, when tested in binding assays, reacted primarily with melanomas and which proved to be specific for GD3 (Yeh *et al.*, 1982; Nudelman *et al.*, 1982). The reactivity pattern suggested that antibody 4.2 defined the same (or a similar) antigen as an antibody, R_{24}, which had been previously obtained by Dippold *et al.* (1980) and shown to bind to GD3 (Pukel *et al.*, 1982).

We have recently made several IgG1 and IgG3 antibodies to the melanoma-associated GD3 antigen. This was achieved by immunizing mice with SK-MEL 28 cells, which express much of the antigen, and screening the hybridomas for binding to GD3 prepared from melanomas (using a plate assay for the screening). One of the hybridomas, 2B2, makes an antibody which is more specific for melanoma than antibody 4.2 in that it does not bind to any cells in normal brain or kidney, while antibody 4.2 binds to a few cells in these organs (Karlsson *et al.*, 1985).

The melanoma-associated GD3, as defined by antibody 4.2, has a longer ceramide-linked fatty acid side chain than brain GD3 (Nudelman *et al.*, 1982). This may explain why antibody 4.2 binds to melanoma, but not to brain, in spite of the fact that brain contains large amounts of GD3: in brain (and other normal tissues), GD3 may be "hidden" in the cell membrane while the longer fatty acids of the melanoma GD3 makes it protrude from the cell membrane so that it can be detected by antibody. It is also possible, however, that melanoma cells lack some molecule that is present in normal cells and prevents the GD3 from detection by antibody.

The melanoma-associated GD3 antigen is one of the potentially most "useful" tumor antigens so far identified in that it is strongly expressed by most melanomas and very weakly (or not detectably) by normal adult human tissues, and it also appears to be an excellent target for both ADCC and complement-mediated cytotoxicity (see below). These observations stimulate the search for analogous glycolipid antigens in melanomas and other types of neoplasms.

3. Proteoglycan

One of the best characterized and most specific melanoma antigen is a proteoglycan. This antigen was first described by Reisfeld's and Ferrone's groups (see Bumol and Reisfeld, 1982; Imai *et al.*, 1982). Our own involvement with it started when we obtained an IgG1 antibody, 48.7, which reacted primarily with melanoma cell lines and to frozen sections of melanomas, as assessed by binding assays and by immunohistology (Hellström *et al.*, 1983a). SDS–PAGE immunoprecipitation with antibody 48.7 was performed subsequently and revealed two bands which had an approximate MW of 250 kDa as well as a band corresponding to a MW⩾400 kDa, both of which could be detected in most melanomas (Hellström *et al.*, 1983a). In view of the work of Reisfeld's and Ferrone's groups, we tested by sequential immunoprecipitation whether the antigen defined by antibody 48.7 was related to the antigens defined by them (Bumol and Reisfeld, 1982; Imai *et al.*, 1982). The data indicated that this was the case (Hellström *et al.*, 1983a; G. Mosely, unpublished findings), which is why the antigen defined by antibody 48.7 is referred to as a proteoglycan. We have recently obtained additional antibodies which define three different epitopes of the proteoglycan antigen.

D. Antigen Heterogeneity

By studying frozen tissue sections with immunohistological techniques, we have been able to detect the three major antigens in essentially all primary melanomas tested (Garrigues *et al.*, 1982; Hellström *et al.*, 1983a; I. Hellström, unpublished findings). The frequency of antigen expression in metastatic melanomas is lower and has varied between 60% for p97 and 80–85% for the two other antigens. Antigen expression varies among different metastases from the same patient (I. Hellström, unpublished observations), and occasionally even between different parts of the same metastasis.

The expression of each of the three antigens appears to be independently regulated since one melanoma can have much of one antigen and lack detectable amounts of another. At least one major antigen has, however, been detected in all of the more than 100 metastatic melanomas which we have tested, and most melanomas (96%) express at least two of them (K. E. Hellström *et al.*, 1984b).

One cannot conclude from immunohistological studies whether the observed variation in antigen expression relates to the cell cycle or represents true clonal differences. It is important to remember, however, that clonal variation has been observed with respect to the expression of several melanoma-associated antigens (Yeh *et al.*, 1981; Albino *et al.*, 1981); the existence of intercellular variation is indeed, one of the few "common denominators" in cancer and is likely to complicate many diagnostic and therapeutic uses of antibodies.

There are differences with regard to which normal tissues express significant amounts of a given antigen. For example, studies of frozen sections have demonstrated p97 in myoepithelial cells of sweat glands, and, in small amounts, in some parenchymal cells of liver (Garrigues *et al.*, 1982). The proteoglycan antigen is absent from these tissues but is present in some endothelial cells (Hellström *et al.*, 1983a) while the GD3 antigen, dependent on what antibody is used, is either not detectable at all in normal tissues, as is the case when using antibody 2B2 or IF4 (Karlsson *et al.*, 1985), or can be demonstrated in some cells of the brain and kidney (with antibody 4.2).

The heterogeneity in antigen expression in tumors, as well as the fact that different antigens are expressed differently in normal tissues, suggest that a combination of antibodies to several melanoma antigens will be advantageous for most clinical purposes. First, there may be few if any tumor cells that are not recognized when several antibodies are combined. Second, when used as part of a combination, each antibody may be employed at a concentration at which it has negligible reactivity with normal tissues.

III. POTENTIAL DIAGNOSTIC USES OF ANTIBODIES TO MELANOMA ANTIGENS

A. *In Vitro* Diagnosis by Immunohistology

The immunohistological studies referred to in the preceding section have shown that every tested, consecutive sample of histologically diagnosed metastatic melanoma could be stained by antibodies to at least one of the three major melanoma antigens (K. E. Hellström *et al.*, 1984b; I. Hellström, unpublished observations). This implies that if a tumor sample does not stain by antibodies to any of these antigens, it is probably not a melanoma, a conclusion that has diagnostic significance; however, work is needed also with atypical melanomas (particularly such that can be diagnosed by electron microscopy but not by light microscopy).

Antibodies to the three major melanoma antigens have been used to test more than 100 cases of metastatic melanoma. Approximately 50% of these were found to express all three antigens, while none of some 30 non-melanoma tumors did that (K. E. Hellström *et al.*, 1984b), suggesting that the presence of all three antigens on a tumor sample signifies melanoma. This may be diagnostically helpful when dealing with a metastasis from an unidentified primary neoplasm.

Nintey-seven percent of melanomas expressed at least two of the three antigens, as compared to 15% of non-melanoma tumors (K. E. Hellström *et al.*, 1984b). All of these positive non-melanoma tumors were carcinomas. Lymphomas have been negative for all three antigens. Expression of one of the major melanoma antigens in a tumor sample, therefore, argues against the diagnosis of lymphoma.

We conclude this section by pointing out that the greatest clinical value of immunohistological tests with presently available antibodies will probably not be for *in vitro* diagnosis, but for deciding what antibodies to employ for *in vivo* procedures, such as tumor localization by imaging and therapy with antibody or some "vaccine" (see below).

B. *In Vitro* Diagnosis by Serum Assays

Molecules released from tumor cells into the bloodstream as a result of secretion (Abelev, 1983), antigen "shedding" (Alexander, 1974; Black, 1980) or, simply, as a consequence of tumor cell death, may provide clues about both the presence of a tumor and its size. A prerequisite for this is, however, that either the released molecules are qualitatively different from any molecules that normally occur in serum or that the increased amount, in serum, of a normally occurring molecule is sufficient to be detected.

As discussed above, the markers so far identified in melanoma appear to be normal differentiation antigens that are expressed in much higher amounts in melanomas than in normal adult tissues. Their use to establish serum assays for early diagnosis will consequently depend on the extent to which the release of an antigen from a small number (10^8 or less) of tumor cells (with much antigen per cell) can be detected above a background level of antigen released from many (of the order of 5–10 $\times 10^{13}$) normal cells (with little antigen per cell). In view of this, it appears unlikely that serum assays can be developed that will reveal a primary melanoma unless the marker is present in melanomas at some five orders of magnitude greater than in normal tissues or is released selectively from melanoma. It is obviously easier to develop assays for monitoring changes in patients with known disease as these patients undergo therapy. Indeed, this has been achieved for certain carcinomas (Koprowski *et al.*, 1981; Bast *et al.*, 1983), and should be feasible for melanomas as well.

One shall, however, also bear in mind that the immune system of a patient may provide the "amplification" needed to detect a relatively early tumor, in the form of an immune response to tumor-associated antigens, as suggested by some of the early work in human tumor immunology. (Hellström and Hellström, 1969). If that is the case, it may become feasible to establish assays detecting cell-mediated and/or humoral anti-tumor responses, in patients using, for example, anti-idiotypic antibodies to well characterized tumor antigens as probes.

C. *In Vivo* Diagnosis by Tumor Imaging

As long as a tumor cell surface antigen is well expressed *in vivo* (as can be revealed by testing biopsy material), one has reasons to assume that a specific, high affinity antibody will localize to tumor when injected intravenously into patients. By labelling the antibody with a radioisotope, or an agent useful for imaging by NMR technology, it might be possible to obtain information of diagnostic and prognostic importance.

In order to test this assumption, pilot studies have been performed in nude mice which were grafted with human melanoma and injected intravenously with ^{131}I-labelled anti-p97 antibody or Fab fragments prepared from such antibody. The specific antibody (Fab) was taken up in tumor 10–20 times better than a control antibody (Fab) which was labelled with ^{125}I and injected in parallel, while both antibodies (Fab) localized equally in normal mouse tissues. The highest relative localization of specific antibody (Fab) in tumor versus normal tissue was seen 24–48 hr after it was injected (Matzku *et al.*, 1982; Larson *et al.*, 1983a; Beaumier *et al.*, 1985). An important disadvantage when using nude mice for this type of study must be borne in mind, however: Normal mouse cells entirely lack p97 (Brown *et al.*, 1981b), while (as repeatedly pointed out in this review) normal human cells have trace amounts of it.

The nude mouse experiments were followed by an investigation in patients, which was conducted similarily to studies which had been done with antibodies to carcinoembryonic antigen (CEA) by Goldenberg *et al.* (1978, 1980) and Mach *et al.* (1980) and employing ^{131}I for labelling. Whole antibody was used in an initial study which was performed on eight patients. Localization to tumor was observed in 88% of known metastases (Larson *et al.*, 1983a,b). There were no appreciable side effects. Lack of localization could be attributed to a metastasis either being too small (less than 1.5 cm in diameter) or expressing only low levels of p97 (Larson *et al.*, 1983a); high levels of circulating p97 could also adversely affect localization.

There is strong evidence that the tumor localization of antibody (Fab) observed by imaging patients is antigen specific. First, pair-labelling experiments were performed in which patients were given a mixture of anti-melanoma and control antibodies, one antibody being labelled with ^{125}I and the other with [131]I: There was higher tumor uptake of the specific than of the control antibody, while there was no difference in their uptake in normal tissues (Larson *et al.*, 1983a). Second, studies were done (Larson *et al.*, 1983a) in which the same patient was "imaged" on different occasions, 3–4 weeks apart, after having been given either specific antibody (which localized in tumor) or control antibody (which did not).

Whole anti-p97 antibody was replaced by Fab fragments following the initial study (Larson *et al.*, 1983c). The Fab fragments were chosen for two reasons. First, and most important, they are less immunogenic than whole immunoglobulin so that patients are less prone to produce anti-mouse antibodies that interfere with further imaging (Larson *et al.*, 1983b). Second, the smaller size of Fab fragments makes them localize more quickly in tumor. Presumably, (Fab)$_2$ fragments may be even better for imaging but have not yet been properly evaluated.

At this time more than 50 patients have been given radiolabelled Fab fragments specific for p97, in an attempt to localize metastases by "imaging." Many of the patients have been injected repeatedly. The degree of antibody localization in tumor has been approximately the same whether whole antibody or Fab fragments were used (Larson *et al.*, 1983a,b).

An additional group of 10 patients has received Fab fragments 48.7 which are specific for the proteoglycan antigen (Larson *et al.*, 1984). The degree of antibody localization to tumor has been similar to that seen for p97. In addition, there has been the important advantage that very little antibody was taken up by the (normal) liver, while considerable amounts of anti-p97 antibodies (Fab) are regularly found in liver. A recent study by Ferrone *et al.* (1983) also indicates that the proteoglycan ("high molecular weight") melanoma antigen is a suitable target for tumor imaging.

Opinions may differ as to the prospects for imaging with radiolabelled antibody fragments to be clinically useful for the diagnosis and management of patients with melanoma. Our belief is that the long-term opportunities are excellent, since the imaging techniques are capable not only of demonstrating a "lump"—which may be detected even better by other methods—but of showing whether a lump expresses some known tumor marker and, therefore, represents a neoplasm. Furthermore, nuclear imaging can provide a basis for immuno-therapy by proving that a given antibody actually localizes into a patient's tumor.

At this time, the procedures for tumor imaging with radiolabelled antibodies (fragments) also have substantial weaknesses as compared to competing technologies such as computerized tomography (CAT) scanning and nuclear magnetic resonance (NMR). Their greatest drawback is probably the fact that tumors of less than approximately 1.5 cm in diameter have not been detected by imaging with ^{131}I (Larson *et al.*, 1983b,c). One reason for this is that the existing equipment in nuclear medicine laboratories is geared towards using other isotopes, particularly technetium. By replacing ^{131}I with ^{123}I and performing tomography, the resolution can be improved (Larson *et al.*, 1983c). However, ^{123}I is not ideal, since it is both expensive and hard to obtain. It would be important, therefore, to develop methods for labelling antibodies (or antibody fragments) with an isotope that has better imaging characteristics than ^{131}I and is both easily available and inexpensive (technetium, for example). An ultimate goal may be to combine the superior resolution of the NMR technique with the ability of the labelled antibody approach to detect tumors by their expression of known tumor markers; it is, however, questionable whether this is feasible.

Another problem with the use of radiolabelled antibodies (fragments) for imaging is that a large amount of the labelled products often localizes in normal tissues, particularly in the liver. Different antigens seem to differ in this respect. For example, Fab fragments 48.7, which are specific for the proteoglycan, do not localize appreciably into the liver, while Fab fragments 96.5 and 8.2, specific for p97, both localize there (Larson *et al.*, 1983a, 1985). One may hope that antibodies to some antigens, which have not yet been tried for the imaging of melanoma (for example, antibodies to the GD3 antigen), may show even higher selectivity than those with which we have so far worked. Combinations of antibodies to different melanoma antigens should also be considered. The reason for this is that the use of antibody combinations should decrease the impact of tumor cell heterogeneity. This may be needed in view of the fact (discussed earlier) that an antigen which is expressed in one metastasis is sometimes absent from another metastasis in the same patient.

IV. POTENTIAL THERAPEUTIC USES OF MONOCLONAL ANTIBODIES TO MELANOMA ANTIGENS

A. Targets

The ideal target for antibody therapy would be one that is entirely specific for tumor cells, intimately associated with their neoplastic behavior and easily accessible to the antibody. TGF-α, a tumor-derived growth factor, may be an example of such a molecule, since many tumors (including most melanomas) produce TGF-α. TGF-α has been reported to be highly specific for tumor (as compared to normal tissues) and it has been hypothesized that some cases of neoplasia are maintained by the release of TGF-α and its subsequent binding to a cell surface receptor (Todaro et al., 1984; Marquardt et al., 1984). Tumor growth may then be inhibited if the TGF-α is either neutralized by specific antibody or prevented from binding to its receptor, for example, by an antibody to the receptor. There are probably other growth factors, in addition to TGF-α, which have (some) specificity for tumor. Furthermore, oncogene products are known which have at least relative tumor specificity and play key roles in maintaining neoplasia. However, we do not, at the present time, know very much about the roles, in melanoma, of TGF-α and other growth factors, and of various oncogene products, how tumor specific they are, and how accessible they are to antibody.

The more immediate therapeutic approach is, therefore, to use as targets those melanoma antigens which have been already identified by monoclonal antibodies. There are at least two reasons why the lack of total tumor specificity of these antigens is not overly worrisome. First, melanoma cells often express 20- to 1000-fold more of an antigen than do normal adult cells. Second, the three major melanoma antigens are present in very large amounts at the tumor cell surface, so that it may be possible to concentrate to the tumor cells a cytocidal number of antibody molecules (using free antibodies or such conjugated with toxins or drugs as needed in the particular situation).

We now discuss some different approaches to monoclonal antibody-based therapy. Most of these should be applicable to more specific tumor markers if such become identified, as long as they are expressed at the cell surface in more than trace amounts.

B. Antibodies Alone

Antibodies may be cytostatic (or cytotoxic) to melanoma cells by binding to some molecule that plays a key role in cellular invasiveness or proliferation (Vollmers and Birchmeier, 1983a,b), and in the presence of complement, they may be cytotoxic, even when the target antigen does not have any important cellular function. In the latter case, the antibodies generally belong to the IgG_{2a}, IgM or IgG3 isotypes (Yeh et al., 1979; Steplewski et al., 1981; I. Hellström et al., 1985a).

A synergistic cytotoxic effect was detected by using two IgG_{2a} antibodies to different epitopes of p97 and attributed to an increased complement-binding ability of two closely adjacent antibodies attached to different epitopes of the same antigen molecule (Hellström *et al.*, 1981b). Synergism was observed also when one of the antibodies was an IgG1 which did not give complement-dependent cytotoxicity by itself (I. Hellström *et al.*, 1983b). By combining two synergistically acting antibodies, tumor cell killing *in vitro* could be detected at antibody concentrations as low as 5 ng/ml, which are concentrations that may be easily obtained *in vivo*. A drawback is, however, that it has in most cases not been possible to obtain significant *in vitro* cytotoxicity by using complement from humans rather than from rabbits or guinea pigs. There is, nevertheless, at least one situation in which the killing of melanoma cells by antibody and rabbit or guinea pig complement may have clinical application. Patients with advanced melanoma are sometimes treated by a protocol according to which an autologous bone marrow sample is stored, an otherwise lethal dose of chemotherapy given, and the patients rescued by transplantation of the stored marrow (Thomas *et al.* 1982). One of the problems with this approach is that the bone marrow sample often contains melanoma cells. These cells may be killed by treatment of the marrow with antibody and complement (Dantas *et al.*, 1983). The greatest problem is to find chemotherapeutic drugs with high ability to kill melanoma cells (at any dose).

It is particularly interesting that there are (a few) melanoma antibodies which are highly cytotoxic to melanoma cells in the presence of human complement. These include MG21, an IgG3 specific for the GD3 antigen (Hellström *et al.*, 1985) and R_{24} (A. Houghton, personal communication), the antibody by which the melanoma-associated GD3 antigen was first discovered (Dippold *et al.*, 1980).

Antibody-dependent cellular cytotoxicity (Perlmann and Holm, 1969; Pollack *et al.*, 1972; Skurzak *et al.*, 1972) against melanoma cells has been observed with several IgG2 antibodies (I. Hellström *et al.*, 1981a, 1985a; Steplewski *et al.*, 1979) as well as with three IgG3 antibodies, 2B2, IF4 and MG21 (I. Hellström *et al.*, 1985a). The latter antibodies, which are specific for the GD3 antigen, were found to kill up to 90% of melanoma cells when tested in a 4-hr ^{51}Cr-release assay (I. Hellström *et al.*, 1985a). The concentration of antibody needed to give ADCC *in vitro* was low ($\geqslant$10 ng/ml).

In view of the high efficiency by which some antibodies can kill melanoma cells by activating human complement and/or by ADCC, it seems worthwhile, for antigens of high tumor specificity, to screen for hybridomas that form antibodies with such abilities; the ^{51}Cr-release assay is suitable for that purpose. Efforts should also be given towards developing ways to activate those cell populations which serve as effectors of ADCC.

It may be immaterial whether the antibody effects are mediated by so-called K cells (or related NK cells) and represent a classical ADCC or by macrophages with cytotoxic, cytostatic, or "opsonizing" activity (Sears *et al.*, 1982). The macrophages are also of interest in view of the fact that neoplastic cells are more commonly inhibited (or killed) by activated macrophages than are their normal counterparts. Procedures should, therefore, be considered for using monoclonal antibodies to attract activated macrophages to the site of a growing tumor; some "biological response modifiers" may be suitable for this, in view of their anti-tumor activity when deposited directly into a tumor mass (Bast *et al.*, 1974).

Antibodies 2B2 and IF4 were also tested for activity against melanoma cells in nude mice. The outgrowth of small transplants of human melanoma was effectively prevented by one of the antibodies, 2B2 (K.E. Hellström *et al.*, 1985), when given in 1-mg amounts every second day, and the original tumor implants (1 × 1 mm pieces) were destroyed. The other anti-GD3 antibody, IF4, had no effect; it is noteworthy that this antibody gave significant ADCC only with human effector cells while antibody 2B2 gave strong ADCC with both human and mouse lymphocytes. It was not possible to eradicate tumors that were 4–5 mm in diameter, even by giving 2 mg of antibody 2B2 per mouse on every second day. There was, however, evidence of necrosis in some of the larger tumors in the treated mice and this was accompanied by an influx of inflammatory cells (K. E. Hellström, unpublished findings).

It may be questioned how well the nude mouse model can predict therapeutic effects of antibodies in human patients, since there are important differences between the two systems. First, mouse cells entirely lack the antigens to which the anti-human melanoma antibodies are directed, while small amounts of these antigens are present on various normal human cells, which poses a risk that an injected antibody may also damage normal human tissues. Second, a mouse antibody is antigenically foreign to human patients and will, therefore, induce an immune response to itself. Such a response may lead to the quick elimination of the injected antibody (Goodman *et al.*, 1985). Alternatively, it may be beneficial to the host. The latter could be the case, if the anti-mouse antibodies bind to mouse immunoglobulin at the tumor cell surface in such a way that they facilitate tumor destruction by K (NK) cells and/or macrophages, or if the antibody-coated tumor cells act as "super-antigens" and induce a host response to the tumors. Antibodies activating human complement may be particularly useful for this purpose. Furthermore, when anti-tumor antibodies are injected to an immunocompetent patient, they may induce the formation of anti-idiotypic antibodies (Koprowski *et al.*, 1984; Goodman *et al.*, 1985); these may, in their turn, induce an active tumor immunity (see below). Although there are some reservations as to how appropriate the nude mouse model is, these should not detract from the fact that studies in that model can help select (for studies in man) those antibodies that can kill melanoma cells *in vivo*.

The most straightforward approach to learn about the *in vivo* effect of anti-tumor antibodies is, obviously, to test them clinically in human patients, preferably using antibodies which on the basis of nude mouse data can be expected to have an anti-tumor effect *in vivo*. As a first step towards this, Phase I trials have been initiated in patients with disseminated melanoma. Besides investigating the side effects of antibody therapy in such patients (the natural goal of a Phase I trial), major efforts have been given towards studying the ability of intravenously infused antibodies to localize selectively to melanoma cells. For this purpose, patients have been given up to 500 mg antibody specific for either the proteoglycan antigen (Bernhard et al., 1983a,b) or p97 (Goodman *et al.*, 1985), or a combination of antibodies to these two antigens (Goodman *et al.*, 1985). No trial has yet been done with antibody 2B2, which is the one that showed a particularly strong ADCC combined with an anti-tumor activity in the nude mouse model (see above), or with MG21, which activates human complement.

No therapeutic benefits have been observed with the antibodies tested. Nevertheless, there have been two encouraging observations. First, large doses of antibodies could be repeatedly given over a 10-day period without unacceptable toxicity. Second, by administering 150 mg or more antibodies over a 10-day period, essentially all melanoma cells in tumor biopsies bound the antibodies while there was no significant binding to normal stroma cells (Goodman *et al.*, 1985). It follows from these findings that neither p97 nor the proteoglycan antigen appear to undergo antigenic modulation (Old, 1968) when exposed to the specific antibodies and that they are, in this respect, different from certain other cell surface antigens, e.g., CALLA (Cote *et al.*, 1983); this agrees with data from a study in which cultured melanoma cells were exposed to antibody to one epitope of p97 and subsequently tested for the expression of another epitope of p97 (Hellström *et al.*, 1983b). The infused mouse immunoglobulins had a plasma half-life ($t_{1/2}$) of 40–50 hr, except in one patient who 3 months earlier had received 2 mg of radiolabelled Fab fragments prepared from the anti-proteoglycan antibody 48.7, in whom it was 21.2 hr (Goodman *et al.*, 1985). This patient had antibodies that could bind specifically to Fab fragments prepared from antibody 48.7 and whose binding to Fab 48.7 could be specifically blocked by antibody 48.7 and by cell lysates containing the proteoglycan antigen (Goodman *et al.*, 1985). This indicates that the patient's antibodies were specific for the idiotype of antibody 48.7 and behaved similarily to an anti-idiotypic antibody that had been raised in rabbits using a monoclonal anti-p97 antibody as the immunogen (Nepom *et al.*, 1984). The findings were analogous to observations of Koprowski *et al.* (1984), who had given a mouse antibody specific for a colon carcinoma antigen to patients with colon carcinoma and found anti-idiotypic antibodies in some of the treated patients' sera.

A study by Houghton *et al.* (1985) was published after this chapter was prepared and indicated that objective, clinical responses could be obtained when patients with metastatic melanomas were infused with antibody R_{24}. This suggests an important role for tumor therapy with certain unmodified antibodies.

C. Radiolabelled Antibodies

As discussed previously, tumor imaging studies have shown that radiolabelled Fab fragments that are specific for melanoma antigens can localize in melanoma tissue when injected intravenously into patients. Based on these findings, the relative localization of ^{131}I-labelled anti-p97 Fab fragments in melanoma, as compared to various normal tissues, was calculated. The data suggested that such fragments can be used to deliver a therapeutic dose of radioactivity to tumor without causing unacceptable damage to normal tissues (Larson *et al.*, 1983b).

A Phase I clinical trial was then started (Larson *et al.*, 1983b; Carrasquillo *et al.*, 1984) in which seven patients with Stage III melanoma were given ^{131}I-labelled Fab fragments intravenously. During the course of the trial, the dose of radioactivity was escalated up to 400–830 mCi for the last three patients. Another two patients were included who received ^{131}I-labelled Fab specific for the proteoglycan antigen (Carrasquillo *et al.*, 1984); this was in view of data indicating that these Fab gave at least as selective delivery of radioactivity to tumor as observed for p97 (Larson *et al.*, 1984). The amount of overall toxicity of the treatment was remarkably low except for a substantial depression of the platelet counts in the one patient who received 840 mCi, which could be overcome by giving two transfusions of platelets. There was a temporary clinical response in two of the three patients who received more than 400 mCi. In one of these, it was seen as stabilization of the growth of rapidly progressing liver metastases, and in the other one as disappearance of some tumor nodules which had been visible on CAT scans of the abdominal area (Carrasquillo *et al.*, 1984). One of the two patients who showed a clinical response had received Fab specific for p97, while the other patient had been injected with Fab specific for the proteoglycan antigen. Although radiolabelled antibodies have been previously used for tumor therapy (Order *et al.*, 1975; Leichner *et al.*, 1983; Order, 1984), the studies by Larson *et al.* were the first with Fab fragments prepared from monoclonal antibodies of well-defined specificity.

One advantage with radiolabelled antibodies (or antibody fragments) for therapy is that imaging techniques can be used to determine how much of the therapeutic agent is taken up in tumor before a patient is treated, and also that this uptake can be related to therapeutic effects. Other advantages are that one can use any antibody as long as it has high tumor specificity, and that one can select for labelling either an isotope which exerts its action in a very limited area or an isotope (such as ^{131}I) which releases particles that can kill cells within a large area (up to several millimeters in diameter). In the latter case, it is possible to destroy cells that are adjacent to those cells which bind the labelled antibody. This may be useful for eliminating tumor cell variants that have lost the antigen to which a given antibody is directed, a likely problem in tumor therapy with antibodies.

^{131}I is being routinely used to treat thyroid carcinoma, the major reason why it was selected for antibody labelling in the first clinical trials with melanoma. However, other isotopes may prove to be more suitable. This may include isotopes which emit α particles. Since these have much higher energy levels than the β particles produced by ^{131}I, they should be able to kill a cell binding only a few molecules of the labelled antibody. There have also been considerations about procedures to attach boron or some similar neutron captor to the antibody so as to make a conjugate that will emit α particles after radiation with slow neutrons (Mizusawa *et al.*, 1983). A problem with this approach is, however, that it may be difficult to introduce a sufficient number of boron atoms per antibody molecule for neutron capture to become effective.

A disadvantage of using radiolabelled antibodies for therapy is that even the most specific antibodies so far tested localize only some 5–10 times better in tumors than in normal tissues (Larson *et al.*, 1983a,b). Consequently, there will be considerable radiation to normal tissues when exposing a tumor to a potentially curative dose, leading to risks for both short-term and long-term damage to bone marrow, intestines, etc. Furthermore, treatment with radiolabelled antibodies may be impractical when dealing with large groups of patients who have to be isolated in shielded rooms, etc. Hopefully, the first and more important of these two problems may be solved by learning more about the kinetics of uptake of radiolabelled antibodies (fragments) and how to influence it.

D. Antibody–Toxin Conjugates

An antibody of a desired specificity may be conjugated with toxic substances, such as ricin A chain, to produce a potent "immunotoxin" which
can bind to, and kill, cells expressing the appropriate antigen (Jansen *et
al.*, 1982). Since studies with immunotoxins are described elsewhere in
this volume, it is sufficient to state here that conjugates have been made
that are specific for either p97 (Casellas *et al.*, 1982) or the proteoglycan
(Bumol *et al.*, 1983) and can effectively kill melanoma cells *in vitro*. In
the studies performed with p97, essentially every cell with approximately
20,000 p97 molecules per cell (or more) was killed while cells expressing
5,000 or fewer p97 molecules were not (Casellas *et al.*, 1982). The latter
observation is encouraging in view of what is known about the relative
amounts of p97 on normal and neoplastic cells (see above).

The rate of tumor cell killing by immunotoxins can be substantially
increased by adding ammonium chloride (Casellas *et al.*, 1982) or certain
other agents which damage lysosomes, such as chloroquine (Jansen *et
al.*, 1982). Nevertheless, it has been difficult to develop effective tumor
therapy *in vivo* with immunotoxins, and we are not aware of any report
where immunotoxins have been used to successfully treat melanomas
in human patients, although Bumol *et al.* (1983) obtained encouraging
data in nude mice transplanted with human melanoma.

E. Antibody–Drug Conjugates

Rather than using a toxin for conjugation with an anti-tumor antibody,
one may choose a chemotherapeutic drug, as discussed separately in
this volume. A disadvantage of this approach is that many anti-cancer
drugs only kill dividing cells, while toxins kill cells independently of
their state in the cell cycle. An advantage is, however, that one can choose
among many drugs whose anti-tumor activities and side effects in patients are known. Another advantage is that even if a drug-conjugated
antibody would localize only some three to eight times better in tumor
than in normal tissues (degrees of localization which are commonly
achieved when injecting tumor-bearing patients with radiolabelled antibodies in Fab fragments, as discussed previously), this may be sufficient
to reach the tumor selectivity needed for a therapeutic effect (and perhaps
a cure).

The usefulness of antibodies conjugated with drugs is likely to depend
upon the extent to which drugs exist (or can be found) which have a

therapeutic effect on the given tumor; if there is no good drug, its conjugation with an antibody is unlikely to help. Unfortunately, there are no drugs that are very active against melanoma. One of the few drugs that has any anti-melanoma activity at all is vindesine. Rowland *et al.* (1983, 1985) conjugated this drug with anti-p97 antibody. The conjugates were found to inhibit the *in vitro* colony formation of plated melanoma cells that express high to intermediary levels of p97 ($\geqslant$50,000 molecules per cell) without affecting cells expressing little p97 (<10,000 molecules per cell). Furthermore, they inhibited the outgrowth of melanomas in nude mice, while the unconjugated anti-p97 antibody did not. Similar conjugates, which had been made with antibodies to an antigen shared by many sarcomas and carcinomas (Embleton *et al.*, 1981) as well as with antibodies to CEA, were also tumoricidal *in vitro* (Rowland *et al.*, 1983, 1985). When anti-CEA conjugates were tested in nude mice, they had high anti-tumor activity. Since they were much less toxic than free drug to the mice, they were better than the free drug for therapy (Rowland *et al.*, 1985).

There is a need for innovative approaches in this area. Such approaches may take into account the fact that monoclonal antibodies are available to several cell surface antigens that are strongly expressed by the same melanoma cells and often also to different epitopes of the same antigen. It may, for example, become possible to use an antibody to one antigen determinant to bring a substrate to the tumor cell surface which can produce an event lethal to the tumor cell when interacting with an agent brought in by a second antibody.

The problem of antigenic heterogeneity in tumors is likely to be important, irrespective of whether one uses an antibody alone or conjugates it with a toxin, drug, or some other agent. The most straightforward approach to this problem is to use combinations of antibodies (conjugates) that are specific for several different antigens expressed by the same cells.

F. Anti-idiotypic Antibodies

Antibodies to idiotypic determinants play a major role in regulating the immune response to a variety of antigens (Jerne, 1975; Rajewski and Takemori, 1983). These determinants appear to be shared by T cells, B cells, and antibody molecules (Binz and Wigzell, 1975), which is not surprising in view of the substantial homologies which have recently been found between the amino acid sequences of T cell receptors and immunoglobulins (Hedrick *et al.*, 1984a,b; Yanagi *et al.*, 1984).

Injection of anti-idiotypic antibodies has been found to induce both cell-mediated and humoral immune response to a variety of antigens, including alloantigens (Bluestone *et al.*, 1981), viral antigens (Ertl *et al.*, 1982; Kennedy *et al.*, 1984), and tumor antigens (Binz *et al.*, 1982; Forstrom *et al.*, 1983). The immune response is sometimes facilitated (Forstrom *et al.*, 1983) and sometimes inhibited (Binz *et al.*, 1982), depending on several variables, including the dose of the antibody (Rajewski and Takemori, 1983).

Nepom *et al.* (1984) recently made an anti-idiotypic, anti-melanoma serum. It was prepared by immunizing rabbits wih a monoclonal mouse antibody, 8.2, which is specific for p97^c, one of the five epitopes of p97 to which monoclonal antibodies have been made (Brown *et al.*, 1981c). After removal of irrelevant antibodies by absorption, the rabbit antiserum could bind strongly to Fab fragments prepared from antibody 8.2. This binding could be competitively inhibited by antibody 8.2 and, to a lesser extent, by several other anti-p97^c antibodies, but not by antibodies to other antigens, including antibodies to other p97 epitopes. It was completely inhibited by a cell lysate containing high levels of p97 but not by a control lysate containing only trace levels of p97. When injected into mice, the rabbit antiserum induced the formation of antibodies which carried the idiotype of antibody 8.2 and were specific for p97^c. Furthermore, it induced DTH to a melanoma cell line that expressed much p97, but not to a lung carcinoma line with only trace amounts of p97 (Nepom *et al.*, 1984).

Sera from some patients treated with mouse antibodies to antigens of colon carcinoma (Koprowski *et al.*, 1984) or melanoma (Goodman *et al.*, 1985) have been recently observed to contain anti-idiotypic antibodies, which, to the extent they have been tested, appeared to be similar to those found in the rabbit antiserum prepared by Nepom *et al.* (1984). Koprowski *et al.* (1984) suggested that the appearance of these antibodies in patient sera correlates with a good prognosis.

There is evidence from animal experiments which further indicates that anti-idiotypic antibodies may be therapeutically beneficial (K. E. Hellström *et al.*, 1984a). These experiments were carried out on a BALB/c mouse sarcoma, MCA-1490 (Forstrom *et al.*, 1983). A monoclonal mouse antibody, 4.72, was obtained by immunizing BALB/c mice with MCA-1490 cells and was found to induce DTH to MCA-1490 in BALB/c mice (Forstrom *et al.*, 1983). Another monoclonal antibody, 5.96, was derived from a syngeneic immunization with a different BALB/c sarcoma, MCA-1511 (K. A. Nelson *et al.*, unpublished findings). Each antibody was shown to induce DTH that was specific for each tumor. There are several reasons why antibody 4.72 (and by inference antibody 5.96) is likely to be anti-idiotypic (Forstrom *et al.*, 1983). First, its ability to induce DTH is genetically restricted to mice of the same allotype. Second, mice injected with antibody 4.72 were found to contain a population of Thy-1$^+$, Lyt-1$^+$ lymphocytes which could adoptively transfer tumor-specific DTH. Third, the antibody does not bind to the tumor cell surface but binds to a tumor antigen-specific, T cell-derived suppressor factor (Nelson *et al.*, 1985), as well as to a small population of T cells in tumor-immunized mice (K. Nelson, unpublished findings).

Antibodies 4.72 and 5.96 have recently been tested, in a "crisscross" pattern, for anti-tumor effects against transplanted MCA-1490 and MCA-1511 sarcomas (Nelson *et al.*, 1985; K. A. Nelson, unpublished findings). Mice transplanted with sarcoma and injected with the specific antibody developed fewer takes than untreated mice or mice injected with the "non-specific" antibody. Furthermore, some tumors in the mice injected with the specific antibody regressed after a short period of growth. This is noteworthy, since regression of these sarcomas has never been seen otherwise.

The relative value of anti-idiotypic antibodies as immunogens, as compared to "vaccines" such as purified tumor antigens, synthetic peptides, expressed proteins, etc. (see below), needs to be investigated. An argument in favor of using the antibodies is that they are easier to obtain than to prepare vaccines for which one needs detailed knowledge about the respective tumor antigens.

G. Vaccines

Antigens isolated from melanoma cells may be used as vaccines to induce an active immune response *in vivo*. In those cases where the antigen is a protein, synthetic peptides may be chosen for this purpose as may antigens made by recombinant DNA technology.

Since active immune responses generally lead to long-lasting protection against disease-causing organisms, while the immunological effect of passively transferred antibody is most often only temporary, the use of immunogens may be expected to have an advantage over passive immunotherapy also in the cancer area. There are, however, several potential problems when attempting to induce an active immune response to tumor-associated differentiation antigens, and this is irrespective of whether one uses a vaccine or an anti-idiotypic antibody (as described in the preceding section). First, no immunity may be induced, a finding that would not be surprising since the tumor-associated differentiation antigens may be regarded as "self." The patient to be treated may, for example, lack lymphocyte clones that can recognize the respective antigen as foreign (Nossal, 1983) or the immunogen may activate a suppressor cell response (Nepom *et al.*, 1983) rather than a response leading to tumor destruction. Second, there is a potential problem even if an immune response could be induced in that such a response may damage normal tissues which contain appreciable, albeit small, amounts of the various tumor-associated antigens. A third problem is imposed by the fact that tumor cell populations are heterogeneous. That problem, of course, is not unique to the use of active immunization.

In view of both the possible benefits of active immunization and the various problems listed, it would make sense to perform animal studies before active immunization is tried in man, irrespectively of whether vaccines or anti-idiotypic antibodies are to be used. There are at present a few animal models which appear to be suitable for this purpose. For example, monoclonal antibodies have been obtained to differentiation antigens that are preferentially expressed by mouse bladder carcinomas (K. E. Hellström *et al.*, 1982b; I. Hellström *et al.* 1985b). One of these antigens is essentially confined to bladder carcinomas while some other antigens are expressed, albeit more weakly, in normal bladder epithelium. The degree of specificity of these antigens is similar to that of tumor-associated antigens defined by monoclonal antibodies in melanomas.

V. CONCLUSIONS

Melanomas have been extensively investigated with immunological techniques with the view that most of the information obtained should have general applicability.

Early studies indicated that there are cell surface antigens which are expressed preferentially on melanomas and which can induce both cell-mediated and humoral tumor immunity in patients. Some of these antigens appear to be unique to each tumor while others are shared by many melanomas.

The monoclonal antibody technique has allowed the identification and in-depth characterization of several melanoma-associated antigens.

Quantitative assays have been developed for some of these, which makes it possible to detect only a few antigen molecules per cell. It could be demonstrated that antigen specificity is relative rather than absolute with the more specific antigens being expressed in 20-fold or greater amounts in melanomas than in normal adult tissues.

Three of the melanoma-associated antigens which have thus far been studied appear to be of particular interest: p97, a proteoglycan, and a GD3 ganglioside. They are expressed, in large amounts, at the surface of cells from most melanomas and, in smaller amounts, in some carcinomas, while adult human tissues only contain trace amounts. All three antigens are of the oncofetal or differentiation type, i.e., they are relatively strongly expressed in certain embryonic cells. One of the antigens, p97, is a 97,000 MW glycoprotein which is structurally homologous to transferrin, a known growth factor, and, like tranferrin, it binds iron. It is coded by a gene on chromosome 3, the same chromosome that carries the genes for both transferrin and the transferrin receptor. Genomic (and cDNA) clones coding for p97 have been isolated and should be helpful for further, in-depth studies on this antigen (including its function and regulation of expression).

Monoclonal antibodies to melanoma antigens are likely to have diagnostic applications. Immunohistological analyses of sections can be used to get rapid and reliable information as to what antigens a given melanoma expresses, and they may contribute to the diagnosis of metastases in those cases where the primary tumor is unknown. Radiolabelled antibodies can be applied to the *in vivo* localization ("imaging") of melanoma, since more than 80% of clinically known metastases have been detected in a study using ^{131}I-labelled antibodies (or Fab fragments) specific for p97.

There are also several possible uses of monoclonal antibodies for therapy. Promising results have been obtained in a Phase I trial with ^{131}I-labelled Fab fragments specific for either p97 or the proteoglycan antigen in that large doses of radioactivity could be delivered to tumors with few side effects and with some clinical responses. Furthermore, antibodies to p97 and the proteoglycan have been shown to localize throughout metastatic melanomas, if infused in large doses (>200 mg/patient). Antibodies selected on the basis of strong anti-tumor effects alone or in the presence of human complement or effector cells (such as K cells or macrophages) as well as antibodies conjugated with toxins, drugs, or some immunomodulating agents should be considered for therapy. Attention should also be given to immunogens in the form of anti-idiotypic antibodies and vaccines, the latter including tumor antigens and synthetic peptides.

ACKNOWLEDGEMENTS

The work of the authors has been supported by National Institutes of Health grants CA 38011 and CA 29639, by grant IM 241 from the American Cancer Society, and by ONCOGEN. The authors gratefully acknowledge collaboration with Drs. J. P. Brown, J. A. Carrasquillo, P. Casellas, G. E. Goodman, S. M. Larson, G. F. Rowland, R. G. Woodbury, and M.-Y. Yeh during various phases of the studies discussed in this chapter.

REFERENCES

Abelev, G. (1983). *Oncodev. Biol. Med.* **4**, 371–381.

Albino, A. P., Lloyd, K. O., Houghton, A. N., Oettgen, H. F., and Old, L. J. (1981). *J. Exp. Med.* **154**, 1764–1778.

Alexander, P. (1974). *Cancer Res.* **34**, 2077–2082.

Baldwin, R. W. (1975). *J. Natl. Cancer Inst. (U.S.)* **55**, 745–448.

Bast, R. C., Jr., Zbar, B., Borsos, T., and Rapp, H. J. (1974). *N. Engl. J. Med.* **290**, 1413–1420.

Bast, R. C., Jr., Klug, T. L., St. John, E., Jenison, E., Niloff, J. M., Lazarus, H., Berkowitz, R. S., Griffiths, C. T., Parker, L., Zurawski, V. R., and Knapp, R. C. (1983). *N. Engl. J. Med.* **309**, 883–887.

Beaumier, P. L., Krohn, K. A., Carrasquillo, J. A., Eary, J., Hellström, I., Hellström, K. E., Nelp, W. B., and Larson, S. M. (1985). Submitted for publication.

Bernhard, M. I., Foon, K. A., Deltmann, T. N., Key, M. E., Hwans, K. M., Clarke, G. C., Christensen, W. L., Hoyer, L. C., Hanna, M. G., Jr., and Oldham, R. K. (1983a). *Cancer Res.* **43**, 4420–4428.

Bernhard, M. I., Hwans, K. M., Foon, K. A., Keenan, A. M., Kessler, R. M., Frincke, J. M., Tallam, D. J., Hanna, M. G., Jr., Peters, L., and Oldham, R. K. (1983b). *Cancer Res.* **43**, 4429–4433.

Binz, H., and Wigzell, H. (1975). *J. Exp. Med.* **142**, 1231–1240.

Binz, H., Meier, B., and Wigzell, H. (1982). *Int. J. Cancer* **29**, 417–423.

Black, P. H. (1980). *Adv. Cancer Res.* **32**, 75–199.

Bluestone, J. A., Sharrow, S. O., Epstein, S. L., Ozato, K., and Sachs, D. H. (1981). *Nature (London)* **291**, 233–235.

Brown, J. P., Wright, P. W., Hart C. E., Woodbury, R. G., Hellström, K. E., and Hellström, I. (1980). *J. Biol. Chem.* **255**, 4980–4983.

Brown, J. P., Hellström, K. E., and Hellström, I. (1981a). *Clin. Chem. (Winston-Salem, N.C.)* **27**, 1592–1596.

Brown, J. P., Woodbury, R. G., Hart, C. E., Hellström, I., and Hellström, K. E. (1981b). *Proc. Natl. Acad. Sci. U.S.A.* **78**, 539–543.

Brown, J. P., Nishiyama, K., Hellström, I., and Hellström, K. E. (1981c). *J. Immunol.* **127**, 539–546.

Brown, J. P., Hewick, R. M., Hellström, I., Hellström, K. E., Doolittle, R. F., and Dreyer, W. J. (1982). *Nature (London)* **296**, 171–173.

Brown, J. P., Rose, T. M., Forstrom, J. W., Hellström, I., and Hellström, K. E. (1985). In, "Molecular Biology of Tumor Cells" (B. Wahren, S. Hammarstrom, G. Holm, and P. Perlmann, eds.), pp. 157–167. Raven Press, New York.

Bumol, T. F., and Reisfeld, R. A. (1982). Proc. Natl. Acad. Sci., U.S.A. **79**, 1245–1249.

Bumol, T. F., Chee, D. O., and Reisfeld, R. A. (1982). Hybridoma **1**, 283–292.

Bumol, T. F., Wang, Q. C., Reisfeld, R. A., and Kaplan, N. O. (1983). Proc. Natl. Acad. Sci. U.S.A. **80**, 529–533.

Carrasquillo, J. A., Krohn, K. A., Beaumier, P., McGuffin, R. W., Brown, J. P., Hellström, K. E., Hellström, I., and Larson, S. M. (1984). Cancer Treat. Rep. **68**, 317–328.

Carrel, S., Accolla, R. S., Carmagnola, A. L., and Mach, J.-P. (1980). Cancer Res. **40**, 2523–2528.

Casellas, P., Brown, J. P., Gros, O., Gros, P., Hellström, I., Jansen, F. K., Poncelet, P., Vidal, H., and Hellström, K. E. (1982). Int. J. Cancer **30**, 437–443.

Cochran, A. J., Duan-Ren, W., Herschman, H. R., and Gaynor, R. B. (1982). Int. J. Cancer **30**, 295–297.

Cornain, S., de Vries, J. E., Collard, J., Vennegoor, C., Wingerden, I. V., and Rumke, P. (1975). Int. J. Cancer **19**, 981–997.

Cote, R. J. Morrissey, D. M., Houghton, A. N., Beattie, E. J., and Oettgen, H. F. (1983). Proc. Natl. Acad. Sci. U.S.A. **80**, 2026–2030.

Dantas, M. E., Brown, J. P., Thomas, M. R., Robinson, W. A., and Glode, I. M. (1983). Cancer **52**, 949–953.

de Vries, J. E., and Spits, H. (1984). J. Immunol. **132**, 510–519.

Dippold, W. G., Lloyd, K. O., Li, L. T. C., Ikeda, H., Oettgen, H. F., and Old, L. J. (1980). Proc. Natl. Acad. Sci. U.S.A. **77**, 6114–6118.

Embleton, M. J., Gunn, B., Byers, V. S., and Baldwin, R. W. (1981). Br. J. Cancer **43**, 582–587.

Enns, C. A., Suomaliainen, H. A., Gebhardt, J. E., Schröder, J., and Sussman, H. H. (1981). Proc. Natl. Acad. Sci. U.S.A. **79**, 3241–3245.

Ertl, H., Greene, M., Noseworthy, J., Fields, B., Nepom, G. T., Spriggs, D., and Finburg, R. (1982). Proc. Natl. Acad. Sci. U.S.A. **79**, 7479.

Everson, T. C., and Cole, W. H. (1966). "Spontaneous Regression of Cancer." Saunders, Philadelphia, Pennsylvania.

Ferrone, S., Giacomini, P., Natali, P. G., Ruiter, D., Buraggi, G., Callegaro, L., and Rosa, U. (1983). In "Proceedings of the First International Symposium on Neutron Capture Therapy" (R. G. Fairchild and G. L. Brownell, eds.), pp. 174–183. Brookhaven Natl. Lab., Upton, New York.

Forstrom, J. W., Nelson, K. A., Nepom, G. T., Hellström, I., and Hellström, K. E. (1983). Nature (London) **303**, 627–629.

Galfre, G., Howe, S. C., Milstein, C., Butcher, G. W., and Howard, J. C. (1977). Nature (London) **266**, 550–552.

Garrigues, H. J., Tilgen, W., Hellström, I., Franke, W., and Hellström, K. E. (1982). Int. J. Cancer **29**, 511–515.

Goldenberg, D. M., DeLand, F., Kim, E., Bennett, S., Primus, F. J., Van Nagell, J. R., Estes, N., DeSimone, P., and Rayburn, P. (1978). N. Engl. J. Med. **298**, 1384–1388.

Goldenberg, D. M., Kim, E. E., DeLand, F. H., Bennett, S., and Primus, F. J. (1980). Cancer Res. **40**, 2984–2992.

Goodfellow, P. N., Banting, G., Sutherland, R., Greaves, M., Solomon, E., and Povey, S. (1982). Somatic Cell Genet. **8**, 197–209.

Goodman, G. E., Beaumier, P. L. Hellström, I., Fernyhough, B. and Hellström, K. E. (1985). J. Clin. Oncol. **3**, 340–352.

Goubin, G., Goldman, D. S., Luce, J., Neiman, P. E., and Cooper, G. M. (1983). *Nature (London)* **302,** 114–119.

Halliday, W. J., Maluish, A. E., Little, J. H., and Davis, N. C. (1975). *Int. J. Cancer* **16,** 645–658.

Hedrick, S. M., Nielson, E. A., Kavaler, J., Cohen, D. I., and Davis, M. M. (1984a). *Nature (London)* **308,** 149–152.

Hedrick, S. M., Nielson, E. A., Kavaler, J., Cohen, D. I., and Davis, M. M. (1984b). *Nature (London)* **308,** 153–158.

Hellström, K. E., and Brown, J. P. (1979). In "The Antigens" (M. Sela, ed.), Vol. 5, pp. 1–82. Academic Press, New York.

Hellström, K. E., and Hellström, I. (1969). *Adv. Cancer Res.* **12,** 167–223.

Hellström, I., and Hellström, K. E. (1983). *J. Biol. Response Modif.* **2,** 310–320.

Hellström, I., Hellström, K. E., Pierce, G. E., and Yang, J. P. S. (1968). *Nature (London)* **220,** 1352–1354.

Hellström, I., Hellström, K. E., Sjögren, H. O., and Warner, G. A. (1971). *Int. J. Cancer* **8,** 185–191.

Hellström, I., Hellström, K. E., and Yeh, M.-Y. (1981a). *Int. J. Cancer* **27,** 281–285.

Hellström, I., Brown, J. P., and Hellström, K. E. (1981b). *J. Immunol.* **127,** 157–160.

Hellström, I., Garrigues, H. J., Cabasco, L., Mosely, G. H., Brown, J. P., and Hellström, K. E. (1983a). *J. Immunol.* **130,** 1467–1472.

Hellström, I., Brown, J. P., and Hellström, K. E. (1983b). *Int. J. Cancer* **31,** 553–555.

Hellström, I., Brankovan, V., and Hellström, K. E. (1985a). *Proc. Natl. Acad. Sci. U.S.A.* **82,** 1499–1502.

Hellström, I., Hellström, K. E., Rollins, N., Lee, V. K., Hudkins, K., and Nepom, G. T. (1985b) *Cancer Res.* **45,** 2210–2218.

Hellström, K. E., Brown, J. P., and Hellström, I. (1980). *Contemp. Top. Immunobiol.* **10,** 117–137.

Hellström, K. E., Hellström, I., and Brown, J. P. (1982a). In "Mechanisms of Host Resistance in Cancer" (R. W. Baldwin, ed.), Springer Semin. Immunopathol. Ser., pp. 127–146. Springer-Verlag, Berlin and New York.

Hellström, K. E., Hellström, I., Kohwi, Y, Rollins, N., and Settle, S. (1982b). *Protides Biol. Fluids* **30,** 317–329.

Hellström, K. E., Hellström, I., Nelson, K., and Nepom, G. T. (1984a). *Trans. Proc.* **16,** 470–473.

Hellström, K. E., Hellström, I., Brown, J. P., Larson, S. M., Nepom, G. T., and Carrasquillo, J. A. (1984b). *Contrib. Oncol.* **19,** 121–131.

Hellström, K. E., Hellström, I., and Brown, J. P. (1985). In "Monoclonal Antibodies and Cancer" (G. L. Wright, ed.), pp. 375–379. Dekker, New York.

Herberman, R. B., ed. (1980). "Natural Cell-Mediated Immunity Against Tumors." Academic Press, London.

Herberman, R. B., and Oldham, R. K. (1975). *J. Natl. Cancer Inst., (U.S.)* **55,** 749–753.

Hersey, P., Honeyman, M., Edwards, A., Adams, E., and McCarthy, W. H. (1976). *Int. J. Cancer* **18,** 564–573.

Hersey, P., Edwards, A., Murray, E., McCarthy, W. H., and Milton, G. W. (1983). *JNCI, J. Natl. Cancer. Inst.* **71,** 45–53.

Houghton, A. N., Eisenger, M., Albino, A. P., Cairncross, J. G., and Old, L. J. (1982). *J. Exp. Med.* **156,** 1755–1766.

Houghton, A. N., Mintzer, D., Cordon-Cardo, C., Welt, S., Fliegel, B., Vadham, S., Carswell, E., Melamed, M. R., Oettgen, H. F., and Old, L. J. (1985). *Proc. Natl. Acad. Sci. U.S.A.* **82,** 1242–1246.

Imai, K., Wilson, B. S., Bigotti, A., Natali, P. G., and Ferrone, S. (1982). *JNCI, J. Natl. Cancer Inst.* **68,** 761.

Jansen, F. K., Blythman, H. E., Carriere, D., Casellas, P., Gros, O., Gros, P., Laurent, J. C., Paolucci, F., Pau, B., Poncelet, P., Richer, G., Vidal, H., and Voisin, G. A. (1982). *Immunol. Rev.* **62,** 185–216.

Jerne, N. K. (1975). *Harvey Lect.* **70,** 93–110.

Johnson, J. P., Holzmann, B., Kaudewitz, P., and Riethmuller, G. (1984). *Contrib. Oncol.* **19,** 132–138.

Karlsson, K.-A., Strömberg, N., Thurin, J., Brodin, T., Sjögren, H. O., Hellström, I., and Hellström, K. E. (1985). Submitted for publication.

Kennedy, R. C., Melnick, J. L., and Dreesman, G. R. (1984). *Science* **223,** 930–931.

Kodera, Y., and Bean, M. A. (1975). *Int. J. Cancer* **16,** 579–592.

Kohler, G., and Milstein, C. (1975). *Nature (London)* **256,** 495–497.

Koprowski, H., and Steplewski, Z. (1981). In "Monoclonal Antibodies and T-Cell Hybridomas" (G. J. Hammerling, U. Hammerling, and J. F. Kearney, eds.), pp. 161–173. Elsevier/North-Holland, Amsterdam.

Koprowski, H., Steplewski, Z., Herlyn, D., and Herlyn, M. (1978). *Proc. Natl. Acad. Sci. U.S.A.* **75,** 3405–3409.

Koprowski, H., Herlyn, M., Steplewski, Z., and Sears, H. (1981). *Science* **212,** 53–55.

Koprowski, H., Herlyn, D., Lubeck, M., DeFreitas, E., and Sears, H. F. (1984). *Proc. Natl. Acad. Sci. U.S.A.* **81,** 216–219.

Larson, S. M., Brown, J. P., Wright, P. W., Carrasquillo, J. A., Hellström, I., and Hellström, K. E. (1983a). *J. Nucl. Med.* **24,** 123–129.

Larson, S. M., Carrasquillo, J. A., Krohn, K. A., Brown, J. P., McGuffin, R. W., Ferens, J. M., Graham, M. M., Hill, L. D., Beaumier, P. L., Hellström, K. E., and Hellström, I. (1983b). *J. Clin. Invest.* **72,** 2101–2114.

Larson, S. M., Carrasquillo, J. A., Krohn, K. A., McGuffin, R. W., Hellström, I., Hellström, K. E., and Lyster, D. (1983c). *JAMA, J. Am. Med. Assoc.* **249,** 811–812.

Larson, S. M., Carrasquillo, J. A., McGuffin, R. W., Krohn, K. A., Ferens, J. M., Hill, L. D., Beaumier, P. L., Hellström, K. E., and Hellström, I. (1985). *Radiology* **155,** 487–492.

Leichner, P. K., Klein, J. L., Siegelman, S. S., Ettinger, D. S., and Order, S. E. (1983). *Cancer Treat. Rep.* **67,** 647–658.

Lewis, M. G., Ikonopisov, R. L., Nairn, R. C., Phillips, T. M., Hamilton-Fairly, G., Bodenham, D. C., and Alexander, P. (1969). *Br. Med. J.* **3,** 547–552.

Liao, S.-K., Kwong, P. C., Khosravi, M., and Dent, P. B. (1982). *JNCI, J. Natl. Cancer Inst.* **68,** 19–25.

Loop, S. M. Nishiyama, K., Hellström, I., Woodbury, R. G., Brown, J. P., and Hellström, K. E. (1981). *Int. J. Cancer* **27,** 775–781.

McAlpine, P. J., and Bootsman, D. (1982). *Cytogenet. Cell Genet.* **32,** 121–129.

McCoy, J. L., Jerome, L. F., Dean, J. H., Perlin, E., Oldham, R. K., Char, D. H., Cohen, M. H., Felix, E. L., and Herberman, R. B. (1975). *J. Natl. Cancer Inst. (U.S.)* **55,** 19–24.

Mach, J. P., Carrel, S. Forni, M., Ritschard, J., Donath, A., and Alberto, P. (1980). *N. Engl. J. Med.* **303,** 5–10.

Marquardt, H., Hunkapiller, M. W., Hood, L. E., and Todaro, G. J. (1984). *Science* **223,** 1079–1982.

Matzku, S., Mattern, J., George, P., and Hellström, I. (1982). In "Gasteiner Internationales Symposium" (Höferm Geknar Bergnabbm, ed.), pp. 295–301. Verlag.

Miller, R. A., Maloney, G. G., Warnke, R., and Levy, R. (1981). *N. Engl. J. Med.* **306,** 517–522.

Mizusawa, E., Serino, M., Hawthorne, M. F., Sharkey, R. M., and Goldenberg, D. M. (1983). In "Proceedings of the First International Symposium on Neutron Capture Therapy" (R. G. Fairchild and G. L. Brownell, eds.), pp. 215–224. Brookhaven Natl. Lab., Upton, New York.

Morton, D. L., Malmgren, R. A., Holmes, E. C., and Ketcham, A. S. (1968). *Surgery (St. Louis)* **64**, 233–240.

Nelson, K. A., Hellström, I., and Hellström, K. E. (1985). *In* "T-Cell Hybridomas" (M. J. Taussig, ed.), pp. 129–138. CRC Press, Boca Raton, Florida.

Nepom, G. T., Hellström, I., and Hellström, K. E. (1983). *Experientia* **39**, 235–242.

Nepom, G. T., Nelson, K. A., Holbeck, S. L., Hellström, I., and Hellström, K. E. (1984). *Proc Natl. Acad. Sci. U.S.A.* **81**, 2864–2867.

Nossal, G. J. V. (1983). *Annu. Rev. Immunol.* **1**, 33–62.

Nudelman, E., Hakomori, S., Kannagi, R., Levery, S., Yeh, M.-Y. Hellström, I., and Hellström, K. E. (1982). *J. Biol. Chem.* **257**, 12752–12756.

Old, L. J. (1981). *Cancer Res.* **41**, 361–375.

Old, L. J., Stockert, E., Boyse, E. A., and Kim, J. H. (1968). *J. Exp. Med.* **127**, 523–539.

Order, S. E. (1984). *Compr. Ther.* **10**, 9–18.

Order, S. E., Bloomer, W. B., Jones, A. G., Kaplan, W. D., Davis, M. A., Adelstein, J., and Hellman, S. (1975). *Cancer* **35**, 1487–1492.

Perlmann, P., and Holm, G. (1969). *Adv. Immunol.* **11**, 117–195.

Plowman, G. D., Brown, J. P., Enns, C. A., Schröder, J., Nikinmaa, B., Sussman, H. H., Hellström, K. E., and Hellström, I. (1983). *Nature (London)*, **303**, 70–72.

Pollack, S., Heppner, G., and Brawn, R. G. (1972). *Int. J. Cancer* **9**, 316–323.

Pukel, C. S., Lloyd, K. O., Trabassos, L. R., Dippold, W. G., Oettgen, H. F., and Old, L. J. (1982). *J. Exp. Med.* **155**, 1133–1147.

Raejewski, K., and Takemori, T. (1983). *Annu. Rev. Immunol.* **1**, 569–607.

Reisfeld, R. A., Morgan, A. C., Jr., and Bumol, T. F. (1982). *In* "Hybridomas in Cancer Diagnosis and Treatment" (M. S. Mitchell and H. F. Oettgen, eds.), pp. 183–186. Raven Press, New York.

Rowland, G. F., Simmonds, R. G., Corvalan, J. R. F., Baldwin, R. W., Brown, J. P., Embleton, M. J., Ford, C. H. J., Hellström, K. E, Hellström, I., Kemshead, J. T., Newman, C. E., and Woodhouse, C. S. (1983). *Protides Biol. Fluids* **30**, 375–379.

Rowland, G. F., Axtan, C. A., Baldwin, R. W., Brown, J. P., Corvalan, J. R. F., Embleton, M. J., Gore, V. A., Hellström, I., Hellström, K. E., Jacobs, E., Marsdan, C. H., Pimm, M. V., Simmonds, R. G., and Smith W. (1985). *Cancer Immunol. Immunother.* **19**, 1–7.

Schimke, R. T. (1984). *Cancer Res.* **44**, 1735–1742.

Schultz, G., Bumol, T. F., and Reisfeld, R. A. (1983). *Proc. Natl. Acad. Sci. U.S.A.* **80**, 5407–5411.

Sears, H. F., Mattis, J., Herlyn, D. Hayry, P., Atkinson, B., Ernst, C., Steplewski, Z., and Koprowski, H. (1982). *Lancet* **1**, 762.

Shiku, H., Takahashi, T., Oettgen, H. F., and Old, L. J. (1976). *J. Exp. Med.* **144**, 873–881.

Shiku, H., Takahashi, T., Resnick, L. A., Oettgen, H. F., and Old, L. J. (1977). *J. Exp. Med.* **145**, 784–789.

Skurzak, H. M., Klein, E., Yoshida, T. O., and Lamon, E. W. (1972). *J. Exp. Med.* **135**, 997–1002.

Slamon, D. J., DeKernion, J. B., Verman, I. M., and Cline, M. J. (1984). *Science* **224**, 256–262.

Steplewski, Z., Herlyn, M., Herlyn, J. A., Clark, W. H., and Koprowski, H. (1979). *Eur. J. Immunol.* **9**, 94–99.

Steplewski, Z., Chang, T., Herlyn, M., and Koprowski, H. (1981). *Cancer Res.* **41**, 2723.

Sternberger, L. A. (1979). "Immunocytochemistry," pp. 104–169. Wiley, New York.

Sutherland, R., Delia, D., Schneider, C., Newman, R., Kemshead, J., and Greaves, M. (1981). *Proc. Natl. Acad. Sci. U.S.A.* **78**, 4515–4519.

Takasugi, M., and Mickey, M. R. (1976). *J. Natl. Cancer Inst. (U.S.)* **57**, 255–261.

Thomas, M. R., Robinson, W. A., Glode, L. M., Koeppler, H., Morton, N., and Sutherland, J. (1982). *Am. J. Clin. Oncol.* **5**, 611–622.

Todaro, G. J., Marquardt, H., Twardzik, D. R., Reynolds, F. H., Jr., and Stephenson, J. R. (1984). *In* "Biological Responses in Cancer" (E. Mihich, ed.), Vol. 1, pp. 1–18. Plenum, New York.

Trowbridge, I. S., and Omary, M. B. (1981). *Proc. Natl. Acad. Sci. U.S.A.* **78**, 3039–3043.

Vollmers, H. P., and Birchmeier, W. (1983a). *Proc. Natl. Acad. Sci. U.S.A.* **80**, 3729–3733.

Vollmers, H. P., and Birchmeier, W. (1983b). *Proc. Natl. Acad. Sci. U.S.A.* **80**, 6863–6867.

Woodbury, R. G., Brown, J. P., Loop, S. M., Hellström, K. E., and Hellström, I. (1980). *Proc. Natl. Acad. Sci. U.S.A.* **77**, 2183–2186.

Woodbury, R. G., Brown, J. P., Loop, S. M., Hellström, K. E., and Hellström, I. (1981). *Int. J. Cancer* **27**, 145–149.

Wybran, J., Hellström, I., Hellström, K. E., and Fudenberg, H. H. (1974). *Int. J. Cancer* **13**, 515–521.

Yanagi, Y., Yoshika, Y., Leggett, K., Clark, S. P., Aleksander, I., and Mak, T. W. (1984). *Nature (London)* **308**, 145–148.

Yeh, M.-Y., Hellström, I., Brown, J. P., Warner, G. A., Hansen, J. A., and Hellström, K. E. (1979). *Proc. Natl. Acad. Sci. U.S.A.* **76**, 2927–2931.

Yeh, M.-Y., Hellström, I., and Hellström, K. E. (1981). *J. Immunol.* **126**, 1312–1317.

Yeh, M.-Y., Hellström, I., Abe, K., Hakomori, S., and Hellström, K. E. (1982). *Int. J. Cancer* **29**, 269–275.

Zinkernagel, R. M., and Doherty, P. C. (1974). *Nature (London)* **251**, 547–548.

CHAPTER 3

Improvement of Colon Carcinoma Imaging: From Polyclonal Anti-CEA Antibodies and Static Photoscanning to Monoclonal Fab Fragments and ECT

Jean-Pierre Mach,* F. Buchegger,* J.-Ph. Grob,*
V. von Fliedner,* S. Carrel,* L. Barrelet,*,†
A. Bischof-Delaloye*,† and B. Delaloye*,†

*Ludwig Institute for Cancer Research
Epalinges, Lausanne, Switzerland
† Policlinique Médicale Universitaire and Division of Nuclear Medicine
Lausanne, Switzerland

I. EARLY RESULTS WITH POLYCLONAL ANTI-CEA ANTIBODIES

Following the pioneer work of Pressman and Korngold (1953) and Bale *et al.* (1955), we introduced into this field the model of nude mice bearing grafts of human colon carcinoma to test the *in vivo* tumor localization of affinity-purified antibodies against carcinoembryonic antigen (CEA)

53

(Mach *et al.*, 1974). We showed that purified ^{131}I-labeled goat anti-CEA antibodies could reach up to a 9 times higher concentration in the tumor than in the liver, while the concentration of control normal IgG in the tumor was never higher than 2.3 times that in the liver. We observed, however, great variations in the degree of specific tumor localization by the same preparation of labeled antibodies when colon carcinoma grafts derived from different patients were tested. This is probably due to the fact that human tumors keep their initial histologic properties and degree of differentiation after transplantation into nude mice, and these two factors appear to affect the ease with which circulating antibodies gain access to the CEA present in tumors. The detection of ^{131}I-labeled antibodies in tumors by external scanning also gave variable results. With colon carcinoma grafts from certain donors, we obtained scans with good tumor localization, whereas with colon carcinoma grafts from other donors the antibody uptake was not sufficient to give satisfactory scanning images. In this context, we think that results in the nude mouse model are a good reflection of the clinical reality observed in patients.

Independently, Goldenberg *et al.* (1974) showed specific tumor localization and detection by external scanning with ^{131}I-labeled IgG fractions of anti-CEA serum, using two human carcinomas which had been serially transplanted into hamsters for several years. Using the same experimental model, Hoffer *et al.* (1974) also demonstrated tumor localization with radiolabled IgG anti-CEA by external scanning.

Goldenberg *et al.* (1978, 1980) reported the first detection of carcinoma in patients obtained by external photoscanning following injection of purified ^{131}I-labeled anti-CEA antibodies. They claimed that almost all the CEA-producing tumors could be detected by this method and that there were no false positive results. However, our experience (Mach *et al.*, 1980a, b), using highly purified goat anti-CEA antibodies and the same blood pool subtraction technology as Goldenberg, was that only 42% of CEA-producing tumors (22 out of 53 tested) could be detected by this method. Furthermore, we found that in several patients the labeled anti-CEA antibodies localized non-specifically in the reticuloendothelium, particularly in the liver. Despite the use of the subtraction technology, these non-specific antibody uptakes were difficult to differentiate from the specific uptakes corresponding to liver metastases. The quality of our polyclonal anti-CEA antibodies did not seem to be the limiting factor, since we showed by direct measurement of the radioactivity in resected tumors that they were capable of giving excellent tumor localization. Furthermore, in a few patients scheduled for tumor resection, we injected simultaneously 1 mg of goat anti-CEA antibodies labeled with 1 mCi of ^{131}I and 1 mg of control normal goat IgG labeled with 0.2 mCi of [125]I. By this paired labeled method adapted to the patient situation, we could demonstrate that the antibody uptake in tumors was four times higher than that of control normal IgG (Mach *et al.*, 1980a, b).

These results were very encouraging in terms of specificity of tumor localization. However, the direct measurement of radioactivity in tumors also showed that only 0.05–0.2% of the injected radioactivity (0.5–2 μCi out of 1000 μCi) was recovered in the resected tumors 3–8 days after injection.

II. FIRST MONOCLONAL ANTI-CEA ANTIBODY USED IN PHOTOSCANNING

The obvious advantage of monoclonal antibodies (Mab) are their homogeneity and their specificity for the immunizing antigen. Another advantage of Mab is that they each react with a single antigenic determinant and thus should not be able to form large immune complexes with the antigen (provided that the antigenic determinant is not repetitive).

The first Mab used for immunoscintigraphy in patients was Mab 23 anti-CEA (Mach *et al.*, 1981). The well-characterized Mab 23 (Accolla *et al.*, 1980) was injected intravenously to 26 patients with large bowel carcinomas and 2 patients with pancreatic carcinomas. Each patient received 0.3 mg of purified Mab labeled with 1–1.5 mCi of [131]I. The patient's premedication included lugol 5% iodine solution, promethazine, and prednisolone, as previously described (Mach *et al.*, 1980a). The patients had no personal history of allergy. They were also tested with an intracutaneous injection of normal mouse IgG and found to have no hypersensitivity against this protein. None of the patients showed any sign of discomfort during or after the injection of labeled mouse antibodies. The patients were studied by static external photoscanning 24, 36, 48, and 72 hr after injection. In 14 of the 28 patients (50%), a radioactive spot corresponding to the tumor was detected 36–48 hr after injection. In 6 patients the scans were doubtful and in the remaining 8 patients they were entirely negative.

The photoscanning results were slightly better than those obtained with polyclonal anti-CEA antibodies; i.e., there was less background radioactivity in the liver, but the method was not yet considered as clinically useful in comparison with the most modern other methods of tumor diagnosis. The ratio of antibody radioactivity in resected tumors as compared to normal mucosa was 4.1 in average for 4 patients (range 2.7–7.5) and the ratio of tumor to normal serosa (= normal bowel wall without the mucosa) was 6.1 (range 4.0–10.1) (Mach *et al.*, 1981).

III. DETECTION OF COLORECTAL CARCINOMA BY ECT WITH ^{131}I-LABELED Mab 23

A logical approach to improve tumor detection by immunoscintigraphy is the use of emission computerized tomography (ECT). As we have seen, static photoscanning is limited in part by the presence of radio-labeled antibodies or free ^{131}I released from them, in the circulation, the reticuloendothelial system, the stomach, intestine, and urinary bladder. Increased radioactivity in these compartments may give false positive results. Specific tumor sites may be masked by non-specific radioactivity. These problems cannot be resolved entirely by the presently available subtraction methods using ^{99m}Tc-labeled HSA and free [99m]TcO$_4^-$ (Deland *et al.*, 1980). Axial transverse tomoscintigraphy is a method initially developed by Kuhl and Edwards (1963) with the potential to resolve some of these problems. This method, also called single photon *emission* computerized tomography (SPECT) or ECT, corresponds to the application of the tomographic technique used in *transmission* computerized axial tomography (CT-scan) to scintigraphic data. Mathematical techniques similar to those used in positron and X-ray tomographies allows the reconstruction of transverse sections as well as frontal, saggital, or oblique sections of patients. In collaboration with Ch. Berche and J. -D. Lumbroso from the Institut Gustave Roussy in Villejuif, we have shown that ECT can improve the sensitivity and specificity of tumor detection using ^{131}I-labeled Mab 23 anti-CEA (Mach *et al.*, 1981; Berche *et al.*, 1982). With this method, 15 out of 16 carcinoma tumor sites studied (including 10 colorectal carcinomas, 1 stomach, 1 pancreas, and 4 medullary thyroid carcinomas) were detectable. These results were encouraging in term of sensitivity. However, it should be noted that numerous non-specific radioactive spots, sometimes as intense as the tumors, were observed. Thus, the problem of non-specific accumulation of antibodies remained, but the three dimensions localization of radioactive spots by ECT helped to discriminate specific tumor uptakes from the non-specific ones (Berche *et al.*, 1982).

IV. STUDY OF Mab FRAGMENTS IN EXPERIMENTAL ANIMALS

In order to further improve this method, we produced a series of 26 new hybridomas secreting anti-CEA antibodies and selected them first,

Mab 202

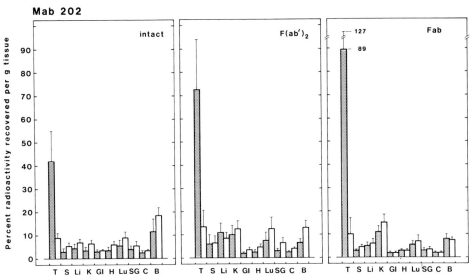

Fig. 1. Distribution of Mab 202 or its fragments (shaded bars) and control IgG or fragments (open bars) injected simultaneously into nude mice bearing grafts of a human carcinoma (CO-112) (Mach *et al.* 1974). The vertical lines represent the standard deviations calculated from groups of four to seven animals per Mab or fragment. T, Tumor; S, spleen; Li, liver; K, kidneys; GI, gastrointestinal tract; H, heart; Lu, lungs; SG, salivary glands; C, carcass and head; B, blood. (From Buchegger *et al.*, 1983. Reproduced from the *Journal of Experimental Medicine*, 1983, Vol. 158, pp. 413–427, by copyright permission of the Rockefeller University Press.)

in vitro, by criteria of high affinity for CEA (Haskell *et al.*, 1983) and low cross-reactivity with glycoproteins present on the surface of granulocytes, termed NCA-55 and NCA-95 (Buchegger *et al.*, 1984). Furthermore, F(ab')$_2$ and Fab fragments were prepared from two selected Mab and tested for their capacity to localize, *in vivo*, in human colon carcinoma heterotransplanted in nude mice (Buchegger *et al.*, 1983). Groups of four to seven mice were injected simultaneously with ^{131}I labeled Mab or fragments and with normal IgG or their corresponding fragments labeled with ^{125}I. The mice were dissected 2–5 days later (2–3 days for both types of fragments and 4–5 days for intact Mab). The results of antibody and normal IgG concentration per gram of tumor and normal organ obtained with Mab 35 and expressed in percentage of the total radioactivity recovered for each isotope are shown in Fig. 1 for Mab 202 and Fig. 2 for Mab 35.

It is evident that the ratios of tumor to normal organ antibody concentration is increased dramatically with the use of fragments. For Mab 202, the ratios of tumor to normal organs antibody concentration (average

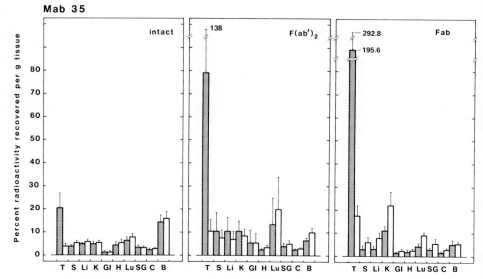

Fig. 2. Distribution of Mab 35 or its fragments (shaded bars) and control IgG or fragments (open bars) injected simultaneously into nude mice bearing grafts of a human carcinoma. (See legend of Fig. 1 for abbreviations.)

from all normal organs) were 15 for intact Mab, 23 for F(ab')$_2$, and 34 for Fab. The specificity indices obtained by dividing each tumor to normal organs ratio obtained for antibody by the corresponding ratio obtained for control IgG were 6.8 for intact Mab, 7.9 for F(ab')$_2$, and 11.9 for Fab. For Mab 35, the tumor to normal organs ratio were 7 for intact Mab, 25

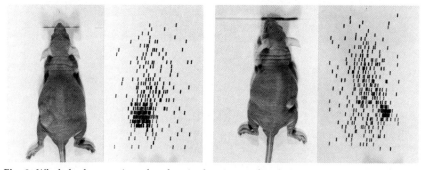

Fig. 3. Whole body scanning of nude mice bearing grafts of a human carcinoma (CO-112), obtained after injection of ^{131}I-labeled Fab fragment of Mab 202 (left panel) or Mab 35 (right panel). Scans shown at the right of the corresponding mice represent raw data without any background subtraction.

for F(ab')$_2$, and 82 for Fab; the specificity indices were 3.4 for intact Mab 8.2 for F(ab')$_2$ and 19 for Fab.

The scanning results obtained with these experimental animals paralleled those obtained by direct measurement of radioactivity. With intact Mab, tumor grafts of 0.5–1 g gave contrasted positive scans only 3 days after injection, whereas fragments of Mab allowed the detection of smaller tumors at an earlier time. Representative scanning results obtained 48 hr after injection of Fab fragments from Mab 202 and 35 demonstrate the clear detection of tumor grafts of 0.3 and 0.1 g, respectively (Fig. 3).

V. DETECTION OF COLON CARCINOMA USING ^{123}I-LABELED Mab FRAGMENTS AND ECT

Based on the foregoing experimental results, we tested a series of 24 patients with colorectal carcinoma after injection of fragments of Mab 202 or 35 labeled with ^{123}I. Only one patient received F(ab')$_2$ of Mab 202, 13 patients F(ab')$_2$ of Mab 35, and 10 patients Fab of Mab 35. The patients were controlled to have no personal history of allergy. The patient's premedication included lugol 5% iodine solution, promethazine, and prednisolone as previously described (Mach et al., 1980a). None of the patients showed any sign of discomfort during or after the injection of antibodies. ^{123}I is an isotope with a very favorable energy of 159 keV and a relatively short physical half-life of 13.2 hr, which proved to be excellent for ECT with Mab fragments. It had been used previously by Epenetos et al. (1982) to label intact Mab for immunoscintigraphy. ^{123}I was prepared from the ^{127}I(p, 5n) ^{123}Xe reaction by the Schweizerisches Institut für Reaktorforshung at Würenlingen, Switzerland. Emission computerized tomography studies of the pelvis and upper abdomen were performed in all patients at 6 and 24 hr after injection and in the majority of patients at 48 hr, using a Searle–Siemens double-head rotating camera. Other parts of the body such as thorax and bones were studied only when there was a clinical suspicion of tumor in these areas or when an abnormal radioactive uptake was detected on whole body scanning (systematically performed before the ECT studies). No subtraction techniques were used, but additional ECT studies of the liver with ^{99m}Tc sulfur colloid were regularly performed after the last ^{123}I analysis with the patient remaining in the same position. Sulfur colloid scintigraphy allowed identification of anatomical landmarks and in some cases comparison of filling defects of ^{99m}Tc colloid with area of increased ^{123}I antibody uptake.

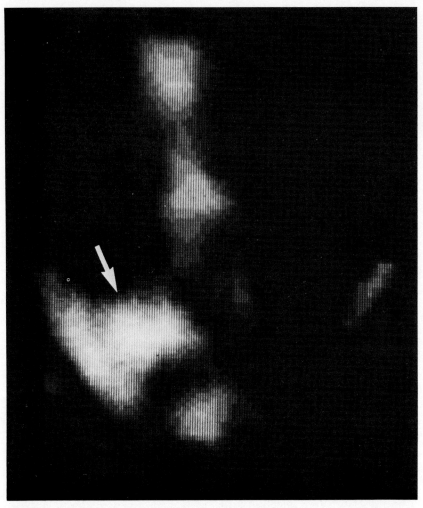

Fig. 4. Coronal ECT section of the posterior part of the pelvis in a patient with a caecum carcinoma of 3–3.5 cm in diameter, taken 24 hr after injection of 1.5 mg of F(ab')$_2$ fragment from Mab 202 labeled with 4 mCi of ^{123}I. The major radioactive spot (arrow) in the center of the right iliac fossa corresponds to the tumor.

One of the first ECT studies, using F(ab')$_2$ of Mab 202, is shown in Fig. 4. The patient was a 80-yr-old male with a caecum carcinoma detected by barium enema. He was injected with 1.5 mg of F(ab')$_2$ from Mab 202 labeled with 4 mCi of ^{123}I and 0.3mCi of ^{125}I. Figure 4 shows a coronal (= frontal) ECT section of the posterior part of the pelvis taken 24 hr

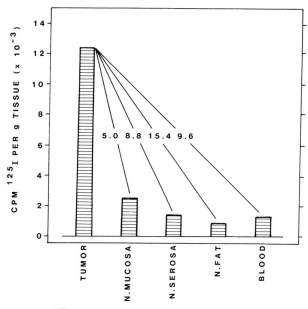

Fig. 5. Concentration of ^{125}I radioactivity per gram (ordinate) in tumor, adjacent normal tissues and blood measured in surgically resected tissue fragments, 5 days after injection of F(ab')2 from Mab 202 labeled with 4 mCi of ^{123}I and with 0.3 mCi [125]I. The results were obtained from the patient with caecum carcinoma studied by ECT as shown in Fig. 4.

after injection. A major radioactive spot localized in the center of the right iliac fossa and corresponding to the position of the tumor can be seen (arrow). Several areas of increased radioactivity corresponding to radioactive uptakes in the bone marrow are detectable in the right iliac wing, in the sacrum, and on two vertebrae. These bone uptakes were not due to the presence of bone metastases, but to a cross-reactivity of Mab 202 with granulocytes and myelocytes present in the bone marrow. Because of this cross-reactivity with granulocytes, we did not use Mab 202 in any of the other patients from this study, despite the fact that this Mab gave excellent tumor uptakes, as demonstrated in Fig. 5. Five days after injection, the patient's tumor was surgically resected and the remaining ^{125}I radioactivity in the tumor and adjacent normal tissues was measured in a gamma-counter as previously described (Mach *et al.*, 1980a, 1981). The tumor was 3.0–3.5 cm in diameter and weighed 29 g. Figure 5 shows that the concentration of radioactivity in tumor divided by that of normal tissues gave ratios of 5.0 with dissected normal mucosa, 8.8 with normal bowel wall without the mucosa (called serosa), 15.4 with normal fat, and 9.6 with blood taken at the time of operation.

The next 23 patients tested with fragments of Mab 35 gave a very high sensitivity of tumor detection by ECT. In the 13 patients injected with $F(ab')_2$ fragments labeled with ^{123}I, 23 out of 28 tumor sites were detected by ECT. This includes 6 of 6 primary or recurrent localized carcinomas, 5 of 8 patients with liver metastases, 0 of 2 lung metastases (of less than 2 cm diameter), and 12 of 12 bone metastases (in 2 patients) (Delaloye *et al.*, 1984). In the 10 patients injected with Fab fragments of Mab 35, 30 out of 31 tumor sites were detected by tomoscintigraphy, including 6 of 7 primary or recurrent carcinomas, 6 of 6 patients with liver metastases, and 18 of 18 bone metastases (in a single patient). We realize that this very high sensitivity is due in part to the selection of patients with known tumors and to the relatively large size of the tumors detected. The smallest primary tumor detected was a carcinomatous polyp of the rectum weighing 4.5 g; the smallest liver metastasis detected had less than 3 cm in diameter as determined by the CT-scan.

VI. DISCUSSION

The major advantage of the use of ECT and ^{123}I-labeled Mab fragment is the high quality of the images which allows distinguishing tumor accumulation of radioactivity from physiological organ concentration and circulating radioactivity without the artifacts inherent in subtraction technology. Our optimistic results in terms of sensitivity should be confirmed in a prospective study in order to determine if such types of immuno-ECT can compete with the most modern morphological diagnostic methods such as CT scan and nuclear magnetic resonance. In any case, we think that ^{123}I-labeled small fragments of Mab with high affinity for CEA represent a definite improvement over previously published results.

Mab against other antigens associated with colorectal carcinoma have been proposed for the detection of this tumor by immunoscintigraphy. We have tested the Mab 17-1A, raised against colon carcinoma in Koprowski's laboratory, with some good results (Mach *et al.*, 1983). Chatal *et al.*, (1984) tested another Mab anti-colon carcinoma, Mab 19-9, also from Koprowski's laboratory, and found it even superior to 17-1A for detection of colon carcinoma by immunoscintigraphy. Farrands *et al.* (1982) from Baldwin's group also obtained good detections of colon carcinoma with their Mab 791T/36, which was raised against human sarcoma cells.

Using intact polyclonal anti-CEA, Begent *et al.*, (1982) reported that they could increase the definition of tumor images by removing circulating radioactive antibodies using liposome-entrapped second antibodies. We think, however, that the use of Mab fragments can resolve the problem of the long half-life in the circulation of labeled intact antibodies without overloading the patient with relatively large amounts of second antibodies.

Finally, the question of the choice of isotope should be mentioned. Among the first, Halpern *et al.* (1983) insisted on the limitations of iodine isotopes, because of their abundant and rapid elimination by the urine presumably due to dehalogenation. For this reason, the authors used antibodies labeled with ^{111}In by chelation using diethylenetriamine pentaacetic acid (DTPA). Fairweather *et al.* (1983), used [111]I-DTPA-labeled anti-CEA antibodies to detect colon carcinoma and reported improvement of the results as compared with ^{131}I-labeling. The non-specific liver uptake of ^{111}In, however, was always very important, thus greatly limiting the method for the detction of liver metastases. Rainsbury *et al.* (1983), using ^{111}In-labeled Mab against the epithelial membrane antigen (EMA) to study breast carcinoma, found that it was capable of detecting only bone metastases.

In conclusion, among the different tracers proposed for diagnosis of colon carcinoma by immunoscintigraphy, we would choose the Fab fragment of Mab 35 labeled with [123]I. This tracer has some limitations—the Fab fragment is too rapidly eliminated through the kidney and the ^{123}I has slightly too-short physical half-life—but the definition of the tumor images obtained at 24 hr appears to be superior to what we have seen with other isotopes and other antibodies.

REFERENCES

Accolla, R. S., Carrel, S., and Mach, J. -P. (1980). *Proc. Natl. Acad. Sci. U.S.A.* **77,** 563–566.

Bale, W. F., Spar, I. L., Goodland, R. L., and Wolfe, D. E. (1955). *Proc. Soc. Exp. Biol. Med.* **89,** 564–568.

Begent, R. H. J., Green, A. J., Bagshawe, K. D., Jones, B. E., Keep, P. A., Searle, F., Jewkes, R. F., Barratt, G. M., and Ryman, B. E. (1982). *Lancet* **2,** 739–742.

Berche, C., Mach, J. -P., Lumbroso, J. -D., Langlais, C., Aubry, F., Buchegger, F., Carrel, S., Rougier, P., Parmentier, C., and Tubiana, M. (1982). *Br. Med. J.* **285,** 1447–1451.

Buchegger, F., Haskell, C. M., Schreyer, M., Scazziga, B. R., Randin, S., Carrel, S., and Mach J. -P. (1983). *J. Exp. Med.* **158,** 413–427.

Buchegger, F., Schreyer, M., Carrel, S., and Mach, J. -P. (1984). *Int. J. Cancer* **33,** 643–649.

Chatal, J. -F., Saccavini, J. -C., Fumoleau, P., Douillard, J. -Y., Curtet, C., Kremer, M., Le Mevel, B., and Koprowski, H. (1984). *J. Nucl. Med.* **25**, 307–314.

Delaloye, B., Delaloye, A., Grob, J. P., Buchegger, F., Barrelet, L., von Fliedner, V., and Mach, J. -P. (1984). *In* "Radioaktive Isotope in Klinik und Forschung," (R. Höfer and H. Bergmann, eds.).Vol. 16, 2. Teil, Proc. Badgastein Symp. H. Egermann, Vienna, Austria.

Deland, F. H., Kim, E. E., Simmons, G., and Goldenberg, D. M. (1980). *Cancer Res.* **40**, 3046–3049.

Epenetos, A. -A., Malther, S., Granowska, M., Nimmon, C. C., Hawkins, L. R., Britton, K. E., Shepherd, J., Taylor-Papadimitriou, J., Durbin, H., Malpas, J. S., and Bodmer, W. F. (1982). *Lancet* **2**, 999–1005.

Fairweather, D. S., Bradwell, A. R., Dykes, Vaugan, A. T., Watson-James, S. F., and Chandler, S. (1983). *Br. Med. J.* **287**, 167–170.

Farrands, P. A., Pimm, M. W., Embleton, M. J., Perkins, A. C., Hardy, J. D., Baldwin, R. W., and Hardcastle, J. D. (1982). *Lancet* **2**, 397–400.

Goldenberg, D. M., Preston, D. F., Primus, F. J., and Hansen, H. J. (1974). *Cancer Res.* **34**, 1–9.

Goldenberg, D. M., DeLand, F., Enishin, K., Bennett, S., Primus, F. J., van Nagell, J. R., Estes, N., DeSimone, P., and Rayburn, P. (1978). *N. Engl. J. Med.* **298**, 1384–1388.

Goldenberg, D. M., Kim, E. D., DeLand, F. H., Bennett, S., and Primus, F. J. (1980). *Cancer Res.* **40**, 2984–2992.

Halpern, S., Stern, P., Hagen, P., Chen, A., Frincke, J., Bartholomew, R., David, G., and Adams, T. (1983). *In* "Radioimmunoimaging and Radioimmunotherapy" (S. W. Burchiel and B. A. Rhodes, eds.), pp. 197–205. Am. Elsevier, New York.

Haskell, C. M., Buchegger, F., Shreyer, M., Carrel, S., and Mach, J. -P. (1983). *Cancer Res.* **43**, 3857–3864.

Hoffer, P. B., Lathrop, K., Bekerman, G., Fang, V. S., and Refetoff, S. (1974). *J. Nucl. Med.* **15**, 323–327.

Kuhl, D. E., and Edwards, R. D. (1963). *Radiology* **80**, 653–662.

Mach, J. -P., Carrel, S., Merenda, C., Sordat, B., and Cerottini, J. -C. (1974). *Nature (London)* **248**, 704–706.

Mach, J. -P., Carrel, S., Forni, M., Ritschard, J., Donath, A., and Alberto, P. (1980a). *N. Engl. J. Med.* **303**, 5–10.

Mach, J. -P., Forni, M., Ritschard, J., Buchegger, F., Carrel, S., Widgren, S., Donath, A., and Alberto, P. (1980b). *Oncodev. Biol. Med.* **1**, 49–69.

Mach, J. -P., Buchegger, F., Forni, M., Ritschard, J., Berche, C., Lumbroso, J. D., Shreyer, M., Girardet, C., Accolla, R. S., and Carrel, S. (1981). *Immunol. Today* **2**, 239–249.

Mach, J. -P., Chatal, J. -F., Lumbroso, J. -D., Buchegger, F., Forni, M., Ritschard, J., Berche, C., Douillard, J. -Y., Carrel, S., Herlyn, M., Steplewski, Z., and Koprowski, H. (1983). *Cancer Res.* **43**, 5593–5600.

Pressman, D., and Korngold, L. (1953). *Cancer* **6**, 619–623.

Rainsbury, R. M., Westwook, J. H., Coombes, R. C., Neville, A. M., Ott, R. J., Kalirai, T. S., McCready, V. R., and Gazet, J. -C. (1983). *Lancet* **2**, 934–938.

CHAPTER 4

Developments in Antibody Imaging

A. R. Bradwell, D. S. Fairweather[1] and P. W. Dykes

Immunodiagnostic Research Laboratory
Department of Immunology
Medical School
University of Birmingham
Birmingham, United Kingdom

I. THEORETICAL CONSIDERATIONS

Many factors are involved in radioimmunodetection (RAID) of cancer, and whilst some have an obvious relationship to the outcome of the scan, others may have a more subtle influence.

Thus, a theoretical understanding of the potential and limitations of the technique allows the most useful avenues to be explored. With this in mind, Rockoff *et al.* (1980) defined the major factors involved and

---

[1]Present address: Department of Geriatric Medicine, University Hospital of South Manchester, Manchester M20 8LR, United Kingdom.

MONOCLONAL ANTIBODIES FOR CANCER
DETECTION AND THERAPY

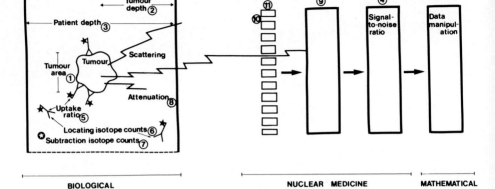

Fig. 1. Parameters used in the model for the radioimmunodetection of tumours. Units: 1, 2 and 3 in square centimeters; 4, signal-to-noise ratio; 5, uptake ratio; 6 and 7, counts per square centimeter; 8, per centimeter; 9, camera resolution, FWHM in millimeters; 10, hole diameter in millimeters; 11, hole depth in millimeters. (From Bradwell, A. R., Fairweather, D. F. and Dykes, P. W., Radioimmunodetection of endocrine tumours, *Advanced Medicine* **19**, 76–92, 1983, by permission of Pitman Publishing Ltd., London.)

used a computer model to show the likely limitations of RAID. We have further adapted this to determine the practical limitations in relationship to the present state-of-the-art (Bradwell *et al.*, 1983d). Figure 1 indicates the 11 parameters that we used. Three of these are patient dependent and therefore fixed: (1) Tumour area (as seen by the camera); (2) tumour depth; and (3) patient depth at the site of the tumour. The signal-to-noise ratio (4) is also fixed and it is generally considered that its minimum recognised value is three.

The uptake ratio (5) of antibody onto the tumour compared with the surrounding normal tissue is the most important single determinant of scan sensitivity. Unfortunately there are a host of factors which reduce antibody uptake *in vivo*; some of these are discussed later. Reported values in patients vary between one and ten (Table I) although animal results have been considerably better (Hedin *et al.*, 1982). The influence of the uptake ratio in detecting different-sized lesions at various depths as determined by the model is shown in Fig. 2.

Calculations indicate that, next to uptake ratios, the most important factor is the absolute count rate of the tumour-locating isotope (6). When using ^{131}I, count rates are usually low compared with other methods using isotopes and in our hands often less than 100/cm^2 in the image. A trebling of this rate would be equivalent to doubling the uptake ratio and a tenfold increase equivalent to a threefold rise in uptake ratio (Fig. 3).

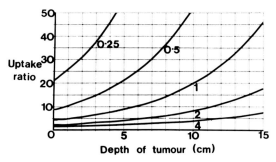

Fig. 2. Relationship between uptake ratio (5) and tumour depth (2) with contours on tumour area (1). Other parameters from Fig. 1: 3 = 20; 4 = 3; 6 = 300; 7 = 300; 8 = 0.127 (^{111}In); 9 = 4.8; 10 = 4.3; 11 = 50.

With regard to the detection system (Fig. 1), the computer model does not suggest that marked benefit is likely to follow from improvements in conventional γ cameras, although for specific areas such as the neck, magnifying collimators may be of value. Computerised tomography (CT) would potentially be advantageous. Most other factors, such as γ-ray scattering in the body, camera blurring and sensitivity are physical limitations inherent in the present systems.

Several techniques of data manipulation have been studied. To reduce subjectivity, scans can be thresholded to display only significant counts and non-linear deconvolution techniques should improve the signal-to-noise ratio (Fairweather *et al.*, 1983c) over the established techniques. Scans should therefore be quantitatively assessed with due regard to the statistical significance of different areas. These techniques are discussed later.

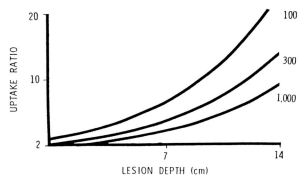

Fig. 3. Demonstrates the relationship between count rates and uptake ratio in detecting a 2-cm diameter tumour at different depths. Parameters from Fig. 1: 3 = 20; 4 = 3; 7 = 1000; 8 = 0.11 (^{131}I); 9 ≐ 4.8; 10 = 4.3; 11 = 50. (From Fairweather *et al.*, 1983b.)

As with other new techniques, there are no accepted normal limits for antibody scans. Poor count rates and a low uptake ratio both contribute to an image that contains artefacts and the distinction between true signal and noise can seem arbitrary.

II. RADIOIMMUNODETECTION PROCEDURES

A. Antisera

The polyclonal antisera used in these studies were prepared in sheep by immunising with purified human proteins. Non-specific antibodies were adsorbed on glutaraldehyde polymers of human serum and normal tissues until specific reaction on tissue sections were obtained using the peroxidase anti-peroxidase technique (Sternberger, 1979). The titre and affinity of the antibodies were tested in radioimmunoassays. An IgG-rich fraction of each antiserum was prepared by ion-exchange chromatography on DEAE-52 cellulose, sterilised by filtration and tested for pyrogens (European Pharmacopoeia, 1971) by an independent laboratory.

We have tended to label the antiserum without further processing although most workers have added an affinity purification step (Goldenberg *et al.*, 1978). This latter process may, however, have some undesirable effects (see below). In the case of mouse monoclonal antibodies, protein A is a useful material for effecting separation of the immunoglobulin sub-classes (Ey *et al.*, 1978; Dykes *et al.*, 1980).

B. Radiolabelling

Until recently, only iodine isotopes have been suitable for simple attachment to proteins and are appropriate for external scanning with γ cameras. The chloramine-T method is usually employed for iodination (Watson-James *et al.*, 1981) since it can be shown to cause little or no detectable change in the biological behaviour of immunoglobulin molecules. The most frequently used iodine isotope has been ^{131}I although studies with ^{123}I have been successful (Epenetos *et al.*, 1982). In addition, [124]I has been used for positron tomography but is unlikely to find wide application (Bateman *et al.*, 1983).

[111]In has been suggested as a useful alternative to ^{131}I for several reasons; first, because of its lower energy (241 and 171 keV), but higher

abundance photons; second, the lack of high radiation β particles; and third, the half-life (2.83 days) is ideal for antibody scanning. There are several technical difficulties in preparing ^{111}In-labelled antibodies of high specific activity but these have recently been overcome (Sundberg et al., 1974; Krejcarek and Tucker, 1977) and the results indicate greater sensitivity than comparable ^{131}I-labelled antibodies (Fairweather et al., 1983c). The details are discussed later in section IV,B.

Most workers have attempted to remove aggregated immunoglobulin after labelling because it may cause false positive localisation in the liver and other reticuloendothelial sites. Gel filtration or centrifugation may be used but we have favoured the latter because it is simple and sterility is easy to maintain.

C. Preparation of the Patient

Uptake of radioactive antibody by the thyroid and stomach is blocked by giving 420 mg of potassium iodide (KI) and 400 mg of potassium perchlorate ($KClO_3$) 30 min before the ^{131}I-labelled antibody (Bradwell et al., 1983a), followed by 120 mg KI, every 6 hr and 200 mg $KClO_3$ every 6 hr for 2 days. After the second scan, only the KI is continued at 120 mg every 8 hr (Fairweather et al., 1983b).

Prior to injecting the labelled antibody, a small amount is given intracutaneously to test for hypersensitivity and, providing there is no reaction, the remainder is given slowly. The documented side effects are remarkably few. Of 80 patients scanned, pyrexia has only occurred twice, which required no treatment. Fifteen patients have had two or more scans with no adverse reactions. This experience is similar to that reported by other investigators (Begent et al., 1983).

D. Nuclear Medicine Techniques

When ^{131}I is used as the radiolabel, at least 18.5 MBq (0.5 mCi) must be injected to obtain sufficient counts for imaging. In general, the higher the dose the better, and 37–74 MBq is preferable. In our experience, the whole body adsorbed dose from ^{131}I-labelled sheep IgG is 0.135 mSi/MBq (500 mrem/mCi). This compares favourably with other imaging techniques (e.g., 1 rem/CT examination).

Images are obtained with a large field of view (LFOV) γ camera (although rectilinear scanners have been used) usually 24 and 48 hr postinjection. As mentioned previously, less than 1% of the injected antibody

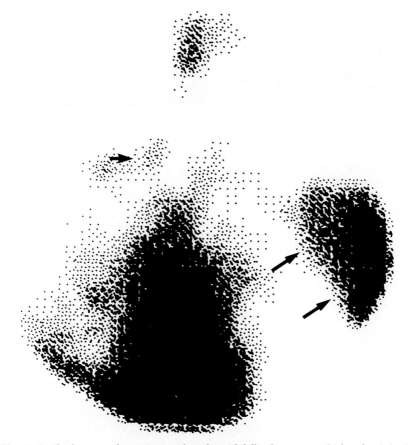

Fig. 4. Antibody scan of a patient with a thyroid follicular tumour 24 hr after injection with ^{131}I-labelled anti-thyroglobulin. (A) Total ^{131}I counts with left shoulder and clavicle lesion arrowed. (B) Subtraction scan showing the enhanced lesions plus pulmonary deposits but also a ring artefact and a silhouette. (From Fairweather *et al.*, 1983a.)

accumulates in any one tumour site. (Mach *et al.*, 1980), and the distribution of antibody in the body is not uniform (about 50% remaining in the vascular compartment). With experience, it is possible to gauge the expected background pattern and therefore pick out small abnormal areas, but this is very subjective.

Computer Subtraction

The addition of a subtraction isotope has caused considerable controversy and attempts have been made to avoid its use (Mach *et al.*, 1980;

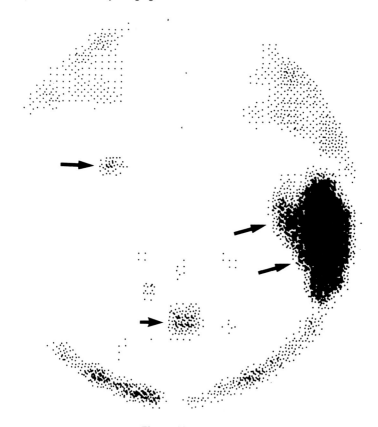

Fig. 4. *(Continued.)*

Begent *et al.*, 1982). On theoretical grounds such a process must add noise (Bradwell *et al.*, 1983d). However, its advantage is that it masks the variation in vascular supply to different tissues, thereby allowing small tumours, with low uptake ratios, to be detected. Indeed, it was the use of this subtraction scanning procedure that enabled Goldenberg to obtain the first convincing results in patients (Goldenberg *et al.*, 1978).

This subtraction technique made use of a second isotope to mimic the distribution of normal immunoglobulin (Fig. 4). In practice, 20 MBq each of ^{99m}Technetium (^{99m}Tc)-labelled pertechnetate and [^{99m}Tc]-albumin are injected 30 and 5 min, respectively, before each scan. A camera and computer with a dual isotope facility are required to record the 141 keV ^{99m}Tc photons and 364 keV ^{131}I photons simultaneously and effect the subtraction.

Although this improves contrast, it does so at the expense of adding artefacts and introducing further statistical fluctuations without increasing the signal, i.e., reducing the signal-to-noise ratio (Bradwell *et al.*, 1983d). Goldenberg used the blood pool (the heart) for normalisation and although this is reported to improve contrast twofold (DeLand *et al.*, 1980), it is subject to bias on exactly which area is taken. An alternative approach is to correlate the ^{99m}Tc and ^{131}I image pixels using the 'least squares' method, where the normalising factor is given by the slope of the regression line (Fairweather, *et al.*, 1983c).

Other problems with subtraction are that the technetium pharmaceuticals do not distribute in exactly the same way as normal IgG and the large difference between ^{99m}Tc and ^{131}I γ energies leads to differences in attenuation and scattering, dependent on the area being scanned. These effects can be compensated to some extent by the use of local subtraction (Goldenberg *et al.*, 1981) where the factor is calculated separately for each organ of interest. This may improve contrast 20-fold, but it is both time consuming and open to greater bias.

Noise (random fluctuation in the background) is a feature of all nuclear medicine techniques but especially antibody scans when ^{131}I is used, since count rates are usually low (typically less than 200/cm^2). Since this fluctuation is given by a Poisson distribution, the variance for each pixel in the subtraction picture can be calculated and the significance of counts in the subtraction picture assessed by replotting after subtracting two standard deviations from each pixel; any counts remaining are regarded as highly significant (Fairweather *et al.*, 1983c). [See Fig. 4 where the lesion arrowed in (A) is shown to be highly significant (B).]

However, regardless of the subtraction technique used it is not possible to equalise the counts in all areas. Thus, the bladder always contains an excess of free iodine or technetium, as many other parts of the urinary tract, which lead to hot or cold areas. Inequalities may also occur around the heart or stomach although the latter can usually be blocked with KI and KClO$_3$. Thus, intelligent assessment of the scans is always required.

III. CLINICAL RESULTS

Overall results of the published series are given in Table I. In general, a >70% positivity rate is achieved with a low (approximately 10%) false positive rate. Similar results are reported by different groups using different antisera and in different situations. Although tumour-to-normal tissue ratios in surgically excised specimens have not been routinely measured, those available indicate similar localising abilities *in vivo* for

TABLE I

CLINICAL STUDIES WITH RADIOLABELLED ANTIBODIES[a]

Authors and antigen detected	Antibody type	Tumour type	No. of lesions scanned	Positive rate (%)	Uptake ratio (U)	Smallest lesion found (cm)
CEA						
Goldenberg *et al.*, 1978	AP	Mixed	40	85	2.5	?
Dykes *et al.*, 1980	PC	Colon	14	80	2.5	2
Mach *et al.*, 1980	AP	Colon	21	58	3.6	?
Mach *et al.*, 1981	Mab	Mixed	28	50	4	?
DeLand *et al.*, 1982	AP	Mixed	156	75	?	?
Berche *et al.*, 1982	Mab	Mixed	17	94	?	1 +
Smedley *et al.*, 1983	Mab	Mixed	27	60	?	?
Fairweather *et al.*, 1983a	PC	Mixed	31	90	?	?
Goldenberg *et al.*, 1983	AP	Colon	65	88	?	?
AFP						
Goldenberg *et al.*, 1980a	PC	Mixed	13	85	?	?
Halsall *et al.*, 1981	PC	Germ cell	15	80	?	2
HCG						
Begent *et al.*, 1980	AP	Germ cell	21	72	?	0.5
Goldenberg *et al.*, 1980b	PC	Germ cell	18	100	40£	?
Thyroglobulin						
Fairweather *et al.*, 1983b	PC	Thyroid	40	85	?	1.7
Insulin						
Fairweather *et al.*, 1982a	PC	Insulinoma	3	66	2.2	2
Others						
Ghose *et al.*, 1980	Mab	Renal	28	95	2.3	2
Farrands *et al.*, 1982	Mab	Colon	10	90	2.3	?
Epenetos *et al.*, 1982	Mab	Mixed	32	75	?	?
Larson *et al.*, 1983	Mab	Melanoma	25	88	4.3	1.5
Rainsbury *et al.*, 1983	Mab	Breast	102	52	4	?

[a]Abbreviations: PC = polyclonal; AP = affinity-purified polyclonal; Mab = monoclonal; U = tumour-to-normal tissue ratio in surgically resected samples; + = using photon emmission tomography; £ = one sample only; ? = unknown.

all types of antisera; conventional, affinity purified and monoclonal. Apart from one group (Berche *et al.*, 1982) who used single photon emission tomography (SPET), most claim that the smallest tumours detectable are 1.5–2 cm in diameter, depending on the site. This may in part be related to the difficulty in confirming smaller areas by conventional tests. However, most patients scanned have had lesions much bigger and large masses are easy to localise by many techniques.

A number of recurring problems have emerged. First, as with any new technique, interpretation of the image may be subjective and difficult to quantify, and the 'picture quality' is poor. Second, there is always some difficulty in establishing the true extent of a patient's disease in order to define false positives and false negatives. Third, different centres pursue conventional investigations with varying vigour, and comparisons with established techniques may be difficult.

IV. RECENT DEVELOPMENTS

The tantalising feature of RAID is that antibodies are highly specific probes for *in vitro* use and in some animal/tumour models. What, therefore, are the promising avenues that might be explored to help realise the potential indicated by the experimental data and the theoretical considerations?

A. Uptake Ratios

A small lesion only receives a minute proportion of the cardiac output and this limits the percentage uptake since antibody will inevitably be catabolised elsewhere. A good analogy is the detection of differentiated thyroid carcinoma with ^{131}I where a very high dose may have to be given to disclose small lesions, despite a specific- and high-affinity uptake mechanism. Access may also be limited by circulating antigen which can form complexes and block antibody-binding sites. Further restrictions are the slow rate of immunoglobulin diffusion out of the normal vascular tree (50% always remains intravascular), and antigenic sites in the tumour may be limited.

There is conflicting evidence regarding the actual site of antibody binding (Mach *et al.*, 1981; Lewis *et al.*, 1982; Moshakis *et al.*, 1981). Antigen may be present within the cells, on the surface, or externally, either soluble or immobilised on cell debris or in phagocytic cells. Accumulation in any, or more, of the above areas will contribute to a positive scan (Fairweather *et al.*, 1982b).

Even when antibody has attached to antigen on the tumour cell surface, it may be rapidly lost. Cross-linking of cell surface components may induce movements in the membrane (Unanue and Karnovsky, 1974) which can lead to the shedding of the antibody–antigen complexes (antigenic modulation) or rapid endocytosis and catabolism (patching and capping). Carcinoembryonic antigen (CEA) is known to cap (Hirai *et al.*, 1980), and there is circumstantial evidence that cell surface bound anti-CEA is lost rapidly (Stern *et al.*, 1982).

Potential areas for improvement include increasing the titre and affinity of the antisera and finding tumour antigens of greater specificity. Monoclonal antibodies (Mab) may seem the ideal answer. There is impressive *in vitro* and animal work to show they can be superior to polyclonal antisera and uptake ratios of over 200—more than 10 times those achieved with conventional antisera—have been achieved (Hedin *et al.*, 1982). However, human studies have been disappointing (see Table I). Some aspects of Mab which should be born in mind are:

1. Their extreme specificity may reduce tumour accumulation if the quantity of antigen is limited, especially if the Mab can only recognise one binding site (epitope) per antigen molecule. In contrast, several polyclonal antibody molecules may attach to each antigen.

2. An apparently specific Mab may bind unexpectedly to other antigens, e.g., a Mab against a segment of CEA may recognise a similar segment in a quite different antigen.

3. The affinity of the antiserum may have to be high (as well as the titre). This has not been easy to achieve.

4. Mouse immunoglobulins may interact with human Fc receptors and produce false positive localisation unless fragments are prepared. The value of antibody fragments has yet to be determined. Nevertheless, it is likely that further studies will show considerable improvements.

There are also problems associated with affinity-purified antisera: It is likely that the highest affinity antibodies are not eluted from the affinity column and it is known that agents capable of breaking the antibody–antigen bond may disrupt the whole molecule sufficiently to alter its biological properties (Searle *et al.*, 1981). These factors may explain why it has proved difficult to improve on high-grade polyclonal antisera.

An alternative approach to increasing the uptake ratio is to use a second antibody to clear the circulation of the unbound first (radiolabelled) antibody. This was initially proposed encapsulated in a liposome, with good results (Krejcarek and Tucker, 1977), but it has since been shown that this may be unnecessary. A seven-fold increase in clearance of unbound localising antibody has been achieved in animals by using a second antibody (Bradwell *et al.*, 1983b). In patients given a second antibody, blood counts have fallen more than twice as quickly as control subjects yet tumour counts have been maintained (Bradwell *et al.*, 1983c).

This second antibody technique could be applied to whatever antibody system is being used providing it does not generate spurious uptake in reticuloendothelial sites. The optimal system has yet to be evaluated.

A further refinement is the use of immunoglobulin fragments which may gain access to tumours more easily than the whole molecule, but results were not strikingly better in one careful *in vivo* study (Mach *et al.*, 1981).

As regards the relevance of the antigen location, it is logical to aim the antibody at a cell surface antigen, although we have successfully scanned patients with antibodies directed against antigens that are not primarily cell surface components, i.e., α-fetoprotein (AFP) (Halsall *et al.*, 1981) and thyroglobulin (Fairweather *et al.*, 1983b). By this means, particularly with anti-thyroglobulin, we hoped to avoid the "capping" and loss of cell surface bound antibody (modulation) that occurs with divalent antibodies. Overall, the results were similar to those obtained with anti-CEA (Table I), perhaps reflecting the multiple factors that determine scanning success in patients. Studies are presently underway to investigate the value of a monovalent antibody which is known to have enhanced tumour binding because modulation does not occur (Glennie and Stevenson, 1982). Mab also may not induce modulation, but this needs to be investigated. Alternatively, use may be made of modulation by labelling the protein with an isotope that is retained within cells (see below).

B. Count Rates

Higher count rates with iodine labels can obviously be achieved by giving a larger dose to the patient and/or counting for a longer time. Both are subject to practical limitations. 74 MBq of ^{131}I-labelled antibody gives a similar absorbed radiation dose to X-ray CT (1 rem) and a scanning time of 5–10 min per view is comparable to other nuclear medicine techniques.

^{131}I, in particular, is not a good isotope for these studies. First, the high photon energy (364 keV) is poorly detected by present γ cameras and requires the use of a high-energy collimator which reduces sensitivity still further. Second, the β emission contributes to a high radiation dose to the patients, limiting total activity which can be injected. ^{123}I has a more suitable photon energy for detection and delivers a radiation dose only one-tenth that of ^{131}I. Unfortunately, the short half-life (13 hr) is not ideal, and it cannot be used with ^{99m}Tc for background subtraction due to overlapping photon energies. ^{123}I-labelled antibodies have been used successfully (Epenetos *et al.*, 1982) but in this study only large tumours were visualised.

^{111}In has suitable characteristics for γ-camera imaging and also gives a three- to eightfold higher count rate than ^{131}I with our γ camera (Searle LFOV) for a similar administered dose. We have labelled anti-CEA with

TABLE II

COMPARISON OF ^{111}IN- AND ^{131}I-LABELLED ANTI-CEA FOR TUMOUR DETECTION IN FIVE PATIENTS WITH CEA-PRODUCING TUMOURS

	Number of sites revealed	
Scan result[a]	^{111}In	^{131}I
+ +	10	4
+	3	4
−	2	7

[a] + + = Definite; + = probable; − = negative.

^{111}In using a bifunctional chelating agent (Sundberg *et al.*, 1974; Krejcarek and Tucker, 1977). A strong chelating group, diethylenetriamine pentaacetic acid (DTPA), was covalently attached to the antibody (Fairweather *et al.*, 1983a). This modified antiserum was then radiolabeled with ^{111}In by mixing the two in solution, when a chelate bond is formed spontaneously. Although this bond is reversible, it is sufficiently stable for *in vitro* studies.

We have studied five patients with CEA-producing tumours with both ^{111}In-labeled anti-CEA and ^{131}I-labelled anti-CEA for comparison (Table II). Not only did ^{111}In show more sites than the ^{131}I-labelled antibody but did so with greater certainty. This advantage of ^{111}In appears to be due to two factors. First, the improved count rates (the patients received the same dose of each isotope and were scanned for equal times) and second, the greater retention of ^{111}In by tumours (Fairweather *et al.*, 1983a). It appears that since the isotope is a trivalent metal ion, once it has entered the cell it is retained for long periods. This is in contrast to iodine which is rapidly excreted. Thus, modulation may be an advantage with indium-labelled antibodies. This is illustrated in Fig. 5 where the higher contrast with ^{111}In is clearly visible at day 5, whereas with ^{131}I an adequate image could not be obtained after 2 days. Unfortunately, the long biological half-life of indium contributes to an absorbed dose equal to that of ^{131}I (which has a shorter biological half-life), but nevertheless it is clearly a superior isotope for scanning.

C. Alternative Imaging Methods

As indicated previously, improvements to the Anger camera are unlikely to yield strikingly better results. The greatest improvement is likely

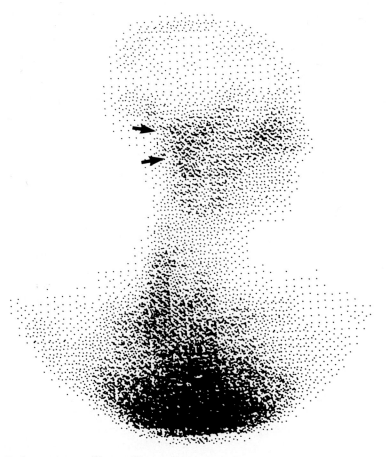

Fig. 5. Comparison of ¹³¹I- and ¹¹¹In-labelled anti-CEA in the same patient. All scans are unsubtracted and the arrows indicate a deposit of CEA-producing squamous carcinoma near the right sub-mandibular joint. A, ¹³¹I scan at 24 hr. B, ¹¹¹In scan at 24 hr. C, ¹¹¹In scan at 5 days. The greater count rates from ¹¹¹In are seen together with its gradual accumulation in the tumour (see pp. 79–80). (From Bradwell, A. R., Fairweather, D. F. and Dykes, P. W., Radioimmunodetection of endocrine tumours, *Advanced Medicine* **19**, 76–92, 1983, by permission of Pitman Publishing Ltd., London.)

to come from tomographic methods. There are two different types of emission tomography, single photon (SPET) and positron (PET). There are important differences between the two techniques (Brownell *et al.*, 1982). The SPET can be implemented with a conventional γ camera detector and established isotopes, but is subject to the limitations inherent in collimated cameras. The PET utilises the paired γ rays produced from the interaction of positrons with electrons in the body. These rays are

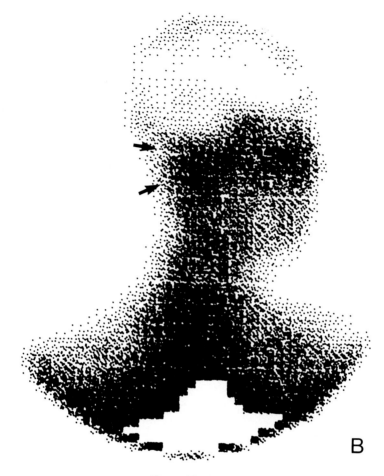

Fig. 5. *(Continued.)*

emitted at 180° to each other, and can be accurately located by two linked detectors opposite one another and without using a collimator.

Berche *et al.* (1982) applied SPET and ^{131}I-labelled Mab to patients with apparently successful results. However, tomographic reconstruction is heavily dependent on good counting statistics which perhaps reflect their need to scan for 40 min. Furthermore, they did not compare SPET with a conventional LFOV γ camera and technetium subtraction.

We have investigated a prototype positron camera (Bateman *et al.,* 1982) which shows promise, and have been able to demonstrate hepatic metastases with a very small injected dose (1 MBq). [123]I or ^{111}In would appear ideal for SPET, particularly ^{123}I because of its favourable dosimetry

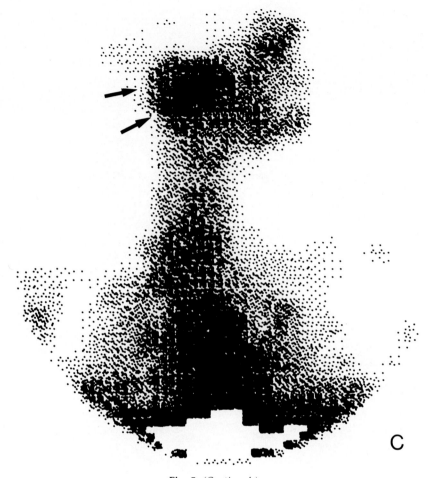

C

Fig. 5. *(Continued.)*

and because with tomography the inability to use technetium subtraction may be less of a drawback.

D. Data Manipulation

The original subtraction method for scan enhancement improved the contrast in the image about twofold (Goldenberg *et al.*, 1978). If an organ-specific pharmaceutical is used for local subtraction (e.g., [^{99m}Tc]-sulphur colloid for the liver), the contrast can be improved 20-fold (23) (see above).

To improve objectivity in the subtraction picture, the variance can be calculated and each point represented as standard deviations above background (see computer subtraction above). Alternatively, statistical noise can be assessed for each point (pixel) in the picture and removed by using a Weiner filter (Fairweather et al., 1983c) for each image before subtraction. Figure 6 shows a resulting image plotted in contours, with each step representing one standard deviation above background. The data can be further improved by deconvolution and contouring in standard deviations above background noise. Initial results indicate that this improves contrast an additional twofold. Furthermore, this approach avoids arbitrary scaling of the image and enables a rapid and quantitative assessment of each area of the scan.

V. CONCLUSION

It is still too early to determine the role of RAID in tumour detection, but some authors suggest its use as a routine procedure and most claim to detect a substantial number of lesions not detected by other imaging techniques. Goldenberg is a keen protagonist (Goldenberg et al., 1983) but we are less enthusiastic (Dykes and Bradwell, 1983), and feel that the main consideration is whether it helps in patient management. There is limited value in locating tumours that cannot be removed or do not respond to therapy and, unfortunately, this is true for most tumours producing CEA. α-Fetoprotein- and human chorionic gonadotrophin (HCG)-producing tumours are usually treated with polychemotherapy based on monitoring the serum concentration, so again, accurate localisation is of restricted use. Many of the other studies described also fall into these categories. Furthermore, RAID has to compete with other techniques in terms of sensitivity and cost. It is unlikely that it will ever compare favourably with CAT scanning of the lungs where density contrast is high. However, in the abdomen the opposite is true, and many workers have detected lesions missed by other methods.

One potential advantage of RAID over all other techniques is that it can determine the tissue type of a known mass. We have scanned a few patients with anti-AFP who had residual masses after chemotherapy, of

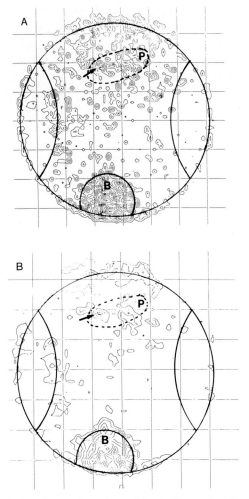

Fig. 6. Data manipulation. Scans of a patient with a malignant insulinoma (arrowed) after injection of ^{131}I-labelled anti-insulin. A, Subtracted image. B, The same data processed through a Wiener filter to remove artefact. C, Same data after deconvolution. Each contour is one standard deviation above the background noise. P = Pancreas; B = bladder.

unknown viability. Results were consistent with the subsequent clinical progress and may have prevented a more risky biopsy. If the sensitivity improves sufficiently to reliably detect lesions half a centimeter in diameter, then a variety of tumours could be usefully located; in particular, relatively benign endocrine tumours could be located prior to surgical excision. This level of sensitivity would also allow accurate staging of a host of tumours prior to surgery or chemotherapy.

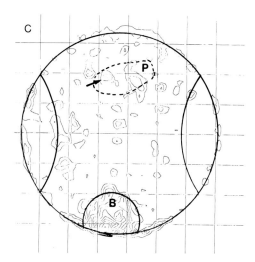

Fig. 6. *(Continued.)*

It must not be forgotten that antibodies can locate in normal, as well as malignant, tissue. Endocrine tissue is characterised by the production of specific substances to which antisera can be raised. The products are highly organ specific, e.g., thyroglobulin for thyroid tissue. We have already shown that antibodies to thyroglobulin and insulin can locate sites of production and it is probable that other endocrine sites can be imaged as well. Myocardial infarcts have also been imaged by antibodies (Brault and White, 1971) as have parasitic cysts (Khaw *et al.*, 1980).

Antibody scans provide functional information (the production and presence of an antigen and its quantity) rather than just structural information. Imaging, combined with the great variety of antisera that can be produced, is likely to find application in diverse fields.

ACKNOWLEDGEMENTS

We would like to thank S. Chandler and Z. Drolc, Department of Nuclear Medicine, Queen Elizabeth Medical Centre; Dr. A. Vaughan, A. Keeling, J. Taylor and S. Watson-James, Department of Immunology, Birmingham Medical School; Dr. E. Bateman, Rutherford Laboratory, Didcot and Dr. M. Irwin, SERC, Institute of Astronomy, Cambridge for their help with these studies; Professors R. Hoffenberg and I. Maclennan for their guidance and encouragement and the many physicians and surgeons whose patients we investigated. D. S. Fairweather was in receipt of a CRC grant.

REFERENCES

Bateman, J. E., Flescher, A. L., Fairweather, D. S., Bradwell, A. R., and Wilkinson, R. (1982). *Sci. Eng. Res. Counc. Rutherford Lab. Rep.* **RL–8L-36.**

Bateman, J. E., Flesher, A. C., Fairweather, D. S., and Bradwell, A. R. (1983). *Clin. Sci.* **65,** 1–18.

Begent, R. H. J., Searle, F., Stanway, G., Jewkes, R. F., Jones, B. E., Vernon, P., and Bagshawe, K. D. (1980). *J. R. Soc. Med.* **73,** 624–630.

Begent, R. H. J., Keep, P. A., Green, A. J., Searle, F., Bagshawe, K. D., Jewkes, R. F., Jones, B. E., Barratt, G. M., and Ryman, B. E. (1982). *Lancet* **2,** 739–742.

Begent, R. H. J., Boultbee, J., Jewkes, R., Katz, D., McIvor, J. (1983). *Clin. Oncol.* **2,** 144–158.

Berche, C., Mach, J. P., Lumbroso, J. D., Langlais, C., Aubrey, F., Buchegger, F., Carrel, S., Rougier, P., Parmentier, C., and Tubiana, M. (1982). *Br. Med. J.* **285,** 1447–1451.

Bradwell, A. R., Dykes, P. W., and Fairweather, D. S. (1983a). *J. Nucl. Med.* **24,** 1081.

Bradwell, A. R., Vaughan, A., Fairweather, D. S., and Dykes, P. W. (1983b). *Lancet* **1,** 247.

Bradwell, A. R., Fairweather, D. S., Keeling, A., Watson-James, S., Vaughan, A., and Dykes, P. W. (1983c). *Clin. Sci.* **65,** 124.

Bradwell, A. R., Taylor, J. R., Dykes, P. W., and Fairweather, D. S. (1983d). *Protides Biol. Fluids* **31,** 313–316.

Brault, J. W., and White, O. R. (1971). *Astron. Astrophys.* **13,** 169–189.

Brownell, G. L., Budinger, T. F., Lauterbur, P. L., and Megeer, P. L. (1982). *Science* **215,** 619–626.

DeLand, F. H., Kim, E. E., Simmons, G., and Goldenberg, D. M. (1980). *Cancer Res.* **40,** 3046–3049.

DeLand, F. H., Kim, E. E., and Goldenberg, D. M. (1982). *In* "Radionuclide Imaging in Drug Research" (C. G. Wilson, J. G. Hardy, M. Frier, and S. S. Davis, eds.), pp. 181–202. Croom Helm, London.

Dykes, P. W., and Bradwell, A. R. (1983). *Gastroenterology* **84,** 651–653.

Dykes, P. W., Hine, K. R., Bradwell, A. R., Blackburn, J. C., Reeder, T. A., Drolc, Z., and Booth, S. N. (1980). *Br. Med. J.* **280,** 220–222.

Epenetos, A. A., Britton, K. E., Mather, S., Shepherd, J., Granowska, M., Taylor-Papadimitriou, J., Nimmon, C. C., Durbin, H., Hawkins, L. R., Malpas, J. S., and Bodmer, W. F. (1982). *Lancet* **2,** 999–1004.

European Pharmacopoeia (1971). **3,** 58–60.

Ey, P. L., Prowse, S. J., and Jenkin, C. R. (1978). *Immunochemistry* **15,** 429–436.

Fairweather, D. S., Bradwell, A. R., and Dykes, P. W. (1982a). *Lancet* **2,** 660.

Fairweather, D. S., Bradwell, A. R., and Dykes, P. W. (1982b). *Br. Med. J.* **284,** 1478.

Fairweather, D. S., Bradwell, A. R., Dykes, P. W., Vaughan, A. T., Watson-James, S. F., and Chandler, S. (1983a). *Br. Med. J.* **287,** 167–170.

Fairweather, D. S., Bradwell, A. R., Watson-James, S. F., Dykes, P. W., Chandler, S., and Hoffenberg, R. (1983b). *Clin. Endocrinol. (Oxford)* **18,** 563–570.

Fairweather, D. S., Irwin, M., Bradwell, A. R., Dykes, P. W., and Flinn, R. M. (1983c). *Protides Biol. Fluids* **31,** 285–288.

Farrands, P. A., Perkins, A. C., Pimm, M. V., Hardy, J. D., Embleton, M. J., Baldwin, R. W., and Hardcastle, J. D. (1982). *Lancet* **2,** 397–400.

Ghose, T., Norvell, S. T., Aquino, J., Belitsky, P., Tai, J., Guclu, A., and Blair, A. H. *Cancer Res.* **40,** 3018–3031.

Glennie, M. J., and Stevenson, G. T., (1982). *Nature (London)* **295,** 712–713.

Goldenberg, D. M., DeLand, F. H., Kim, E., Bennett, S., Primus, F. J., Van Nagell, J. R., Jr., Estes, N., and Rayburn, P. (1978). *N. Engl. J. Med.* **298,** 1384–1388.

Goldenberg, D. M., Kim, E. E., DeLand, F. H., Spremulli, E., Nelson, M. O., Cockerman, J. P., Primus, F. J., Corgan, R. L., and Alpert, E. (1980a). *Cancer* **45,** 2500–2505.

Goldenberg, D. M., Kim, E. E., DeLand, F. H., Van Nagell, J. R., and Javadpour, N. (1980b). *Science* **208,** 1284–1286.

Goldenberg, D. M., Kim, E. E., and DeLand, F. H. (1981). *Proc. Natl. Acad. Sci. U.S.A.* **78,** 7754–7758.

Goldenberg, D. M., Kim, E. E., Bennett, S. J., Nelson, M. O., and DeLand, F. H. (1983). *Gastroenterology* **84,** 524–532.

Halsall, A. K., Fairweather, D. S., Bradwell, A. R., Blackburn, J. C., Dykes, P. W., Howell, A., Reeder, A., and Hine, K. R. (1981). *Br. Med. J.* **283,** 942–944.

Hedin, A., Wahren, B., and Hammerström S. (1982). *Int. J. Cancer* **30,** 547–552.

Hirai, T., Yamamoto, H., and Hamoaka, T. (1980). *J. Immunol.* **124,** 2765–2771.

Khaw, B. A., Fallon, J. T., Strauss, H. W., and Harbe, E. (1980). *Science* **209,** 295–297.

Krejcarek, G. E., and Tucker, K. L. (1977). *Biochem. Biophys. Res. Commun.* **77,** 581–585.

Larson, S. M., Brown, J. P., Wright, P. W., Carrasquillo, J. A., Hellström, I., and Hellström, K. E. (1983). *J. Nucl. Med.* **24,** 123–129.

Lewis, J. C. M., Bagshawe, K. D., and Keep, P. A. (1982). *Oncodev. Biol. Med.* **3,** 161–168.

Mach, J. P., Carrel, S., Forni, M., Ritschard, J., Donath, A., and Alberto, P. (1980). *N. Engl. J. Med.* **303,** 5–10.

Mach, J. P., Buchegger, F., Forni, M., Ritschard, J., Berche, C., Lumbroso, J.-D., Schreyer, M., Girardet, C., Accola, R. S., and Carrel, S. (1981). *Immunol. Today* **2,** 239–249.

Moshakis, V., Bailey, M. J., Ormerod, M. G., Westwood, J. H., and Neville, A. M. (1981). *Br. J. Cancer* **43,** 575–581.

Rainsbury, R. M., Ott, R. J., Westwood, J. H., Kalirai, T. S., Coombes, R. C., McCready, V. R., Neville, A. M., and Gazet, J.-C. (1983). *Lancet* **2,** 934–938.

Rockoff, S. D., Goodenough, D. J., and McIntire, K. R. (1980). *Cancer Res* **40,** 3054–3058.

Searle, F., Boden, J., Lewis, J. C. M., and Bagshawe, K. D. (1981). *Br. J. Cancer* **44,** 137–144.

Skromne-Kadlubik, G., Celis, C., and Ferez, A. (1977). *Ann. Neurol.* **2,** 343–344.

Smedley, H. M., Finan, P., Lennox, E. S., Ritson, A., Takei, F., Wraight, P., and Sikora, K. (1983). *Br. J. Cancer* **47,** 253–259.

Stern, P., Hagan, P., Halpern, S., Chen, A., David, G., Adams, T., Desmond, W., Brautigam, K., and Royston, I. (1982). *In* "Hybridomas in Cancer Diagnosis and Treatment" (M. S. Mitchel and H. F. Oettgen, eds.), pp. 245–253. Raven Press, New York.

Sternberger, L. (1979). "Immunocytochemistry," 2nd ed., pp. 104–169. Wiley, New York.

Sundberg, M. W., Mears, C. F., Goodwin, D. A., and Diamanti, C. I. (1974). *J. Med. Chem.* **17,** 1304–1307.

Unanue, E. R., and Karnovsky, M. J., (1974). *J. Exp. Med.* **140,** 1207–1220.

Watson-James, S. F., Fairweather, D. S., and Bradwell, A. R., (1980). *Med. Lab. Sci.* **40,** 67–68.

CHAPTER 5

Digital Superimposition of X-CT and Tomoscintigraphy Images Providing Anatomical Landmarks for a Comprehensive Interpretation of Immunoscintigraphy

Jean Lumbroso,* Bernard Aubert,* Robert Di Paola,*
Jean-Pierre Mach,[+] Jean Pierre Bazin,* Marcel Ricard,*
Jean Daniel Piekarski,* Philippe Rougier,* Jean Claude
Saccavini,[‡] Florent Aubry,* Claude Parmentier* and
Maurice Tubiana*

*Institut Gustave-Roussy
and Unité de Recherches de Radiobiologie Clinique
INSERM U66
Villejuif, France
[+]Ludwig Institute for Cancer Research
Epalinges, Lausanne, Switzerland
[‡]Office des Rayonnements Ionisants
Gif-sur-Yvette, France

MONOCLONAL ANTIBODIES FOR CANCER
DETECTION AND THERAPY

I. INTRODUCTION

Immunoscintigraphy was first successfully performed on man by Goldenberg *et al.*, (1978) and Mach *et al.* (1980) using polyclonal antibodies directed against carcinoembryonic antigen (CEA). The method was then improved by the introduction of monoclonal antibodies (Mab) (Accola *et al.*, 1980) and their fragments by Mach *et al.* (1981), and the use of tomoscintigraphy (TS) (Berche *et al.*, 1982; Lumbroso *et al.*, 1983). However, a major limitation of the method is the low uptake of radiolabelled antibodies which results in low-contrast images. The area corresponding to the uptake in the tumour site coexists with an important background level and with areas of non-specific uptake due to the metabolism of the Mab.

A uniform background may produce heterogeneous artifacts on the images reconstructed by tomoscintigraphy (Todd-Pokropek and Soussaline, 1982). It is not uncommon that the tumour site is not the area of higher uptake in the studied radioactive distribution. The final images produce hot spots with no identifiable anatomical structure. These factors result in a low clinical specificity of the method. This parameter, related to the risk of false positive diagnoses, was estimated to be from 63 to 84% (Berche *et al.*, 1982).

We present a method here based on the transfer of X-CT scan data to the computer nuclear medicine system performing the TS which allows the computer-assisted superimposition of the respective images. The clinical data are obtained from a series of 22 patients studied with an anti-CEA Mab.

II. MATERIAL AND METHODS

A. Tomoscintigraphy, X-CT Scan, Transfer of Images

Tomoscintigraphy was performed with a 40-cm field diameter γ-camera (Acticamera, CGR), attached to a mechanical device allowing a continuous axial rotation (20 min for 360°) and connected to a nuclear medicine computer system (Infogam, Sopha Médical). The distance between the collimator and the rotation axis was 28 cm. Before the acquisition of the tomographic data, an anterior view was recorded with radioactive landmarks along the Y axis. The position of the radioactive sources was noted on the patient's skin. Transversal slices of 4 pixel thickness were reconstructed from 100 projections (64 × 64 matrix size) using Fourier transform and resolution correction (Berche *et al.*, 1978). When the slices demonstrated hot spots which could correspond to a tumour site, complementary X-CT scan was indicated and performed on a whole body scanner (CE10000, CGR) in an adjacent floor. The patient was positioned in the same way as the TS bed. The Y coordinates of the X-CT slices were chosen to correspond to those of the TS slices using the marks left on the patient's skin. Three to ten slices were performed, with or without intravenous contrast media, with a 380-mm field in a 256 × 256 matrix size. The X-CT images were stored on a magnetic tape and later transferred to the nuclear medicine computer. X and Y shifts of the images were sometimes necessary to allow the coincidence of the marks recorded in the two methods.

B. Digital Superimposition

Briefly, a 256 × 256 × 8 bit color TV display was used. Each image was converted into a 128 × 128 size to occupy one quadrant of the screen. Up to three images could be coded in a fundamental color with 16 levels. The X-CT image was usually the green one, and the TS image the red one; the blue image was set to zero and could be used in the case of dual isotope TS. After superimposition, the resulting image was coded on 80 levels and the overlapping areas were processed to obtain a color as near as possible as would be obtained with three transparent images.

C. Phantom Studies

An abdomen-like lucite phantom was studied. Its dimensions were 35 × 20 × 8 cm and was filled with a radioactive solution representing the background level. Three spheres of 5,3 and 2 cm diameter were filled with a solution of the same radionuclide to obtain a ratio of concentration to that of background of 2,4 and 8 respectively. For a first set of measurements, the phantom was filled with ^{131}I solutions to reproduce the actual patient-study conditions described below: medium energy collimator (FWHM of 29.6 mm in air at the rotation axis); low count statistics (60,000–100,000 counts for one slice). The uniformity of the camera in the useful field of view (UFOV) was 11% (NEMA). A second set of meas-

TABLE I

DATA ON PATIENTS REFERRED FOR IMMUNOSCINTIGRAPHY AND RESULTS

Case	Tumour sites	Type[a]	CEA[b]	TS[c]	D. sup.[d]	T. size[e]
A. Gastrointestinal cancers						
1	Liver	M	48	d	d	E 2.5d
2	Liver	M	33	−	x	E 2.3d
3	Rectum	P	2.7	−	x	S 5×5
5	Left colon	P	8.6	+	+	S 5h
6	Sigmoid	P	45	−	x	S 4h
6	Liver	M	45	−	x	x
7	Stomach	P	8	+	d	S 3d
8	Recto-sigmoid	P	3.4	−	x	S 4.5h
9	Sigmoid	P	50	−	x	x
9	Liver	M	50	−	x	E 3.5d
11	Liver	M	57	+	+	S 7×6×5
13	Lungs	M	22.6	−	x	S 1.2d
14	Liver	M	656	+	+	x
15	Unknown	X	12	−	x	x
18	Liver	M	520	d	+	E 5d
19	Transverse colon[f]	P	173	−	x	S 3d
20	Liver, coeliac nodes	M	325	−	x	x
B. Medullary thyroid carcinomas						
4	Unknown	X	13	−	x	x
10	Liver	M	27	d	d	R 3.5d
12	Unknown	X	22	−	x	x
C. Breast carcinomas						
21	Liver	M	40	−	x	L 0.5d
22	Unknown	X	1[g]	−	x	x
D. Unknown primary tumours						
16	Pleura	X	245	−	x	x
17	Unknown[h]	X	180	−	x	

[a]P = primary tumour; M = metastasis; X = no data.

[b]CEA blood level in nanograms per millilitre; normal is less than 5 ng/ml. For patients 4, 10 and 12, the blood calcitonin level was, respectively, 40, 24 and 5.8 ng/ml for a normal less than 0.25 ng/ml.

[c]Result of TS: + = positive; − = negative; d = doubtful.

[d]Digital superimposition. The same code as TS, with an x when not done.

[e]Tumour size. First letter indicates the method which allowed the measurement (E for echotomography, S for surgery, R for radiology); the dimensions are given in centimeters. If only one dimension is available, it is followed by h for height, d for diameter; x means no data.

[f]Mab labelled with [123]I.

[g]Patient referred because her CEA blood level was estimated to be 45 ng/ml in another institution.

[h]Patient referred for a paraneoplastic disease.

urements were made in the best possible conditions: the phantom was filled with ^{99m}Tc allowing the use of a very high-resolution, low-energy tomography collimator (FWHM of 11.2 mm in water at the rotation axis) and providing higher statistics (250,000 counts for one slice). In addition, an on-line microprocessor corrected the uniformity of the camera in the UFOV to 8% (NEMA).

D. Patients, Antibodies and Imaging Schedule

Twenty-two patients were referred for immunoscintigraphy (Table I). Fifteen patients had gastrointestinal cancers, three patients had medullary thyroid cancers (MTC), two patients had breast carcinomas and two patients an unknown primary cancer. Seventeen patients had known tumour sites. For five patients, the existence of tumour sites was only suspected from other morphological examinations or from biological results. Of these five patients, two (cases 15 and 22) were classified as free of disease 8 and 3 months, respectively, after immunoscintigraphy, and three (cases 4, 12 and 17) showed no change in their clinical and biological data. Data that were available to estimate the tumour size are included in Table I.

According to a previously described protocol (Lumbroso *et al.*, 1983), 200–500 µg of an anti-CEA Mab (mouse IgG) named "202" (Haskell *et al.*, 1983) was labelled (Iodogen° method) with 37 MBq (1 mCi) or ^{131}I; after purification as well as sterility and pyrogenicity controls, they were intravenously infused to the patient for 1 hr under anti-allergic drugs and clinical monitoring. In one case, the Mab was labelled with ^{123}I.

Whole body images were recorded at days 1, 2, 6, or 7 after injection, and TS was performed at days 1 and 2.

III. RESULTS

A. Phantom Studies

The images obtained in the patient-study conditions with ^{131}I are represented in Fig. 1. The 2-cm diameter sphere, which presented the highest (eight) ratio of radionuclide concentration to background, is easy to identify. The spheres two and four times more radioactive than the background are not easily identified.

The images obtained in the best possible conditions with ^{99m}Tc are represented in Fig. 2. The relative position of each sphere is different from that in Fig. 1. The identification of each sphere is very clear, although their respective size cannot be estimated on TS.

B. Patient Studies

The results are summarized in Table I. The superimposition of X-CT and TS images was indicated in seven cases; it was not done when TS did not demonstrate hot spots which could correspond to a tumour uptake.

Patient 5 had a colon cancer situated near the left colon angle. The superimposition of TS and X-CT images (Fig. 3) allowed the identification of the two major uptake sites seen on TS, one corresponding to the bone marrow of the vertebral body and the second to the tumour; the minor uptake spots corresponded to the background and to free iodine uptake by the normal colon mucosa coinciding with the X-CT air density images. The patient was operated on 5 days after injection: The ^{131}I contrast between tumour and normal colon was 6.4; tumour and fat, 7.6, tumour and blood, 2. The specificity index calculated according to Pressman *et al.* (1957), comparing the Mab tumour uptake to the uptake of a control IgG labelled with ^{125}I was 4.8.

For patient 7, the uptake area which could correspond to the gastric cancer included on digital superimposition a large part of the normal stomach and could not be differentiated from a non-specific uptake of free iodine by the gastric mucosa.

Patient 11 was referred for a high CEA blood level with negative hepatic echotomography. Tomoscintigraphy demonstrated (Fig. 4) an uptake focus in the right abdominal side, and superimposition with X-CT (Fig. 5)

Fig. 1. Phantom study with ^{131}I in patient-study conditions. A, Tomoscintigraphy, standard color scale; B, tomoscintigraphy, 16 levels red scale; C, X-CT in the same plane as TS, 16 levels green scale; D, digital superimposition of B and C.

Fig. 2. Phantom study with ^{99m}Tc in the best possible conditions. Presentation as in Fig. 1.

Fig. 3. Immunoscintigraphy patient (case 5) presenting a left colon cancer. Presentation as in Fig. 1.

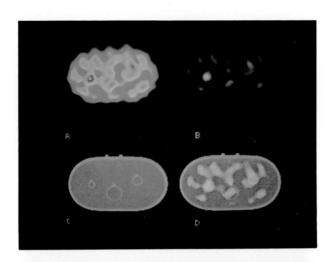

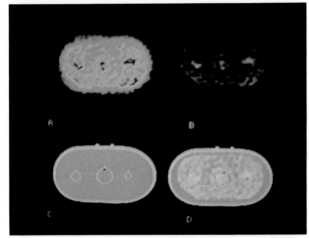

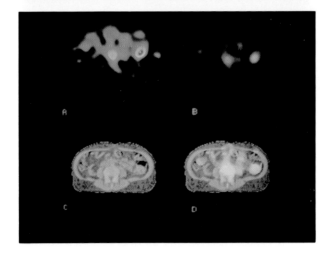

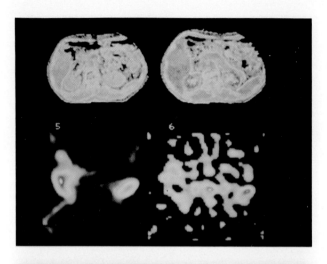

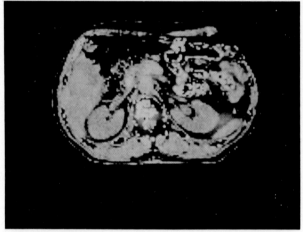

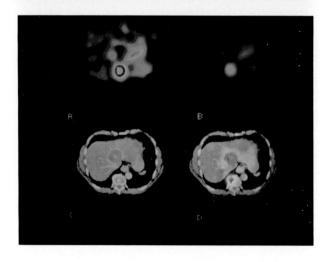

allowed us to differentiate this tumour uptake from a non-specific uptake of free iodine by the right colon angle. This metastasis was missed by echography because it was situated in an atypic extension of the lower part of the right lobe of the liver. The diagnosis was confirmed by surgical removal of the metastasis.

Patient 14 had multiple metastases of the right lobe of the liver. An uptake of the radiolabelled Mab was visualized in this part of the liver, principally around the largest metastases.

Similar images are well illustrated by the results of patient 18 (Fig. 6). He presented a large metastasis of the upper part of the liver, near the suprahepatic veins. The TS was equivocal, but the digital superimposition clearly demonstrated a superficial Mab uptake ring around the metastasis. In this case, the major uptake areas corresponded to the vertebral body, to the spleen and, due to free iodine, to the stomach.

Patient 10 was referred for a hypervascular liver metastasis of MTC. After TS and X-CT superimposition of the images, the radio-isotope uptake in the tumour was not found to be significantly different from the blood background level, especially at the level of the suprahepatic veins.

For patient 1, X-CT demonstrated a heterogeneous hepatic steatosis precluding the identification of the liver metastases and no conclusion could be drawn from the superimposition with TS.

IV. DISCUSSION

In any transverse plane, X-CT provides accurate anatomical information, whereas TS tends to give functional information about the same structures. Digital superimposition of images provided by two different techniques is subject to limitations. X-CT images have a millimetric definition and no appreciable geometric distortion; TS images have a res-

Fig. 4. Liver metastasis discovered by immunoscintigraphy, case 11. On the first line, X-CT before (left) and after (right) intravenous contrast medium. On the second line, TS in the same plane, performed with ^{99m}Tc sulphur-colloid (left) and with radiolabelled Mab (right).

Fig. 5. Full screen display of digital superimposition of the X-CT and the TS images separately shown in Fig. 4.

Fig. 6. Immunoscintigraphy patient (case 18) presenting a liver metastasis. Presentation as in Fig. 1.

olution of about 20 mm and are affected by the spatial distortions inherent in γ cameras and induced by auto-attenuation, statistical noise, reconstruction filters and finally by the display characteristics.

These reasons explain why the apparent size of an uptake area on TS is often larger than the X-CT image of the corresponding structure. This is illustrated by both phantom- and patient-study images. Furthermore, filtering and background subtraction cause a degradation of the external contours of the TS images: This is particularly clear on the phantom study where the TS images seem to be smaller than the X-CT images. This does not affect the coincidence of the barycentre of each radioactive sphere on TS and X-CT images.

For the interpretation of TS, care has to be taken to differentiate significant uptake areas from background heterogeneous artifacts, especially when the statistics of the counting is poor. The comparison of adjacent slices is useful for this first step. A second step is the differentiation between non-specific uptake areas due to the metabolism of the Mab and specific uptake areas due to the presence of a tumour site. The bone marrow, the spleen, the large vessels and, due to free iodine, the stomach, are known to be areas of non-specific uptake. In addition, they are often adjacent to suspected tumour sites, and contain a comparable or higher level of radioactivity.

Summarily, digital superimposition of X-CT and TS images is a useful tool for a more specific clinical interpretation of immunoscintigraphy. Furthermore, in the case of large tumours, it provides information about the distribution of the Mab in the tumour and its periphery.

ACKNOWLEDGEMENTS

This work was supported in part by an INSERM PRC 129033 research grant. We are indebted to Mireille Benetiere for her technical assistance and to Ingrid Kuchenthal who reviewed the manuscript.

REFERENCES

Accola, R. S., Carrel, S., and Mach, J. P. (1980). *Proc. Natl. Acad. Sci. U.S.A.* **77**, 563–566.
Berche, C., Aubert, B., Bethencourt, A., and Di Paola, R. (1978). *In* "Information Processing in Medical Imaging" (A. B. Brill, R. R. Price, W. J. McClain, and M. W., Landay, eds.), Vol. 2, pp. 214–251. ORNL/BCTIC, Oak Ridge, Tennessee.

Berche, C., Mach, J. P., Lumbroso, J., Langlais, C., Aubry, F., Buchegger, F., Carrel, S., Rougier, P., Parmentier, C., and Tubiana, M. (1982). *Br. Med. J.* **285,** 1447–1451.

Goldenberg, D. M., Deland, F., Kim, E., Bennet, S., Primus, J., Van Nagell, J. R., Estes, N., Desimone, P., and Rayburn, P. (1978). *N. Engl. J. Med.* **298,** 1384–1388.

Haskell, C. M., Buchegger, F., Schreyer, M., Carrel, S., and Mach, J. P. (1983). *Cancer Res.* **43,** 3857–3864.

Lumbroso, J., Berche, C., Mach, J. P., Rougier, P., Aubry, F., Buchegger, F., Lasser, P., Parmentier, C., and Tubiana, M. (1983). *Bull. Cancer* **70,** 96–102.

Mach, J. P., Carrel, S., Forni, M., Ritschard, J., Donath, A., and Alberto, P. (1980). *N. Engl. J. Med.* **303,** 5–10.

Mach, J. P., Buchegger, F., Forni, M., Ritschard, J., Berche, C., Lumbroso, J. D., Schreyer, M., Girardet, C., Accola, R. S., and Carrel, S. (1981). *Immunol. Today* **2,** 239–249.

Pressman, D., Day, D., and Blau, M. (1957). *Cancer Res.* **17,** 845–850.

Todd-Pokropek, A., and Soussaline, F. (1982). "Nuclear Medicine and Biology" (C. Raynaud, ed.), Vol. I, pp. 1018–1021. Pergamon, Oxford.

CHAPTER 6

Localization of an Anti-tumour Monoclonal Antibody in Human Tumour Xenografts: Kinetic and Quantitative Studies with the 791T/36 Antibody

M. V. Pimm and R. W. Baldwin

Cancer Research Campaign Laboratories
University of Nottingham
Nottingham, United Kingdom

I. INTRODUCTION

Advances in hybridoma technology which led to the production of monoclonal antibodies recognising tumour-associated products have provided new potential approaches for detection and therapy of primary and metastatic tumour deposits. A major component of this development was the demonstration of *in vivo* localization of parenterally administered anti-tumour monoclonal antibody within tumour deposits. Now that this can be achieved, it has become feasible to investigate the efficiency and benefits of both diagnostic external imaging of the tumour localization of antibody labelled with appropriate radionuclides, and tumour therapy using antibody conjugated to conventional cytotoxic agents or plant or bacterial toxins. Antibody localization in this context is reflected in a greater level of antibody in malignant tissue than in normal tissue on a weight basis. This uptake must be shown to be a specific immunological recognition of tumour-associated antigen by the antibody and not to be due to only non-specific accumulation of immunoglobulin at tumour sites. This degree of specificity can be assessed in parallel studies using normal immunoglobulin, or an unrelated monoclonal antibody, preferably of the same isotype as the antibody in question. Virtually all monoclonal antibodies examined for localization into human tumours have been of mouse or rat origin, and prior to clinical trials experimental evaluation of antibodies for tumour localization has relied heavily on the use of human tumours developing as xenografts, principally in congenitally athymic or immuno-deprived mice. Using these model systems, and the foregoing criteria for localization, it has been firmly established that anti-human tumour monoclonal antibodies can localize in human tumour xenografts. These antibodies have included those to carcinoembryonic antigen (CEA) (Hedin *et al.,* 1982; Buchegger *et al.,* 1983; Wahl, *et al.,* 1983), colorectal carcinoma (Herlyn *et al.,* 1983; Zaloberg *et al.,* 1983); (Pimm *et al.,* 1982), melanoma (Ghose *et al.,* 1982), breast carcinoma (Colcher *et al.,* 1983) and teratoma (Moshakis *et al.,* 1981b); this experimental confirmation of the potential of these antibodies for tumour localization has formed the basis for a number of clinical trials of the diagnostic application of monoclonal antibodies (Epenetos *et al.,* 1982; Farrands *et al.,* 1982; Rainsbury *et al.,* 1983; Fairweather *et al.,* 1983; Chatal *et al.,* 1984; Mach *et al.,* 1981, 1983).

Following the initial empirical observation of tumour localization of radiolabelled monoclonal antibodies in both tumour xenografts and clinically, further development and optimization of this localization now requires attention to be focussed on parameters limiting the degree of this localization. Thus a consideration of the *rate* of antibody localization is necessary to optimize the time of external imaging of localization of radiolabelled antibody, and for the design of dosing schedules for the administration of antibody drug conjugates. In addition to rate, the *extent* of localization which can be achieved needs examination. The absolute amount of antibody deposited in tumour will clearly depend on the administered dose, but tumour tissue will eventually become 'saturated' with antibody at a level dictated by the degree of antigen expression within the tumour and its availability to antibody. Excess antibody will remain in the circulation and any increase in antibody dose will not increase absolute tumour levels, and indeed tumour levels relative to blood or whole body burden will decline. In this situation, excess antibody will obscure tumour-localized antibody in diagnostic imaging, and in therapeutic trials leave drug–antibody conjugate potentially capable of non-specific systemic toxicity.

In addition to the extent of localization the, intratumoural *site* of antibody deposition needs to be considered. Even supposing all malignant cells express equally the target antigen for the antibody, intratumoural variations in vascularity and necrosis may influence levels of antibody in different parts of the tumour. Moreover some, or possibly the majority, of antibody will be complexed with antigen shed into extravascular space within the tumour. This potential non-uniform distribution of localized antibody may have little or no influence on imaging of the tumour with radiolabelled antibody, but clearly could be a deciding factor in the success of therapy with antibody–drug conjugates.

The parameters governing the rate, extent and site of specific antibody deposition in tumours are as yet poorly explored. Clearly, tumour localization following passive transfer of an antibody potentially reactive with antigens expressed on malignant cells will be governed by a complex series of interacting events involving a balance between the rate of specific tumour uptake and the rate of catabolism of the antibody. It can be envisaged that the rate of catabolism of any one antibody will be relatively constant, being governed by normal physiological processes, but these processes will be disturbed if antibody complexes with tumour-derived antigen in the circulation. The rate of specific antibody uptake into the tumour will depend on such factors as the affinity of the antibody, rate of blood flow through the tumour, and its level of vascularisation and necrosis, these latter being partly dependent on the anatomical site of the tumour. Presumably the initial extravasation of antibody and its diffusion into tumour tissue will also be controlled by normal physiological processes, but again these processes will be disturbed by interaction of the antibody with tumour antigen on tumour cell surface and/or in the extra- and intravascular compartments of the tumour.

It is clear that the overall kinetic and quantitative aspects of tumour localization of monoclonal antibody will be a result of complex dynamic interactions, but these need to be understood if the full potentials of tumour localization of antibody, particularly as carriers of therapeutic agents, are to be realised. Consequently, studies have been carried out in this Department with an anti-tumour monoclonal antibody and human tumour xenografts to examine some of the quantitative and kinetic aspects of tumour localization (Pimm et al., 1982; Pimm and Baldwin, 1984). The influence of variations in tumour size and site and antibody dose on the extent and rate of specific antibody localization have been examined, together with the site of intratumoural deposition of the antibody. The findings from these studies will be discussed to illustrate some of the approaches directed at an understanding of events leading to tumour localization.

II. ANTI-OSTEOGENIC SARCOMA MONOCLONAL ANTIBODY 791T/36

The antibody 791T/36, a mouse IgG_{2b} antibody, is produced by a hybridoma following fusion of splenocytes from a mouse immunized against cells of an osteogenic sarcoma cell line designated 791T and mouse myeloma P3NS1 (Embleton et al., 1981). The initial screening of this antibody showed it to react with 7 of 13 osteogenic sarcoma cell lines, but it is not osteogenic sarcoma specific, since cells from 6 of 26 other, unrelated, tumours were also reactive (Embleton et al., 1981). It does not react with a range of normal human fibrobalsts, or erythrocytes, but the antigen is expressed during phytohemagglutinin (PHA)-induced blastogenesis of human T (and B) cells (Price et al., 1983a). Biochemical studies have identified the antigen on osteogenic sarcoma cells and blast cells as a glycoprotein of 72,000 Da (Price et al., 1983b). Clinically, localization of radiolabelled 791T/36 antibody has been shown by external imaging techniques in primary osteogenic sarcomas (Farrands et al., 1983), in primary ovarian carcinomas (Symonds et al., 1985) and primary and metastatic deposits of mammary (Williams et al., 1984) and colorectal (Farrands et al., 1982; Armitage et al., 1984) carcinomas. In the latter situation at least, the target antigen is expressed in tumour stroma and/or gland sections rather than intimately associated with malignant cell surfaces, but here, too, the antigen complexed with antibody has been confirmed to be the 72,000-Da glycoprotein (Price *et al.* 1984). In a therapeutic context, conjugates of this antibody and a number of anti-cancer and immunomodulating agents have been prepared and are being evaluated for *in vitro* and *in vivo* therapeutic effectiveness. Thus, conjugates of 791T/36 antibody with vindesine (Embleton *et al.*, 1983) and methotrexate (Garnett *et al.*, 1983) show selective cytotoxicity toward 791T target cells and retard growth of 791T xenografts (Pimm *et al.*, 1984). In addition, conjugates with interferon retain antibody activity and interferon potency, and can localise in appropriate tumour xenografts (Pelham *et al.*, 1983).

In view of the potential importance of the 791T/36 antibody for diagnostic and therapeutic applications, it was selected for examination of quantitative aspects of its localization. These studies have been carried out in immuno-deprived mice with osteogenic sarcoma 791T xenografts.

III. DEMONSTRATION OF SPECIFIC ANTIBODY LOCALIZATION WITHIN XENOGRAFTS

The tumour localization property of 791T/36 antibody has been evaluated by studying the organ distribution of radioiodine-labelled purified preparations in xenografts of human tumours in CBA mice immuno-deprived by thymectomy, and whole body irradiation with cytosine arabinoside protection (Pimm *et al.*, 1982). Since an initial limiting factor in the successful localization of parenterally administered antibody into tumours is the circulation of the antibody in the blood in a chemically undergraded and biologically active form, blood samples were taken from 791T xenograft-bearing mice 2 days following intraperitoneal injection of ^{131}I-labelled antibody and examined for the nature of the circulating radioactivity-labelled material. Sephacryl S-300 gel filtration of the serum (Fig. 1) showed radioactivity in a discrete peak, coincident with the second serum protein peak, well recognised as containing serum IgG. There was no grossly aggregated or degraded radiolabelled material in the serum. Further confirmation that radiolabel was associated with mouse IgG was obtained by precipitation of the radiolabel from the serum with rabbit anti-mouse IgG antibody (92% precipitation). Furthermore, it was demonstrated that the radiolabelled antibody in the circulation was still in a biologically active form, since it bound specifically to target cells ex-

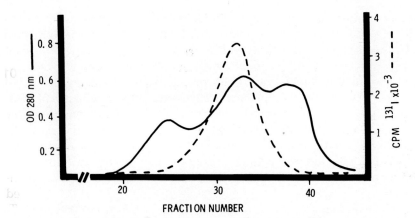

Fig. 1. Gel filtration on Sephacryl S-300 of serum from 791T xenografted mouse injected 3 days previously with 20 µg ^{131}I-labelled 791T/36 antibody; 1 ml serum, column dimensions 90 cm × 1.5 cm.

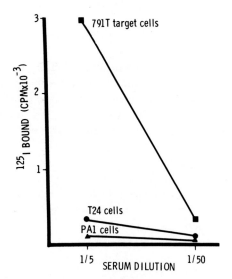

Fig. 2. Cell-binding activity of radiolabel in serum of mice injected 3 days previously with 10 µg ^{125}I-labelled 791T/36 antibody. Serum (0.1 ml) incubated with 2×10^5 cells, washed and counted for bound radioactivity. Target cells: 791T osteogenic sarcoma, T24 bladder carcinoma, PAI ovarian carcinoma.

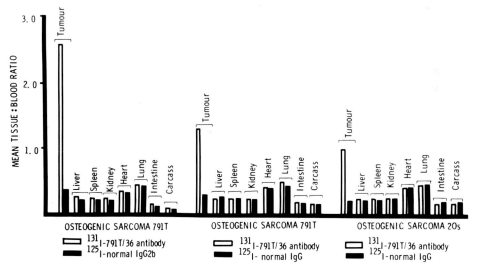

Fig. 3. Organ distribution study of ^{131}I-labelled 791T/36 antibody and ^{125}I-labelled normal IgG (5 μg of each) injected 3 days previously into mice with 791T xenografts. Mean, four mice. (From Pimm *et al.*, 1982.)

pressing the 791T/36-defined antigen, but not to cells deficient in this antigen (Fig. 2).

Organ distribution studies following injection of ^{131}I-labelled 791T/36 antibody demonstrated that there was a preferential localization of radioactivity in 791T xenografts compared with normal tissues. This can be conveniently illustrated by normalizing the count rates of ^{131}I per gram of tumour and normal organs with respect to the ^{131}I count of blood [tissue : blood ratio (T : B)] (Fig. 3). This localization is clearly not due to an abnormal blood level in the tumour, since simultaneously injected ^{125}I-labelled normal mouse IgG_{2b} (the same isotype as the 791T/36 antibody) did not preferentially localize in tumour tissue. This simultaneous injection of labelled antibody and corresponding normal, control, immunoglobulin allows the calculation of the extent of specific:non-specific tumour levels. This is conventionally expressed as a specificity of localization index (LI), calculated as the ratio of T:B ratio of antibody and T:B ratio of control immunoglobulin. In the experiment illustrated in Fig. 3, the LI for antibody in the tumour is 6.1 : 1, but virtually 1 : 1 for all normal organs. Further confirmation of immunological nature of the localization of 791T/36 in osteogenic sarcoma xenografts came from parallel studies with xenografts of other tumours, some expressing and some

lacking the 791T/36-defined antigen (Fig. 4). There was clear-cut localization of antibody only in xenografts derived from target cell lines expressing the antigen (e.g., osteogenic sarcomas 788T, 20S, but not into
xenografts not expressing the antigen (e.g., bladder carcinoma T24, colon
carcinoma HCT8).

The conclusion from these initial studies is that 791T/36 antibody can
localize specifically in tumour xenografts that express the appropriate
antigen, and this model system should be amenable for assessment of
quantitative aspects of this localization.

IV. SITE OF ANTIBODY LOCALIZATION IN XENOGRAFTS

The intratumoural site of deposition of ^{125}I-labelled 791T/36 following
its specific xenograft localization was determined by autoradiography of
tissue sections. Essentially the site of deposition of the antibody was
mainly in the periphery of the tumour. Although some scattered silver
grains were visible throughout the tumour, most dense grains were visible at the interface between the sub-capsular connective tissue and
malignant cell areas (Fig. 5). Where connective tissue was invaginated
into malignant cell areas, there was also a dense development of silver
grains. However, there was little or no development of silver grains
within the connective tissue itself, except at the interface with tumour
cells.

From the autoradiographical studies, it is probable that 791T/36 antibody localized in tumour xenografts is complexed, at least in part, with
tumour-derived antigen, and not firmly attached to tumour cell surfaces.
Further indication that 791T/36 antibody which had localized in 791T
xenografts was complexed with antibody came from gel filtration studies
on saline extracts of tumour containing radiolabelled antibody (Fig. 6).
Thus, mincing of tumour tissue in pH72 phosphate buffered saline eluted
radioactivity in soluble form (i.e., not sedimented by 100,000 g centrifugation). A high proportion of this radioactivity was in a form with a
higher molecular weight than IgG, so that about 50% was excluded from
Sephacryl S-300. Similar gel filtration at pH3, which would be expected
to dissociate antibody–antigen complexes, showed only one peak of radioactivity, within the IgG-containing region of the profile (Fig. 6), indicating that the radiolabelled antibody in the eluate was in an acid-
labile complex form.

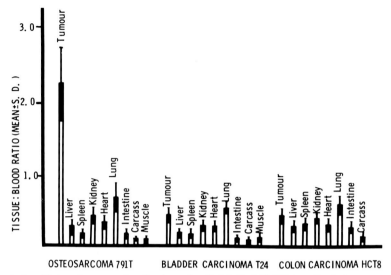

Fig. 4. Specificity of tumour localization of radiolabelled 791T/36 antibody in mice with human tumour xenografts; 10 μg of labelled 791T/36 per mouse, four mice per group, killed 3 days after injection.

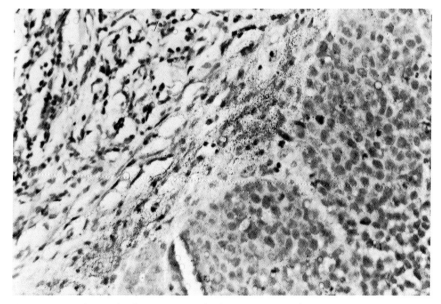

Fig. 5. Autoradiograph of 791T xenografted tumour tissue from mouse injected 2 days previously with 500 μCi ^{125}I-labelled 791T/36 antibody. Silver grains are seen mainly in the sub-capsular region. ×360. (From Pimm *et al.*, 1982.)

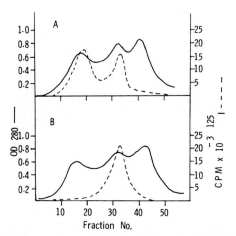

Fig. 6. Sephacryl S-300 chromatography profile of ^{125}I-labelled 791T/36 antibody. (A) PBS-eluate of 791T xenograft tissue from mouse injected 24 hr previously with ^{125}I antibody, mixed with normal mouse serum and run in PBS. (B) PBS eluate of 791T xenograft tissue from mouse injected 24 hr previously with ^{125}I antibody, mixed with normal mouse serum and column run in pH3 citrate–phosphate buffer.

V. QUANTITATIVE EVALUATION OF LOCALIZATION IN XENOGRAFTS

A. Rate and Extent of Antibody Localization

The majority of antibody localization experiments in xenografted animals involve examination of the tumour levels of radiolabelled antibody several days after its administration. For precise analysis of the rate of localization, groups of mice with 791T/36 xenografts were injected with a mixture of ^{131}I-labelled 791T/36 antibody and ^{125}I control IgG$_{2b}$, and the tumour and blood levels of radiolabels examined between 6 hr and 7 days later. Initially the data from this experiment were analysed to determine what proportions of the two radiolabels present in the body as a whole were present per unit weight of tumour and blood. This normalization of data allows simple representation of the change of distribution within the mice of the radiolabels, irrespective of their continual excretion. As shown in Fig. 7, ^{131}I-labelled antibody was detected in the blood 6 hr after intraperitoneal injection (the earliest time examined) at 22% of the whole body count per gram. This level was maintained virtually constant throughout the whole 7-day time course of the experi-

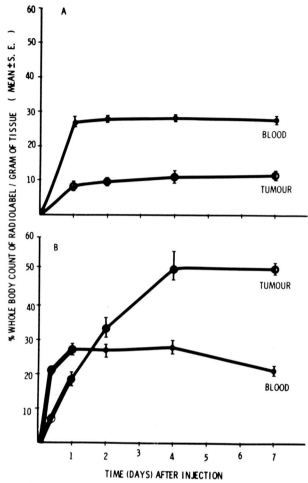

Fig. 7. Time course of tumour and blood levels of (A) ^{125}I-labelled normal IgG$_{2b}$ and (B) ^{131}I-labelled 791T/36 antibody in 791T xenografted mice. Mean, four to five mice per point. Results expressed with respect to whole body counts of radiolabels. (Reprinted with permission from *Europ. J. Cancer Clin. Oncol.*, Vol. 20, M. V. Pimm and R. W. Baldwin, Copyright 1984, Pergamon Press.)

ment, i.e., the blood level of radiolabel relative to the mouse as a whole remained virtually constant over the time period examined. Although radiolabelled antibody was detectable also in the tumour 6 hr after administration, its level, relative to the whole body survival, continued to increase for the first 4 days after injection time, its level only exceeding that of the blood after the first 36 hr. The maximum level achieved, 50%

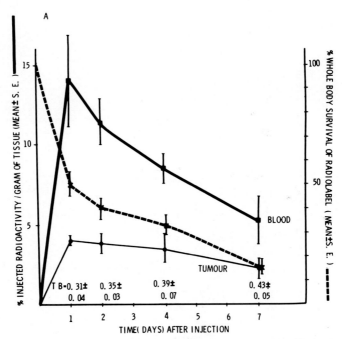

Fig. 8. Time course of tumour, blood and whole body levels of (A) ^{125}I-labelled normal IgG$_{2b}$ and (B) ^{131}I-labelled 791T/36 antibody in 791T xenografted mice. Mean, four to five mice per time point. Results expressed with respect to initial injected dose. (Reprinted with permission from *Europ. J. Cancer Clin. Oncol.*, Vol. 20, M. V. Pimm and R. W. Baldwin, Copyright 1984, Pergamon Press.)

of the whole body level per gram of tumour was maintained to day 7, the last time point of analysis. Simultaneous studies wiith ^{125}I normal IgG$_{2b}$ showed a similar pattern of blood level to that seen with antibody, at about 28% of the whole body count per gram, but in distinction to the antibody, tumour levels of normal IgG$_{2b}$ remained virtually constant at no more than 10% per gram for the 7-day observation period. This type of analysis shows that specific antibody localization into subcutaneous tumour xenografts is a slow process and is not completed until at least 4 days after injection.

A further analysis of the data from this experiment was carried out to determine the proportion of the originally injected radiolabelled materials in tumour and blood (Fig. 8). This showed that with 791T/36 antibody, 8% of the original injection material, was present per gram of tumour at a peak of 2–4 days after injection. The relative changes in tumour and blood levels produced an increase in T : B ratio from 0.67 at day 1 to 2.8

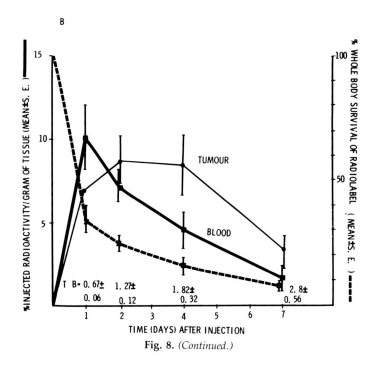

Fig. 8. *(Continued.)*

at day 7; however, this was partly due to a decline in blood levels rather than increased uptake of antibody into xenografts. With normal IgG$_{2b}$, T : B ratios increased from 0.31 at day 1 to only 0.43 at day 7.

B. Influence of Varations in Tumour Site and Size on Efficiency of Specific Antibody Localization

1. Tumour Site

Many experimental systems for the evaluation of xenograft localization of radiolabelled anti-tumour antibodies rely on xenografts developing subcutaneously. To examine whether improved localization could be achieved with tumours at another site, tumour levels of ^{131}I-labelled 791T/36 and ^{125}I-labelled normal IgG$_{2b}$ were examined in groups of mice with subcutaneous or intramuscular 791T xenografts. Overall, there was no difference in the T : B ratios in the two groups of mice (Fig. 9). Thus

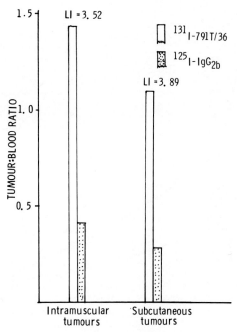

Fig. 9. Localization of ^{131}I-labelled 791T/36 antibody compared with [113]I-labelled normal IgG$_{2b}$ (2 μg of each) in intramuscular and subcutaneous 791T xenografts. Mean, three mice per group.

with subcutaneous tumours the mean T : B ratio of antibody was 1.09, and of control IgG$_{2b}$, 0.28 (mean LI, 3.89). With intramuscular tumours, the mean T : B ratios of antibody and control IgG$_{2b}$ were 1.41 and 0.41, respectively (mean LI, 3.43). From this limited study, the implication is that intramuscular 791T xenografted tumours would not be a better target than subcutaneous growths for 791T/36 antibody for evaluation of imaging procedures or therapy with drug–antibody conjugated.

2. Tumour Size

To examine whether uptake of 791T/36 antibody is proportional to tumour size, mice with xenografts of a range of sizes were similarly injected with mixtures of ^{131}I-labelled 791T/36 antibody and ^{125}I-normal IgG$_{2b}$ and tumour and blood levels examined 3 days later. Since this analysis required assays in individual mice, it would be inappropriate to examine directly the correlation between the proportion of the injected dose of antibody localized and xenograft size, since if individual mice showed

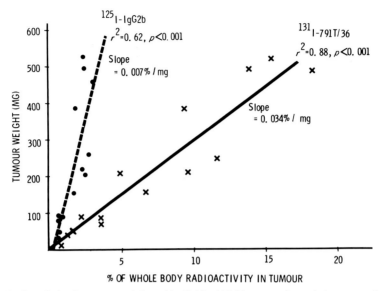

Fig. 10. Correlation between weights of individual 791T xenografts and the proportion of the total body count of ^{131}I-labelled 791T/36 antibody and ^{125}I-labelled normal IgG$_{2b}$ localized in the tumours. Mice killed 3 days after injection of 10 µg of each preparation.

differences in the rate of clearance of radiolabelled antibody they would have different amounts of antibody potentially capable of tumour localization. This was overcome by normalizing the tumour radioactivity counts with respect to the whole body count of radiolabel. Figure 10 illustrates one such experiment. There was a statistically significant correlation ($r^2 = 0.88$, $p<0.001$) between the proportion of the total body count of ^{131}I (the 791T/36 label) present within the tumours and their weights. From the slope of the regression line, it was calculated that 34% of the total body radioactivity was present per gram of tumour 3 days after injection. This was remarkably reproducible, the mean from six separate experiments being 36 ± 3% of the total body load of ^{131}I antibody per gram of tumour. There was also a significant correlation between the proportion of the total body count of control IgG$_{2b}$'s ^{125}I label within tumours and their weights. Here, however, only 7% of the total body count was present per gram of tumour, about one-fifth of the antibody level and in keeping with the LI derived from the data in Fig. 7. The main implication from these data is that antibody concentrates in tumour tissue at a constant level, only the size of tumour influencing what proportion of the body load of antibody will be within the tumour, and the amount of antibody per unit weight of tumour being constant.

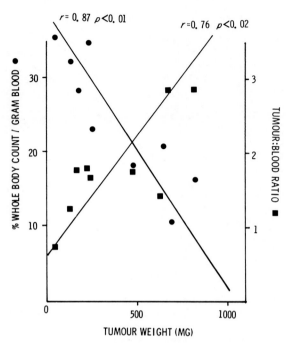

Fig. 11. Correlations between weights of individual 791T xenografts and the proportion of the total body count of ^{131}I-labelled 791T/36 antibody per gram of blood and the T : B ratio. Analysis of the proportion of the whole body count and tumour weight showed significant correlation, $r = 0.92$ with 36% per gram; mice killed 3 days after injection.

This finding would indicate, therefore, that T : B ratio would be a fairly standard parameter for any given antibody tumour system, since this T : B ratio is a ratio between percentage of whole body count per gram tumour and percentage of whole body count per gram of blood. It is clear, however, that factors tending to reduce the blood level of antibody, even without influence on the tumour level of antibody, would increase the T : B ratio. The indication from this is that antibody with a short biological half-life (e.g., IgM) or Fab or F(ab')$_2$ fragments would give high T : B ratios, provided tumour levels could be achieved rapidly and maintained during rapid excretion of antibody or fragments (see below).

A further implication from the present work would be that large tumours might take up sufficient radiolabelled antibody to produce a significant decrease of blood levels and corresponding increase in T : B ratios, even though the proportion of the whole body count per gram of tumour was remaining constant. One such case is illustrated by the data in Fig. 11. Here there is a significant correlation between the blood level of radiolabelled antibody (normalized to whole body level) and size of tumour, i.e., animals with larger tumours had a significantly lower blood level of radiolabel. Consequently the T : B ratio of radiolabel was significantly higher in animals with largest tumours, even though the proportion of the whole body count per gram of tumour was constant throughout at 36% per gram. One implication from this consideration is that although the T : B ratio is a convenient indication of the localization of a particular antibody, comparison of localization potential of different antibodies should not be judged only on this T : B ratio, unless it is clear that tumours of comparable sizes were used.

C. Influence of Variations in Antibody Administration on Specific Localization into Xenografts

1. Influence of Route of Administration

Since antibody localization in tumours can only occur following extravasation of antibody from the circulation, it would seem to be most appropriate to inject antibody for localization intravenously. This would almost certainly be the preferred route clinically, but in experimental animals this is technically more laborious than simple intraperitoneal injection, particularly if repeated injections are to be given. Although as already shown, intraperitoneally administered antibody does enter the circulation rapidly and subsequently tumour localizes, the possibility that greater localization could be achieved by intravenous injection should be explored. However, as shown in Fig. 12, 3 days following a single dose of radiolabelled 791T/36 antibody, there was virtually no difference in tumour or other organ levels whether the antibody had been injected intravenously or intraperitoneally. Moreover, there was no significant effect on the whole body survival of the radiolabel (ip injected, 23%; iv injected, 29%), and therefore on the proportion of the injected dose per gram of tumour. From these data, it is concluded that intraperitoneal injection of antibody is as efficient as intravenous to achieve tumour localization.

2. Influence of Antibody Administration Regime on Tumour Levels

Many studies on tumor localization of monoclonal antibodies have employed a single administration of antibody. From kinetic considerations already discussed, it can be concluded that tumour levels of an-

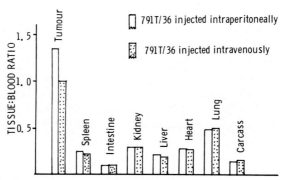

Fig. 12. Comparison of 791T xenograft localization of labelled 791T/36 antibody (4 μg/ mouse) injected intraperitoneally or intravenously. Mean, three mice per group, killed 4 days after injection.

tibody should be maintained longer if antibody was administered repeatedly or continuously and this would be most attractive in therapy of tumours with antibody or antibody–drug conjugates. What is not clear, however, is whether higher *absolute* levels of antibody can be achieved in tumours by repeated rather than single injection since the levels of antibody localization achieved by repeated administration seems to have undergone little or no experimental evaluation. Consequently, with the 791T xenograft system, the tumour levels achieved following single or multiple doses of 791T/36 antibody have been examined. Here, mice with 791T xenografts were given 40 μg of radiolabelled 791T/36 either as a single intraperitoneal administration, followed by dissection and organ counting 3 days later, or divided between three daily doses, followed by examination 3 days after the first dose (Fig. 13).

The proportion of the injected dose of radiolabelled antibody in the tumour was higher in the group given antibody in divided doses, but this was a reflection of the higher overall body survival of antibody in these mice (36%) compared with those given a single injection (25% whole body survival). Thus, with a single dose of antibody, tumour levels were 7.8 ± 0.8% of the injected dose per gram; blood levels were 5.3 ± 0.66% per gram. These figures were in good agreement with those seen 3 days after injection in the kinetic studies (Fig. 8). With repeated administration, the tumour level was 11.8 ± 1.38% injected dose per gram ($p = 0.05$) but blood levels were also increased to 7.7% of the injected dose per gram. The result of this higher blood level, as well as tumour level, in mice given repeated rather than single injections of labelled antibody was that there was virtually no difference in tumour, or normal organ, levels between the two groups when compared in relation to blood levels (Fig. 13).

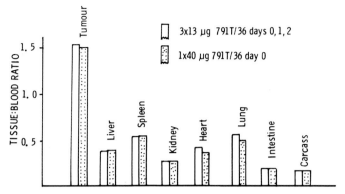

Fig. 13. Comparison of 791T xenograft localization of labelled 791T/36 antibody given as a single dose (40 μg) on day 0 or three doses (3 × 13 μg) on days 0, 1 and 2. Groups of four mice, killed 3 days after first injection.

The major implications from these findings is that while higher tumour levels of antibody can be achieved by repeated administration, greater discrimination between tumour and normal tissues is not obtained.

3. Relationship between Antibody Dose and Localization in Xenografts

Small doses of antibody are generally used to demonstrate localization into tumour xenografts and, in the tests discussed so far, mice with 791T xenografts received only limited (i.e., microgram) doses of radiolabelled 791T/36 antibody, and there was evidence that tumours were saturated. However, for delivery of therapeutic agents, conjugated to antibody, saturation of the tumour would be preferred. Therefore, to determine the maximum level of 791T/36 antibody which could be deposited in 791T xenografts, groups of mice were injected with between 10 μg and 2 mg of labelled antibody and killed after 3 days. Analysis of the data from these mice showed that, as would be expected, blood levels of antibody increased in proportion to the administered dose, but tumour levels did not increase proportionally; this resulted in a decline in the T : B ratio (Fig. 14). Thus, the T : B ratio was 1.6 : 1 at 10 μg of antibody per mouse, but only 0.51 : 1 at 2 mg per mouse, barely higher than that achieved with control immunoglobulins (cf. Fig. 3). Calculation of the absolute level of radiolabelled antibody in the tumours showed that with a dose of 10 μg (i.e., 0.5 mg/kg), there was 0.76 μg/g of tumour, i.e., 7.6% of the injected dose per gram, comparable to that previously seen. With the highest dose of antibody (2 mg, i.e., 100 mg/kg), there was 70 μg/g of tumour i.e., 3.5% per gram. This particular test was carried out

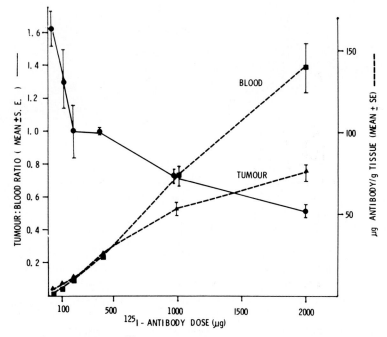

Fig. 14. Influence of dose of ^{125}I-labelled 791T/36 antibody on tumour and blood levels in 791T xenografted mice. Groups of four mice, killed 3 days after injection. (Reprinted with permission from *Europ. J. Cancer Clin. Oncol.*, Vol. 20, M. V. Pimm and R. W. Baldwin, Copyright 1984, Pergamon Press.)

with tumours weighing 100–300 mg but it is probable from the tumour size–antibody localization relationship already established that 'saturation' levels of smaller tumours would also be at about 70 μg/g of tissue. From these data, and that derived from kinetic studies, it is suggested that to maintain antibody saturation in tumours, relatively large doses of antibody (100 mg/kg) body weight would have to be given at 3- to 4-day intervals.

D. Equilibrium between Tumour-localized and Blood-borne Antibody

In addition to a consideration of the maximum level of antibody which can be deposited in tumour, it is also important to consider whether this antibody is in dynamic equilibrium with blood-borne antibody. Only if

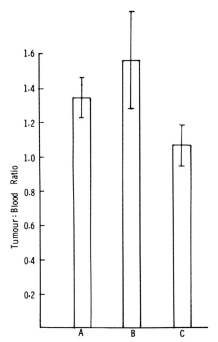

Fig. 15. Attempted displacement of 791T xenograft localized 791T/36 antibody by a larger dose of unlabelled antibody. (A) 10 μg ^{125}I-labelled 791T/36 injected on day 0, killed day 3. (B) 10 μg ^{125}I-labelled 791T/36 day 0, killed on day 5. (C) 10 μg ^{125}I-labelled 791T/36 day 0, 2 mg unlabelled 791T/36 day 3, killed on day 5. Four to five mice per group, all injections intraperitoneally. No statistical significance between groups.

this is the case could antibody which had delivered an anti-tumour agent at the tumour site be replaced by further antibody–drug conjugate.

To examine whether 791T/36 antibody which had localized in 791T xenografts was in a state of dynamic equilibrium with antibody in the blood, an attempt was made to displace radiolabelled antibody, already localized in xenografts with a further, larger dose of antibody. Groups of mice injected with 10 μg of ^{125}I-labelled 791T/36 antibody and killed 3 or 5 days later showed effective localization of radiolabel in xenografts (T : B ratios 1.35 and 1.56) (Fig. 15). Mice also injected with 10 μg of ^{125}I-labelled 791T/36 antibody, but which had received a further 2 mg of unlabelled antibody 3 days later, were killed after a further 2 days, i.e., 5 days after the initial ^{125}I-labelled 791T/36. These mice still had radiolabelled 791T/36 antibody in the xenografts at levels comparable (mean T : B ratio 1.06) to that in mice injected with the labelled antibody.

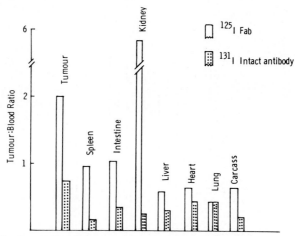

Fig. 16. Distribution of ^{131}I-labelled 791T/36 antibody and ^{125}I Fab fragment in mice with 791T xenografts; 10 μg of each preparation. Mean, three mice, examined 1 day after injection.

E. Kinetics of Localization of 791T/36 Fab Fragments in 791T Xenografts

Theoretically, clearer localization of antibody in tumours should be achieved using Fab or F(ab')$_2$ fragments rather than intact antibody. The removal of the Fc part of the molecule should prevent non-specific interactions with Fc receptor-bearing cells, and the rapid blood clearance and excretion of fragments should reduce blood and normal tissue levels, allowing tumour localization to be more clearly seen. Consequently, the feasibility of preparing fragments from the 791T/36 antibody for *in vivo* localization studies has been assessed. Conventional pepsin digestion of 791T/36 antibody failed to yield F(ab')$_2$ fragments, and this is in keeping with the established difficulty in preparing F(ab')$_2$ fragments from mouse immunoglobulin of the IgG$_{2b}$ isotype (Parham, 1983). Papain digestion, however, yielded Fab fragments and this was assessed for localization into 791T xenografts compared with intact antibody. Initial distribution studies that compared Fab with intact antibody in mice with 791T xenografts showed clear localization of the Fab fragment in tumour tissue (T : B ratio 2 : 1), compared with all normal organs examined with the exception of the kidneys, where T : B ratios were up to 6 : 1 (Fig. 16).

Kinetic studies showed that the accumulation of Fab fragments into 791T xenografts was much faster than that seen with intact antibody but both tumour and blood levels, in relation to the whole body level, were

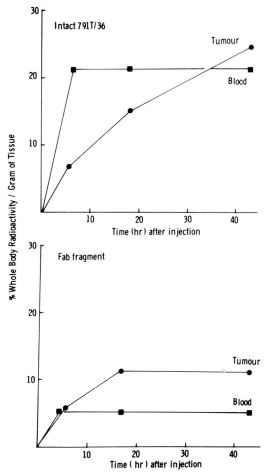

Fig. 17. Time course of tumour localization of intact 791T/36 and its Fab frgment in 791T xenografts. Groups of three mice were injected with 10 μg of ^{131}I-labelled 791T/36 and 10 μg ^{125}I Fab.

lower than intact antibody (Fig. 17). Here, tumour and blood levels were examined up to 40 hr after injection with ^{131}I-labelled intact 791T/36; blood levels had stabilized within 6 hr of intraperitoneal injection. Although labelled 791T/36 was detectable in tumour tissue within 6 hr, it continued to rise throughout the 40-hr observation period, in keeping with the previous, longer term kinetic study (cf. Fig. 7). With the Fab fragment also, blood levels had also stabilized within 6 hr but at only 5% of the whole body count per gram compared with 22% for intact antibody,

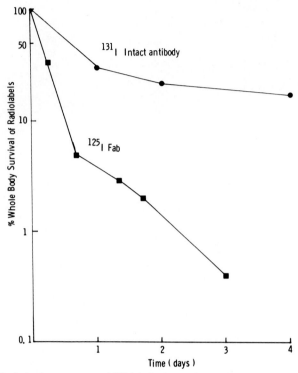

Fig. 18. Whole body retention of ^{131}I-labelled 791T/36 antibody compared with ^{125}I Fab fragment. Mean, six mice per group.

presumably reflecting the greater extent of extravasation of the fragment. In contrast to intact antibody, tumour levels of the fragment had reached maximum level by 17 hr, when the T : B ratio was 2 : 1. Although the Fab fragment showed faster localization into xenografts than the intact antibody, the whole body survival of the fragment was much shorter (Fig. 18). One consequence of this was that the tumour level of Fab, although greater than that of intact antibody when expressed as a T : B ratio, was much lower when calculated as a proportion of the injected dose per gram of tumour (Fig. 19).

VI. DISCUSSION

The objective of the studies reviewed here was to examine some of the kinetic and quantitative aspects of 791T/36 antibody localization into

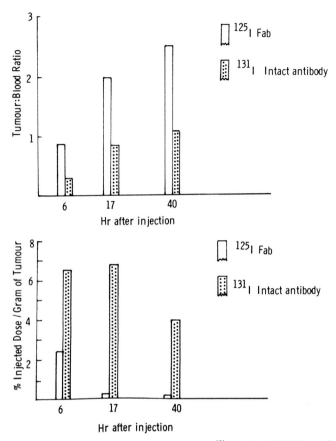

Fig. 19. Time course of blood and tumour levels of ^{131}I-labelled 791T/36 antibody and [125]I Fab fragment in mice with 791T xenografts. Mean, three mice per group.

xenografted tumour. Such quantitative studies with tumour-localizing monoclonal antibodies are essential for rational design of protocols for antibody administration for detection of tumours by external imaging and for treatment with antibody–drug conjugates. The major areas of investigation were the rate and extent of antibody uptake into tumour xenografts and the influence on this uptake of variations in the tumour's size and site, and the antibody's dose, route and time of administration.

Following intraperitoneal administration, antibody entered the circulation and survived in an undegraded, biologically active form for at least several days after injection. There was no evidence that antigen had been shed from the developing xenografts and complexed with antibody in the circulation. If this happened, it is possible that xenograft localization of the antibody might be impaired. In other xenograft situations, formation of complexes between anti-CEA antibody and circulating antigen has been demonstrated, and similar observations have been reported in clinical imaging trials (Primus *et al.*, 1980; Mach *et al.*, 1981) where, surprisingly however, there was no inhibition of effective tumour localization of the antibody.

Organ distribution studies in xenografted mice injected with radiolabelled 791T/36 antibody showed clearly that antibody (but not control immunoglobulin) localized in tumour tissue compared with normal organs. Examination of the kinetics of this localization showed that, although antibody was detectable in tumour tissue within a few hours of injection, the rate of localization was such that the maximum deposition of antibody in tumour with respect to the initial dose of antibody was not seen until 2 days. Moreover, the greatest discrimination between tumour and normal tissue was not seen until 4 days after injection; this improved discrimination was due partly to faster loss of antibody from normal tissues than that from the tumours. This requirement for several days to have elapsed before maximal localization is a feature of many other solid xenograft systems (Moshakis *et al.*, 1981b; Hedin *et al.*, 1982; Levine *et al.*, 1980; Gaffar *et al.*, 1981; Ghose *et al.*, 1982). This rate is probably a reflection of the degree of vascularity of these tumours, since other, more vascular tumours, show more rapid antibody uptake. Thus, with a Rauscher murine erythroleukaemia, maximum uptake into spleens of leukaemic mice was seen within 6 hr of injection of radiolabelled monoclonal antibody (Scheinberg and Strand, 1983). A more rapid uptake of antibody into tumours is not, however, necessarily accompanied by a higher level of localization nor a greater discrimination between the target tumour and normal organs. For example, with the Rauscher leukaemia, the maximum spleen to blood ratio was 1.6 : 1, not as high as that often seen in the 791T xenograft model.

In an attempt to achieve even greater discrimination between tumour and normal tissue than was seen with intact 791T/36 antibody, a Fab fragment of antibody was examined for localization into 791T xenografts. One of the most marked differences between Fab and intact antibody was the faster rate of localization of the fragment, this being completed within 18 hours, compared to 4 days for intact antibody. This difference is presumably a reflection of the faster and greater extravasation of Fab compared with intact antibody. This greater degree of extravasation was also reflected in the present studies in the proportion of whole body count of radiolabelled material present in the blood, being only 5% of the whole body count per gram compared to 22% per gram with intact antibody. In addition to faster localization of the fragment, the present tests show that the discrimination between tumour and normal tissues was at least as great, and on some occasions greater, than that seen with intact antibody. However, the major disadvantage of Fab fragment rather than intact antibody, which is emphasized by the present studies, is the much faster whole body clearance of the fragment. This resulted first in high kidney levels of the fragment and second, and most importantly, in much lower absolute levels of fragment deposited in tumour compared with intact antibody.

The findings of the present studies are in agreement with several other reports where it has been shown that xenografted mice injected with radiolabelled antibody fragments have shown rapid excretion of the fragment, lower absolute levels of tumour localization and high levels of radiolabel in kidney and bladder (Herlyn et al., 1983; Wahl et al., 1983; Colcher et al., 1983). In some situations (e.g., Wahl et al., 1983) it was concluded that $F(ab')_2$ was the more suitable of the two for tumour imaging, but with some anti-CEA antibodies Fab fragments were superior to $F(ab')_2$ (Buchegger et al., 1983). Clearly, for improved tumour imaging, greater and faster discrimination between tumour and normal tissues is necessary, and in this situation antibody fragments might be more suitable than intact antibody. For therapeutic applications, however, the use of fragments might require much higher doses compared with intact antibody to achieve tumour saturation, and the rapid clearance of the fragment might also necessitate more frequent administration to maintain high tumour levels.

With intact 791T/36 antibody, the extent of localization into 791T xenografts was up to 8% of the injected dose of antibody per gram of tumour tissue. Although this figure is comparable to that achieved in several other systems (e.g., Levine et al., 1980; Gaffar et al., 1981; Hedin et al., 1982), one question which arises from this observation is why does not more of the antibody localize in the tumour, particularly when only small, non-saturating doses of antibody are given. The extent of localization will depend, however, partly on how fast the antibody is being catabolized and is, therefore, becoming unavailable for tumour localization. Thus in the present situation, when 8% of the injected dose of antibody was present per gram of tumour tissue 2–3 days after injection, the whole body survival was only about 20% of the injected dose, i.e., about 40% of the total body load of antibody had localized per gram of tumour. There was a good correlation between tumour size and the proportion of the whole body count per gram of tissue, and extrapolation of these data would suggest that large tumours (of 2 g or over) would contain virtually all of the radiolabelled antibody surviving in the mouse, particularly at later time points where 50% of the body load of antibody was present per gram of tumour. It is probable that this relationship would break down with large tumours, due to necrosis and/or poor vascularization, but nevertheless these considerations indicate that a substantial proportion of the body burden of radiolabelled antibody can localize in solid tumour deposits. In the present tests, tumours growing intramuscularly were compared with subcutaneous xenografts for extent of localization but overall there was no increased uptake of antibody; the ratio of antibody radioactivity in tumour compared with blood was virtually identical. Tumours at other sites have not been examined, but it is most likely that even if these showed a greater rate of localization of antibody, the extent would not be significantly different from that seen with subcutaneous tumours.

One observation from the present studies was that, with very large tumours, so much antibody was taken into tumour tissue that there was a detectable decrease in blood levels and a corresponding increase in T : B ratios, although the level of activity in the tumour, on a weight basis, remained virtually constant. One implication from this is that although the T : B ratio is a convenient indication of the localization of a particular antibody, comparison of localization potential of different antibodies should not be judged only on this T : B ratio, unless it is clear that tumours of comparable sizes were used. In addition, simply a decline in blood levels due to rapid catabolism of antibody could increase the T : B ratio. To take one example, Hedin *et al.*, (1982) found a whole body survival of anti-CEA monoclonal antibody of 7.6–9% of the injected dose 4 days after injection (in contrast to the 15% of the present study) an a T : B ratio of 7 : 1, although the absolute level of antibody deposited in the tumours was no higher than with the 791T/36 antibody.

In preliminary tests, mice with xenografts received only a single limited (i.e., microgram) dose of radiolabelled antibody, and there was evidence that tumours were saturated with antibody. In tests designed to assess the degree of tumour localization achieved by repeated, rather than a single, injection of radiolabelled antibody, there was no greater localization, at least as assessed by the discrimination between tumour and normal organs. However, no kinetic studies were undertaken in this situation, and it is probably that repeated administration of antibody could maintain the tumour levels over a more prolonged period than a single injection.

To determine the maximum amount of antibody which could be localized in 791T xenografts by a single administration, mice were given large doses of antibody (<100 mg/kg) in an attempt to saturate tumours; here the maximum tumour level achieved was 70 μg of antibody per gram of tissue. As would be expected, blood levels increased in proportion to the administered dose, but as tumour levels did not increase proportionally, this resulted in a decline in the T : B ratio. Thus, the T : B ratio was 1.6 : 1 at 10 μg of antibody per mouse, but only 0.51 : 1 at 200 μg per mouse; this was barely higher than that generally achieved with control immunoglobulins. This particular test was carried out with tumours weighing 100–300 mg but it is probable from the tumour size–antibody localization relationship already established that 'saturation' levels of smaller tumours would also be at about 70 μg/g of tissue. From these data, and that derived from kinetic studies, it is suggested that to maintain antibody saturation in tumour, relatively large doses of antibody (100 mg/kg) body weight would have to be given at 3- to 4-day intervals. This regime of administration has, for example, been used to treat successfully 791T xenografts with 791T/36 antibody conjugated to vindesine (Pimm et al., 1984). In the therapeutic context, it is also important to consider the intratumour site of antibody deposition and whether it is in dynamic equilibrium with blood-borne antibody. A dynamic equilibrium seems unlikely since antibody already localized, but at levels well below saturation, was not displaced by a larger, saturating dose of antibody. The implication from this is that there is not a simple dynamic equilibrium between antibody deposited in the tumour and that in the blood and therefore it seems unlikely that antibody which had delivered an anti-tumour agent at the tumour site could be replaced by further antibody–drug conjugate. What does eventually happen to antibody deposited in tumour is virtually unknown. Certainly tumour levels ultimately decline (although more slowly than that in the blood and body as a whole) but whether this involves simple release of free, degraded or antigen-complexed antibody has not been explored.

In considering the site of initial antibody deposition in xenografts, it is certain that the localization of 791T/36 antibody in xenografts is immunologically directed, as emphasized by control tests with normal immunoglobulin and distribution studies with 791T/36 antibody in mice with xenografts lacking the 791T/36-defined antigen. This means that deposition of antibody within the tumour results from its combining with the appropriate antigen but the precise nature of the site of this antigen recognition is not fully clear. Analysis of tissue eluates showed antibody in high molecular weight form, putatively as an immune complex but, at least from the limited autoradiography studies, 791T/36 antibody localized in 791T xenografts is seen to be deposited primarily in the periphery of the tumour, and not throughout the whole tumour. This is probably simply a reflection of the diffusion gradients of antibody entering the tumour from the peripheral blood supply, and this type of distribution has been seen with other antibody/xenograft systems (e.g., Moshakis *et al.*, 1981a); however; in others, particularly with anti-CEA antibody, antibody was seen deposited more deeply in tumour tissue, but then was not uniformly distributed, being most concentrated at areas of known high CEA expression (Buchegger *et al.*, 1983). Clearly it would be valuable to know, in the present and similar systems, whether depth of penetration of antibody into tumours is related to the antibody dose, and whether larger doses of antibody result in deeper penetration into tumour tissue.

VII. CONCLUSIONS

These studies have shown that human tumour xenograft models can be used to answer precise kinetic and quantitative questions related to tumour localization of radiolabelled monoclonal antibody. The data so far obtained may be valuable for the design and interpretation of experimental localization studies with other antibodies for both tumour imaging and therapeutic applications. In addition similar studies are clearly warranted in the clinical situation, insofar as they are feasible by analysis of radiolabelled antibody levels in blood and resected tumour sample (see Chapter 7 by Armitage *et al.*, this volume).

A major question not fully resolved, certainly in the present study, is the precise nature of antibody deposited in tumours, and the ultimate fate of this antibody. When further data are available on this and other points of *in vivo* antibody behaviour, then, together with knowledge of *in vitro* characteristics of antibody–antigen interactions with 791T/36 antibody (Roe *et al.*, 1985), it may be feasible to produce mathematical models of antibody distribution, tumour deposition and catabolism, aiding in the choice of antibody and design of administration regimens for any particular antibody-mediated requirement.

ACKNOWLEDGEMENTS

The work was supported by the Cancer Research Campaign, London, U.K.

REFERENCES

Armitage, N. C., Perkins, A. C., Pimm, M. V., Farrands, P. A., Baldwin, R. W., and Hardcastle, J. D. (1984). *Br. J. Surg.* **71**, 407–412.

Buchegger, F., Haskell, C. M., Schreyer, M., Scazziga, B. R., Randin, S., Carrel, S., and Mach, J. -P. (1983). *J. Exp. Med.* **158**, 413–427.

Chatal, J. -F., Saccavini, J. -C., Fumoleau, P., Douillard, J. Y., Curtet, C., Kremer, M., Mevel, B., and Koprowski, H. (1984). *J. Nucl. Med.* **25**, 307–314.

Colcher, D., Zalutsky, M., Kaplan, W., Kufe, D., Austin, F., and Schlom, J. (1983). *Cancer Res.* **43**, 736–742.

Embleton, M. J., Gunn, B., Byers, V. S., and Baldwin, R. W. (1981). *Br. J. Cancer* **43**, 582–587.

Embleton, M. J., Rowland, G. F., Simmonds, R. G., Jacobs, E., Marsden, C. H., and Baldwin, R. W. (1983). *Br. J. Cancer* **47**, 43–49.

Epenetos, A. A., Britton, K. E., Mather, S., Shepherd, J., Taylor-Papadimitriou, J., Nimmon, C. C., Durbin, H., Hawkins, L. R., Malpas, J. S., and Bodmer, W. F. (1982). *Lancet* **2**, 999–1004.

Fairweather, D. S., Bradwell, A. R., Dykes, P. W., Vaughan, A. T., Watson-James, S. F., and Chandler, S. (1983). *Br. Med. J.* **287**, 167–170.

Farrands, P. A., Perkins, A. C., Pimm, M. V., Hardy, J. G., Embleton, M. J., Baldwin, R. W., and Hardcastle, J. D. (1982). *Lancet* **2**, 397–400.

Farrands, P. A., Perkins, A. C., Sully, L., Hopkins, J. S., Pimm, M. V., Baldwin, R. W., and Hardcastle, J. D. (1983). *J. Bone Jt. Surg., Br. Vol.* **65 B**, 638–640.

Gaffar, S. A., Pant, K. D., Schochat, D., Bennett, S. J., and Goldenberg, D. M. (1981). *Int. J. Cancer* **27**, 101–105.

Garnett, M. C., Embleton, M. J., Jacobs, E., and Baldwin, R. W. (1983). *Int. J. Cancer* **31**, 661–670.

Ghose, T., Ferrone, S., Imai, K., Norvell, S., Luner, S. J., Martin, R. H., and Blair, A. M. (1982). *JNCI, J. Natl. Cancer Inst.* **69**, 823–826.

Hedin, A., Wahren, B., an Hammarström, S. (1982). *Int. J. Cancer* **30**, 547–552.

Herlyn, D., Powe, J., Alavi, A., Mattis, J. A., Herlyn, M., Ernst, C., Vaum, R., and Koprowski, H. (1983). *Cancer Res.* **43**, 2731–2735.

Levine, G., Ballou, B., Reiland, J., Solter, D., Gumerman, L., and Hakala, T. (1980). *J. Nucl. Med.* **21**, 570–573.

Mach, J. -P., Buchegger, F., Forni, M., Ritschard, J., Berche, C., Lumbroso, J. -D., Schreyer, M., Giradet, C., Accolla, R. S., and Carrel, S. (1981). *Immunol. Today* **2**, 239–249.

Mach, J. -P., Chatal, J. -F., Lumbroso, J. -D., Buchegger, F., Forni, M., Ritschard, J., Berche, C., Douillard, J. -V., Carrel, S., Herlyn, M., Steplewski, Z., and Koprowski, H. (1983). *Cancer Res.* **43**, 5593–5600.

Moshakis, V., McIlhinney, R. A. J., Raghaven, D., and Neville, A. M. (1981a). *Br. J. Cancer* **44**, 91–99.

Moshakis, V., McIlhinney, R. A. J., and Neville, A. M. (1981b). *Br. J. Cancer* **44**, 663–669.

Parham, P. (1983). *J. Immunol.* **131**, 2895–2902.

Pelham, J. M., Gray, J. D., Flannery, G. R., Pimm, M. V., and Baldwin, R. W. (1983). *Cancer Immunol. Immunother.* **15**, 210–216.

Pimm, M. V., and Baldwin, R. W. (1984). *Eur. J. Cancer Clin. Oncol.* **20**, 313–324.

Pimm, M. V., Embleton, M. J. Perkins, A. C., Price, M. R., Robins, R. A., Robinson, G. R., and Baldwin, R. W. (1982) *Int. J. Cancer* **30**, 75–85.

Pimm, M. V., Rowland, G. F., Simmonds, R. G., Marsden, H., Embleton, M. J., Jacobs, E., and Baldwin, R. W. (1984). *Br. J. Cancer* **49**, 384.

Price, M. R., Campbell, D. G., Robins, R. A., and Baldwin, R. W. (1983a). *Eur. J. Cancer Clin. Oncol.* **19**, 81–90.

Price, M. R., Campbell, D. G., and Baldwin, R. W. (1983b). *Scand. J. Immunol.* **18**, 411–420.

Price, M. R., Pimm, M. V., Page, C. M., Armitage, N. C., Hardcastle, J. D., and Baldwin, R. W. (1984). *Br. J. Cancer* **89**, 809–812.

Primus, F. J., Bennett, S. J., Kim, E. E., DeLand, F., Zahn, M. C., and Goldenberg, M. (1980). *Cancer Res.* **40**, 497–501.

Rainsbury, R. M., Ott, R. J., Westwood, J. H., Kalirai, J. S., Coombes, R. C., McCready, V. R., Neville, A. M., and Gazet, J. -C. (1983). *Lancet* **2**, 934–938.

Roe, R., Robins, R. A., Laxton, R. R., and Baldwin, R. W. (1985). *Mol. Immunol.* **22**, 11–21.

Scheinberg, D. A., and Strand, M. (1983). *Cancer Res.* **43**, 265–272.

Symonds, E. M., Perkins, A. C., Pimm, M. V., Baldwin, R. W., Hardy, J. G., and Williams, D. A. (1985). *Br. J. Obstet. Gynaecol.* **92**, 270–276.

Wahl, R. L., Parker, C. W., and Philpott, G. W. (1983). *J. Nucl. Med.* **24**, 316–325.

Williams, M. R., Perkins, A. C., Campbell, F. C., Pimm, M. V., Hardy, J. G., Wastie, M. L., Blamey, R. W., and Baldwin, R .W. (1984). *Clin. Oncol.* **10**, 375–381.

Zalcberg, J. R., Thompson, C. H., Lichtenstein, M., Andrews, J., and McKenzie, I.F.C. (1983). *JNCI J. Natl. Cancer Inst.* **71**, 801–808.

CHAPTER 7

Monoclonal Antibody Imaging in Malignant and Benign Gastrointestinal Diseases

N. C. Armitage,* A. C. Perkins,† J. D. Hardcastle,*
M. V. Pimm‡ and R. W. Baldwin‡

* Department of Surgery
University Hospital
Queen's Medical Centre
Nottingham, United Kingdom
† Department of Medical Physics
University Hospital
Queen's Medical Centre
Nottingham, United Kingdom
‡ Cancer Research Campaign Laboratories
University of Nottingham
Nottingham, United Kingdom

MONOCLONAL ANTIBODIES FOR CANCER
DETECTION AND THERAPY

I. INTRODUCTION

As early as 1948, Pressman and Keighley were able to show that antibodies could be radiolabelled and retain their immunological characteristics.

With the description of the tumour-associated antigen, carcinoembryonic antigen (CEA), in 1965 (Gold and Freedman, 1965) a suitable target was available for the imaging of gastrointestinal cancers. Carcinoembryonic antigen is a foetal antigen which is normally present in gastrointestinal epithelium in small quantities only, but is found in large quantities in colorectal cancer cells. Thus, it was using antibodies raised against CEA that the first successful tumour imaging in colorectal cancers was achieved by Godenberg *et al.*, in 1978. He used a hyperimmune goat antiserum prepared against CEA; 3 sites of primary colorectal cancer and 4 of secondary sites were successfully imaged. This study was followed up in 1980, and 9 out of 10 primary sites, and 26 out of 31 secondary sites (85%), of colorectal cancer showed localization (Goldenberg *et al.*, 1980). Other gastrointestinal cancers, including gastric and pancreatic, as well as ovarian, uterine, lung and mammary cancers showed localization though less consistently. Using a polyclonal anti-CEA, this time raised in sheep, Dykes *et al.*, (1980) were successful in imaging patients with colorectal cancer. Begent has recently reported a series of patients in whom immunoscintigraphy was part of the follow-up of colorectal cancer (Begent *et al.*, 1983). The scans were prompted by rising serum CEA levels and radiolabelled anti-CEA was used as the agent. In this group of 26 patients, successful localization of recurrent disease was achieved in 21, of whom 5 went on to laparotomy for intraabdominal disease. The use of polyclonal serum, however, is far from ideal; the advantages of using a monoclonal antibody are reduction in the amount of immunoglobulin injected, reduction in potential crossreactions with other proteins, and an increase in the specificity of the localization. Mach *et al.*, (1981) reported the first use of a monoclonal anti-CEA for localizing human colorectal cancers. He achieved good localization in the primary and secondary tumours, with good tumour:normal tissue ratios of uptake of the antibody. Whilst these monoclonal anti-CEA antibodies may have no greater affinity than polyclonal sera, the potential problems should be reduced.

A number of monoclonal antibodies have been raised against colorectal cancer-associated antigens, 17-1A (Herlyn *et al.*, 1979) and YPC2/12.1 (Finan *et al.*, 1982). Mach, using 17-1A intact antibody and F(ab′)₂ fragments of antibody, successfully localized primary and secondary colorectal cancer in 31 of 52 (60%) patients (Mach *et al.*, 1983). Radiolabelled YPC2/12.1 successfully localized areas of known metastatic colorectal cancer in 13 of 16 (81%) patients studied (Smedley *et al.*, 1983).

In 1981, Embleton described a monoclonal antibody raised against a human osteogenic sarcoma cell line, 791T (Embleton *et al.*, 1981). As will be described later, this antibody also showed reactivity against other tumours, including some colorectal cancers. This prompted a pilot study using radiolabelled antibody in patients with primary and disseminated colorectal cancer. Successful localization was achieved in four out of five patients with primary tumours and in six patients with disseminated disease (Farrands *et al.*, 1982). This antibody has been evaluated in the imaging of patients with colorectal cancer, with benign colorectal tumours, and with malignant tumours of other parts of the gastrointestinal tract. The results of clinical imaging have been carefully correlated with clinical findings and direct measurement of the preferential uptake of antibody by the tumours (Armitage *et al.*, 1984).

II. MONOCLONAL ANTIBODIES STUDIED

1. 791T/36

This monoclonal antibody was obtained by immunizing BALB/c mice with osteogenic sarcoma 791T cells. Spleen cells from the immunized mouse were fused with P3-NSI-Ag4 murine myeloma cells in the presence of 50% polyethylene glycol. From this fusion, two hybridomas showed good activity against the immunizing cell line, these being designated 791T/36 and 791T/48 (Embleton *et al.*, 1981).

Antibody 791T/36 has been shown to be of the IgG₂ᵦ subclass and reacts with a 72,000-MW antigen on the cell surface of the immunizing cell line 791T (Price *et al.*, 1983). This antibody showed no reactivity with a range of normal fibroblasts, blood mononuclear cells or red cells. It did, however, show some reactivity with 6 out of 26 tumour cell lines tested by a cell absorbtion assay, including the colon cancer cell line HT29 (Embleton *et al.*, 1981). It was on the basis of the reactivity with colorectal cancer cells that localization studies in patients with this type of tumour were attempted.

2. 791T/36 Fab Fragments

Fab fragments of 791T/36 were studied for their localization in six patients with colorectal cancer. These fragments were prepared from intact 791T/36 by papain digestion at an enzyme:substrate molar ratio of 20 : 1 at pH 7.2 for 3½ hr at 37°C. The mixture was purified to remove undigested 791T/36 and Fc fragments to leave a single protein of 48,000 MW.

3. Normal Mouse Immunoglobulin

In one patient, labelled normal mouse immunoglobulin (NMI) of the IgG_{2b} subclass was simultaneously administered with labelled 791T/36 to compare non-specific with antigen-specific binding of antibody. This NMI was purified from normal mouse serum.

A. Purification

For large-scale production of monoclonal antibody, the hybridomas are maintained as ascites in BALB/c mice. To obtain purified antibody from ascitic fluid, the fluid was diluted 1 : 1 in 0.1 M citrate phosphate buffer pH 7.5 and passed through a Sepharose-protein A column (Pharmacia, Hounslow, Middlesex). The column was washed and the antibody eluted with citrate–phosphate buffer over a pH gradient of 7.5–3.0 using a flow rate of 12 ml/min with an LKB ultragrade gradient mixer (LKB, South Croydon, Surrey). The material eluted at pH 3.0–4.0 was pooled, dialysed against PBS and concentrated by positive pressure membrane ultrafiltration, the yield of purified immunoglobulin being 2.8–3.4 mg/ml ascitic fluid.

To obtain normal mouse IgG_{2b}, a similar procedure was applied to normal mouse serum. Purified antibody was tested for toxicity and the presence of pyrogens by rabbit injection.

B. Labelling

Antibodies were labelled with ^{131}I by the iodogen method (Fraker and Speck, 1978). Three hundred-microlitre aliquots of iodogen (1,3,4,6-tetrachloro-3 α, 6 diphenylglycoluril methylene chloride were evaporated under nitrogen in polypropylene tubes (Sarstedt, Leicester). Antibody at 1 mg/ml and Na [131]I (Amersham International) was added in the coated tubes and incubated at room temperature for 15 min. The reaction mixture was removed from the tubes and passed through a Sephadex G-25 column (Pharmacia) to remove free iodine.

Labelling efficiency was tested by counting the proportion of ^{131}I attached to protein and in most instances was found to be 70% for 791T/36. Two hundred micrograms of 791T/36 antibody was labelled with about 70 MBq (1.5 mCi) for each patient dose.

One patient was infused simultaneously with ^{131}I-labelled 791T/36 and ^{123}I-labelled normal mouse immunoglobulin. To prepare the latter, [123]I (Atomic Energy Research Establishment, Harwell, Oxon) was supplied dry in NaOH. This was dissolved in 5 μl of 0.3 M citrate buffer at pH 3 and 1 μl 0.8 nM potassium iodide/mCi immediately before addition to the immunoglobulin solution for labelling using the iodogen method as above, and then passed down a Sephadex G-25 column (Pharmacia).

The radiolabelled preparations were diluted in normal saline and sterilized by Millipore filtration. Initially, doses were made up into 500 ml saline but this was reduced to 20 ml later in the studies.

III. PATIENTS STUDIED

A total of 74 patients were injected with radiolabelled intact 791T/36 or its Fab fragments. Of these, 38 had primary colorectal cancers, 19 had disseminated disease (2 patients having both primary and disseminated cancers), 4 patients had benign colorectal tumours and 1 had a stricture of the sigmoid colon due to diverticular disease.

Fourteen patients with malignant gastrointestinal tumours in the rest of the gastrointestinal tract were studied.

A. Injection

To block thyroid uptake of ^{131}I, patients were started on 60 mg potassium iodide daily and continued for 10 days. To test for anaphylaxis, a subcutaneous injection of 1 ml of unlabelled antibody was given and the patient observed for 5 min.

Following this the patients were injected slowly with radiolabelled antibody (200 μg immunoglobulin, 70 MBq) into a vein on the dorsum of the hand. The patient's pulse and blood pressure were monitored before, during and following the injection. Blood samples were taken prior to injection and 2 min following the injection. In most patients, a 0.5-ml sample of the dose was saved for counting of radioactivity. In a number of patients, blood samples were taken daily following injection to measure the clearance of the radiolabelled antibody from the bloodstream. In four patients, the urinary excretion of ^{131}I was measured by collection of 24 hr urine samples and counting of these for radioactivity.

Patients were followed up in the outpatient clinic, and blood taken at intervals up to 2 yr to determine the production of anti-mouse antibody.

B. Imaging

Patients were imaged between 6 hr and 5 days following injection of radiolabelled antibody. Those patients undergoing surgery for primary tumours were mostly imaged prior to operation. Only two were imaged post-operatively. Where possible, imaging was timed for the day immediately preceding the operation. Patients with disseminated cancer, or those not undergoing surgery, were mostly imaged 48–72 hr after injection.

Patients were imaged using a IGE400T γ camera (International General Electric) with a 40-cm field of view, and fitted with a high-energy collimator (400 KeV maximum). A 20% window was set on the 364-keV γ-ray emissions of ^{131}I. Counts were acquired on each view for 600 sec and stored by computer (Nodecrest NMS80) (Nodecrest Medical Systems, Byfleet, Surrey) on magnetic tape. The standard views taken were of anterior and posterior, upper and lower abdomen. In addition, for rectal tumours and suspected pelvic recurrences, a 'sitting' view was taken with the patient sitting on the imaging table and with the γ camera positioned below. Where appropriate, skull and thoracic views were taken. All patients were asked to empty their bladders prior to imaging.

A blood pool image was obtained by labelling the patients' red blood cells *in vivo* by the injection of stannous pyrophosphate, the dose calculated by nomogram, followed by 200-MBq [^{99m}Tc]pertechnetate (Pavel *et al.*, 1977) and/or the circulating transferrin labelled by injection of 200-MBq [^{113m}In]chloride (Wochner *et al.*, 1970). Blood pool images were acquired over the same views as the iodine image to simulate the distribution of radiolabelled antibody in the circulation. After normalization of count rates in the images, the ^{99m}Tc or ^{113m}In blood pool images were subtracted from the ^{131}I-labelled antibody images by the technique described by DeLand (DeLand *et al.*, 1980). Dual radionuclide image subtraction is well established in nuclear medicine and was originally applied by Kaplan *et al.*, (1966) for pancreatic imaging using ^{75}Se, which concentrates both in the pancreas and the liver. Following the administration of [^{99m}Tc]sulphur colloid or colloidal ^{198}Ay, the resulting liver image can be subtracted thus removing the background activity. In the present study, the iodine view and the background views contain different numbers of counts within each digital picture cell. It was, therefore, necessary to normalise the counts within the background to view to 100% total counts within the iodine view. The percentage subtraction was obtained by determining the total number of counts within both the iodine and background views, i.e.,

$$\frac{\text{Total counts within the iodine view}}{\text{Total counts within the background view}} \times 100\%$$

The subtracted images show areas of accumulation which can not be accounted for simply by the vascular concentration. Quantitation of antibody localization was then obtained from the images by defining a digital region of interest (ROI) at both the site of antibody accumulation and a site over normal tissues (normally adjacent or contralateral position). The counts per cell in the two regions were used to obtain a target : non-target tatio (T : NT) both for the ^{131}I image and the subtracted image, thus

$$\text{T : NT} = \frac{\text{Counts in target ROI}}{\text{Number of image cells in target ROI}} \div \frac{\text{Counts in non-target ROI}}{\text{Number of image cells in non-target ROI}}$$

The resultant edited image was carefully studied and the distribution of radiolabelled antibody compared with the site of primary and secondary tumours as determined by operation, other imaging techniques and clinical findings. Where a clear 'hot spot' was seen, a T : NT ratio of emitted counts was obtained.

IV. PROCESSING OF RESECTED SPECIMENS

A. Imaging

With those patients coming to surgery the resected specimens were opened, the tumour measured and imaged immediately. They were placed directly onto the face of a IGE400T γ camera with a high-energy collimator. Radioactive counts were acquired for 1000 sec. From the images so obtained, T : NT ratios were calculated in a similar manner to that previously described for the patient images.

B. Counting of Radioactivity

Following the acquisition of the γ-camera images, samples of tumour and normal large bowel were taken for radioactivity counting. From these a value for counts per minute per gram tissue was calculated. This value was obtained for tumour and normal full thickness large bowel. In some, the mucosa and muscle coats of normal large bowel were counted separately. A T : NT ratio was calculated between tumour and full thickness normal bowel. The counts per minute per gram tumour and counts per minute per gram normal colon were compared by the paired *t* test.

One patient was injected simultaneously with ^{131}I-labelled 791T/36 and ^{123}I-labelled normal mouse IgG_{2b} and, in this case, counts were obtained for both isotopes.

V. RESULTS

A. Imaging of Patients

1. 791T/36: Primary Colorectal Cancer

A total of 33 patients with primary colorectal cancer were injected with radiolabelled 791T/36. The details are given in Table I. Of these patients, 24 were imaged pre-operatively from 6 hr to 5 days after injection. In 13 of the 24 patients, the primary tumour was successfully localized. Patient 4 had two primary tumours and for imaging purposes both have been considered separately. If tumours of different parts of the large bowel are considered separately, then the results of imaging are as shown in Table II. If tumours within the pelvis (rectum and rectosigmoid) are considered, then it can be seen that of the 13 patients imaged, only five (42%) tumours were successfully localized. This compares with successful localization on external imaging in 8 (67%) of 11 patients who had lesions outside the pelvis (Fig. 1). [131]I is excreted through the urinary tract and the bladder had a high emission of radioactivity in all patients despite emptying of the bladder immediately before the examination.

The mean T : NT ratios, after subtraction, have been calculated only for those patients who had positive images; this T : NT was 4.4 : 1 overall.

Patient 14 had residual tumour left in the pelvis after resection of his primary tumour; patient 33 had massive hepatic metastases as well as a primary rectal cancer and both have been included in the group of patients studied with recurrent metastatic colorectal cancer as well.

2. 791T/36: Recurrent Metastatic Colorectal Cancer

Eighteen patients were imaged, with a total of 26 sites of metastatic or recurrent colorectal cancer. The details are shown in Table III. In all cases where positive localisation was shown, there was good correlation between the images and the clinical/radiological findings. In 12 patients there was laparotomy/autopsy confirmation of the tumour deposits.

Thirteen patients had liver metastases, in whom 10 had laparotomy or biopsy confirmation. Positive imaging was achieved in 11 patients, the smallest deposits visualised being multiple 1-cm diameter deposits in both lobes in patient 48. Conventional sulphur colloid scans were obtained in 8 patients of which only 5 (65.6%) were considered definitely abnormal. Figure 2a shows the sulphur colloid liver scan of patient 47 with filling defects in both lobes. The subtraction antibody image (Fig. 2b) can be clearly seen to correlate closely with the areas of increased emission corresponding to those 'cold' areas on the conventional scan. Patient 40 was shown at laparoscopy to have almost complete replacement of his liver by secondary tumour, and no operation was performed. Autopsy confirmed the laparascopic findings and showed a primary tumour of the ascending colon. At imaging this could not be distinguished from the extensive liver deposits and this patient has been considered in the disseminated group only.

Seven patients had pelvic/perineal tumour recurrences, of which five were distinctly demonstrated. Two pelvic recurrences failed to image, one of which was a 2-cm diameter nodule in a perineal wound. This is probably below the resolution of the technique in this site at present. All but one of the other seven recurrences were positively identified (Table IV).

In all, there were 26 sites of metastasis and, of these, 21 (85%) were positively identified using this technique.

One patient with a small pre-sacral recurrence after anterior resection had been imaged before removal of her primary tumour (patient 18 of

TABLE I

^{131}I-LABELLED 791T/36 PRIMARY COLORECTAL CANCER

Patient	Age	Sex	Primary site	Size of tumour (cm)	Interval after injection (days)	Imaging result	T : NT ratio Before subtraction	T : NT ratio After subtraction
1	71	M	Sigmoid	5 × 6	1	+ve	1.5 : 1	8.0 : 1
2	57	F	Sigmoid	4 × 4	1	+ve	2.0 : 1	2.0 : 1
3	75	M	Rectosigmoid	4 × 4	2	−ve	—	—
4	64	M	Transverse	3 × 3	1	+ve	—	—
5	64	M	Rectum	4 × 4		+ve	1.5 : 1	2.1 : 1
6	64	M	Sigmoid	6 × 3	3	+ve	1.2 : 1	1.5 : 1
7	30	F	Rectosigmoid	3 × 4	—	Not imaged	—	—
8	72	M	Sigmoid	3 × 4	—	Not imaged	—	—
9	72	F	Sigmoid	5 × 5	1	−ve	—	—
10	72	M	Ascending colon	5 × 4	1	+ve	1.1 : 1	6.6 : 1
11	60	M	Rectum	Unresectable	3	−ve	—	—
12	51	F	Rectosigmoid	4.5 × 5	—	Not imaged	—	—
			Rectosigmoid	3 × 3	3	−ve	—	—

						Not imaged Not imaged	Imaged post-operatively	
13	44	F	Sigmoid	3 × 5	—	} Not imaged		
14	75	M	Rectum	3 × 5	—			
15	72	F	Caecum	4 × 4	3	+ve	1.9 : 1	4.5 : 1
16	78	M	Caecum	6 × 8	2	+ve	1.2 : 1	5.4 : 1
17	73	F	Rectum	5 × 4	3	−ve	—	—
18	67	F	Rectum	3.5 × 4	3	+ve	1.2 : 1	5.4 : 1
19	67	M	Rectum	5.5 × 5.5	6 hr	−ve	—	—
20	62	M	Rectum	4 × 2	2	−ve	—	—
21	63	F	Rectum	3 × 3	—	Not imaged	—	—
22	53	M	Rectum	7.5 × 5	3	+ve	1.3 : 1	2.5 : 1
23	58	F	Sigmoid	3.5 × 2.5	3	−ve	—	—
24	59	M	Rectum	5 × 5	4	−ve	—	—
25	60	M	Rectosigmoid	4.5 × 3.5	3	+ve	1.7 : 1	3.0 : 1
26	78	F	Caecum	3.5 × 3.5	2	+ve	1.6 : 1	2.3 : 1
27	73	M	Rectum	7.0 × 7.5	5	+ve	1.5 : 1	10.0 : 1
28	61	F	Descending colon	2.5 × 2.5	2	−ve	—	—
29	50	F	Rectum	8.5 × 6.0	—	Not imaged	—	—
30	59	M	Rectum	10.0 × 10.0	—	Not imaged	—	—
31	82	M	Rectum	4 × 3	—	Not imaged	—	—
32	71	F	Rectum	4 × 3	—	Not imaged	—	—
33	69	F	Rectum	Not resectable	3	−ve	—	—

139

TABLE II

¹³¹I-LABELLED 791T/36 PRIMARY COLON CANCER

Site	Number of patients	Number imaged	Number positive		Mean T : NT after subtraction
Caecum and ascending colon	4	4	4 ⎫		3.5 : 1
Transverse and descending colon	2	2	1 ⎬ 8 of 11		2.1 : 1
Sigmoid colon	7	5	3 ⎭		3.9 : 1
Rectosigmoid	5	3	1 ⎫ 5 of 13		3.0 : 1
Rectum	15	10	4 ⎭		5.0 : 1
Total	33	24	13		

the primary colorectal cancer group). After giving the subcutaneous test dose of 791T/36 for the repeat injection, she developed a red flare at the injection site and the intravenous dose was not administered. She has subsequently been shown to have developed anti-mouse antibodies.

3. 791T/36: Benign Colorectal Conditions

Four patients with benign colorectal tumours and one patient with a diverticular stricture were injected with radiolabelled 791T/36. The details are shown in Table V; as can be seen, none of these lesions was localized by external imaging.

4. 791T/36: Non-colonic Gastrointestinal Malignancies

A total of 14 patients with malignant disease of the gastrointestinal tract were injected and the details are shown in Table VI. As can be seen from this, only 2 patients (56 and 63) showed positive *in vivo* imaging.

5. 791T/36: Fab Fragments

Six patients with primary and metastatic colorectal cancer were injected with 791T/36 Fab fragments. The details are shown in Table VII. In all patients imaged, a high proportion of the activity was seen in the kidneys. In patient 70 there was increased activity over all of the descending and sigmoid colon but no definite uptake in the tumour. Patient 74 had a pelvic recurrence causing chronic retention of urine; greatly increased activity was seen corresponding to his distended bladder but no distinct tumour uptake could be distinguished. In no patients could tumour uptake of antibody fragments be shown by external scanning.

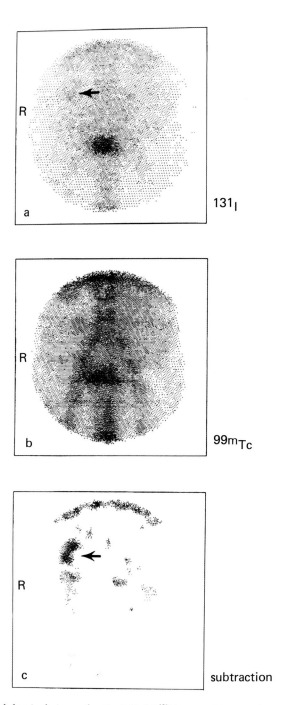

Fig. 1. Anterior abdominal views of patient 16: (a) ^{131}I image with area of increased uptake arrowed; (b) blood pool image; (c) subtracted image showing marked uptake in tumour (caecum) arrowed.

TABLE III

^{131}I-LABELLED 791T/36 METASTATIC RECURRENT COLORECTAL CANCER

Patient	Age	Sex	Secondary sites	Diagnostic criteria	Interval to imaging (days)	Imaging result	T : NT Before subtraction	T : NT After subtraction
34	58	F	Liver	Laparotomy	2 + 3	– ve	2.0 : 1	8.1 : 1
			Intraabdominal			+ ve	0.9 : 1	2.0 : 1
35	71	M	Liver	Laparotomy	2 + 3	+ ve	1.2 : 1	5.8 : 1
			Pelvis			+ ve		
36	50	M	Liver	Liver scan/clinical	2	+ ve	1.5 : 1	4.4 : 1
37	44	M	Liver	Brain scan	2	+ ve	1.5 : 1	2.4 : 1
			Brain	Chest X-ray		+ ve	1.3 : 1	4.0 : 1
			Lung	Autopsy		– ve	—	—
38	60	F	Pelvis	Laparotomy	2	+ ve	1.9 : 1	4.3 : 1
39	68	M	Liver	Clinical	1	+ ve	1.8 : 1	4.0 : 1
40	74	M	Liver	Laparoscopy/liver scan Autopsy	4	+ ve	1.2 : 1	2.4 : 1
41	70	M	Pelvis	Clinical/IVP	3	+ ve	2.0 : 1	6.0 : 1
14	75	M	Pelvis	Laparotomy	4	+ ve	1.4 : 1	1.8 : 1
33	69	F	Liver	Liver scan/liver biopsy	3	+ ve	1.4 : 1	3.3 : 1
42	54	F	Pelvis	CAT scan	2	+ ve	1.4 : 1	2.1 : 1
43	65	M	Liver	Liver scan	2	+ ve	1.2 : 1	3.6 : 1
			Intraabdominal	Clinical		+ ve	1.8 : 1	7.7 : 1
44	61	M	Liver	Laparotomy	3	– ve	—	—
45	63	M	Perineal	CAT scan/biopsy	2	– ve		
46	72	M	Liver	Laparotomy	2	+ ve	1.5 : 1	2.7 : 1
47	56	M	Liver	Liver scan ultrasound	2	+ ve	1.1 : 1	4.5 : 1
48	65	M	Liver	Laparotomy	2 + 9	+ ve	<1cm Not quantitatable	
			Intraabdominal			+ ve	As for liver metastasis	
49	75	M	Lung	Chest X-ray	2	– ve	1.2 : 1	6.6 : 1
			Pelvis	Clinical/biopsy		+ ve	As for liver metastasis	
			Liver			+ ve		

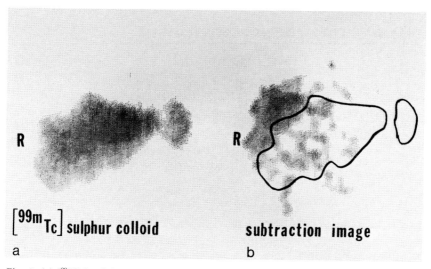

Fig. 2. (a) [^{99m}Tc] sulphur colloid scan of patient 47 showing large filling defect of right lobe; (b) subtraction antibody image showing dense uptake corresponding to filling defect as shown by [^{99m}Tc] sulphur colloid scan (overlay).

B. Imaging and Counting of Resected Specimens

All but two of the patients injected with radiolabelled 791T/36 underwent resection of their primary tumour (patient 10 had an unresectable rectal tumour). Figure 3a shows the resected specimen of patient 16 with its corresponding γ-camera image (Fig. 3b).

In general terms there was fair correlation between the T : NT ratios derived from the specimen images and those from the counted samples. To some extent the former may be influenced by the relative thickness

TABLE IV

^{131}I-LABELLED 791T/36 METASTATIC RECURRENT COLORECTAL CANCER

	Number imaged	Number positive	Mean T : NT ratio after subtraction
Liver	13	11	3.5 ± 1.2 : 1
Pelvis/perineum	7	5	4.0 ± 2.0 : 1
Intraabdominal	3	3	7.4 ± 0.8 : 1
Lung	2	1	Not quantifiable
Brain	1	1	4.0 : 1
Total	26	21	

TABLE V

^{131}I-LABELLED 791T/36 BENIGN COLORECTAL DISEASE

Patient	Age	Sex	Site	Size (cm)	Histology	Interval (days)	Imaging result
50	53	F	Rectum	3 × 1.5	Villous adenoma	2	Not imaged
51	75	F	Rectum	3 × 6	Villous adenoma	3	− ve
52	56	M	Transverse	1 × 1	Tubulo-villous adenoma	4	− ve
53	54	M	Sigmoid	Multiple 3 × 3 largest	Tubulo-villous	3	− ve
54	44	M	Sigmoid	10 × 2	Diverticular stricture	1	− ve

of tumour and normal tissue. This will tend to cause some distortion of the true emitted T : NT ratio, the mean image T : NT being 2.2 : 1 ($\pm$ 0.7)—colon T : NT 2.2 $\pm$ 0.5; rectosigmoid and rectum T : NT 2.3 $\pm$ 0.8. This is comparable with the values obtained from counting of specimens. For this, the overall mean T : NT ratio was 2.5 : 1 $\pm$ 1.1—colon 2.8 $\pm$ 1.3; rectosigmoid and rectum 2.3 $\pm$ 0.9. There is no significant difference between the T : NT ratios for different sites in the large bowel. There is a highly significant difference between the tumour and normal counts per minute per gram ($p < 0.001$).

C. Double Labelling Study

Patient 19 was simultaneously injected with ^{131}I-labelled 791T/36 (15 MBq) and ^{123}I-labelled normal IgG$_{2b}$ (25 MBq) (NMI). This patient came to resection the following day and samples of tumour and normal colon were counted for both isotopes. The results are shown graphically in Fig. 4 with the tissue : blood ratio of radioactivity shown for tumour and normal tissue for both ^{131}I-labelled 791T/36 and ^{123}I-NMI, the T : NT ratios being 3.3 : 1 for ^{131}I-labelled 791T/36 and 1.1 : 1 for ^{123}I NMI. These data indicate that the binding of 791T/36 is antigen related rather than non-specific.

1. Benign Colorectal Disease

Four patients with benign tumours and one patient with a diverticular stricture were studied. Patient 52 underwent endoscopic polypectomy

TABLE VI

^{131}I-LABELLED 791T/36 WITH NON-COLONIC GASTROINTESTINAL MALIGNANCY[a]

Patient	Primary site	Histology	Management	External scan result
55	Floor of mouth	Squamous carcinoma	Radiotherapy	−ve
56	Lower Oesophagus	Anaplastic carcinoma	Radiotherapy	+ve
57	Lower Oesophagus	Poorly differentiated squamous carcinoma	Radiotherapy	−ve
58	Lower Oesophagus (liver metastases)	Anaplastic carcinoma	Intubation	Liver 2° −ve
59	Stomach (recurrent)	Moderately differentiated adenocarcinoma	Gastroenterostomy	−ve
60	Stomach (linitis plastica)	Poorly differentiated adenocarcinoma	Laparotomy/biopsy	−ve
61	Stomach	Poorly differentiated adenocarcinoma	Partial gastrectomy	Not imaged
62	Stomach	Adenocarcinoma	Laparotomy/biopsy	−ve
63	Stomach (2° right lobe of liver)	Moderately differentiated adenocarcinoma	Gastroscopy/biopsy	+ve Stomach +ve Right lobe liver
64	Stomach	Moderately differentiated adenocarcinoma	Gastrectomy	Not imaged
65	Small bowel	Moderately differentiated adenocarcinoma	Small bowel resection	−ve
66	Small bowel	Lymphoma	Small bowel resection	−ve
67	Pancreas (2° left lobe of liver)	Adenocarcinoma	Laparotomy/bypass	−ve Liver 2° −ve
68	Pancreas	Moderately differentiated adenocarcinoma	Laparotomy/bypass	−ve

[a]From Armitage *et al.* (1984).

TABLE VII

^{131}I-LABELLED 791T/36 FAB FRAGMENTS—COLORECTAL CANCER

Patient	Age	Sex	Primary site	Size (cm)	Interval days	Secondary site	Imaging result
69	71	F	Sigmoid	5 × 4	—	Nil	Not imaged
70	69	F	Sigmoid	2 × 2	3	Nil	Non-specific
71	59	M	Rectosigmoid	4.5 × 3	2	Nil	−ve
72	76	M	Rectum	5 × 3	2	Nil	−ve
73	—	F	Ascending colon	Not resectable	6 hr 24 hr	—	−ve
74	74	M	—	—	2	Pelvic	+ve Activity in bladder

and no normal colonic tissue was available for comparison. Patient 53 had a segment of sigmoid colon and upper rectum excised for polyposis coli; two adenomas were taken as representative samples. No increased uptake in any of the four adenomas available for measurement was observed when the radioactivity was counted. Some increased activity was seen on imaging the resected specimen of patient 54 but this was simply due to the greatly thickened bowel wall in the region of the diverticular stricture, counting of radioactivity showing no difference in uptake.

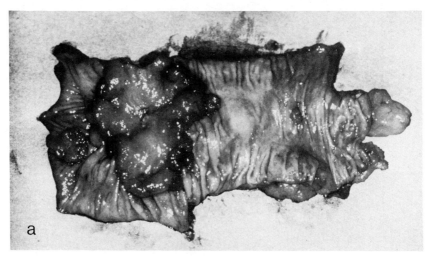

Fig. 3. (a) Resected specimen from patient 16; (b) γ-camera image of resected specimen of patient 16 showing increased uptake in region of tumour.

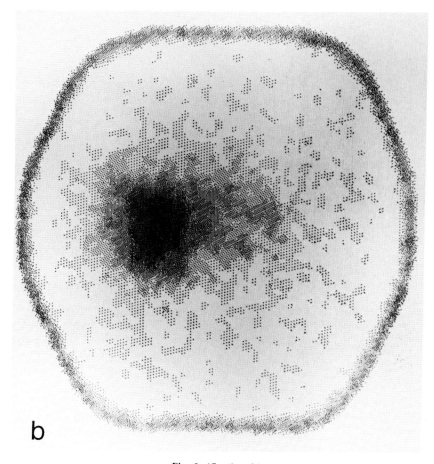

b

Fig. 3. *(Continued.)*

2. Non-colonic Malignant Disease

Due to the nature of the type of malignant disease, few resected specimens were available. Both specimens from patients with stomach cancer failed to give a positive image and the counts per minute per gram for tumour and normal tissue showed no difference. No specimens were available from any of the three oesophageal or two pancreatic cancers. For the two small bowel tumours, one patient with an adenocarcinoma had a positive resected specimen image, with a T : NT of 1.9 : 1. The counts per minute per gram, however, showed no difference. The other

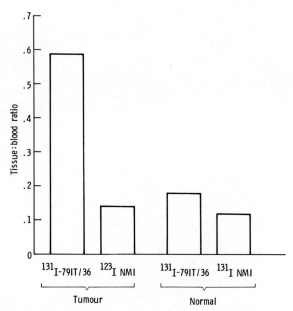

Fig. 4. Double labelling study showing specific preferential uptake of ^{131}I-labelled 791T/36 in rectal tumour. (From Baldwin *et al.*, 1984. *In* "Cancer Invasion and Metastasis, Biologic and Therapeutic Aspects," R. W. Baldwin, M. V. Pimm, M. J. Embleton, N. C. Armitage, P. A. Farrands, J. D. Hardcastle and A. C. Perkins. Copyright 1984, Raven Press, New York.)

patient had a small bowel lymphoma which failed to show a positive image, and the counts per minute per gram ratio was 1 : 1.

3. 791T/36 Fab Fragments

In four patients with primary colorectal cancer injected with 791T/36 Fab fragments, a resected specimen was available. There was no increased uptake in the tumour over normal colon after the injection of 791T/36 Fab fragments either as shown by imaging of the specimens or counting of radioactivity.

D. Kinetics of Radiolabelled Antibody Blood Clearance

In nine patients after injection of radiolabelled 791T/36, and in 3 patients after injection of Fab fragments of 791T/36, serial venous samples were

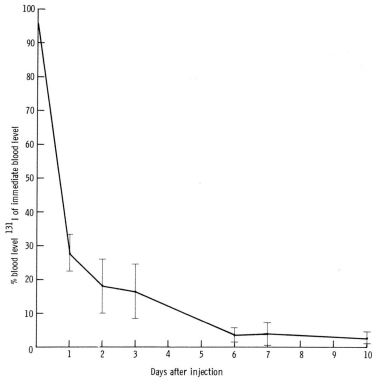

Fig. 5. Clearance of ^{131}I-labelled 791T/36 from blood as a percentage of the level immediately after injection.

taken and the radioactive counts per minute per millilitre blood measured. These were corrected for the decay of ^{131}I and plotted against time as a percentage of the blood level of radiolabelled antibody immediately after infusion; the results are as shown in Fig. 5. It can be seen that there is an early rapid fall in the level of circulating antibody in the first 24 hr to about 30% of the immediate level, which probably corresponds to antibody moving from the vascular to extravascular compartment. Subsequently the fall is more gradual and corresponds to clearance and excretion of the antibody with a half-life of about 2 days. It was established that the radioactivity was still associated with an IgG_{2b} protein and that this protein retained activity against 791T/36 target cells (Baldwin *et al.*, 1984).

Fab fragments of the antibody are cleared very rapidly from the blood and, at 24 hr, less than 10% of the initial level is detectable, falling to below 1% at 3 days.

E. Urinary Excretion

In three patients 24-hr urine samples were collected over the first 24 hr following injection of radiolabelled 791T/36, and in two patients after 791T/36 Fab fragments. In these patients 23.3 ± 6.1% of the injected ^{131}I was excreted in the first 24 hr, whilst in patient 32 a further 9.5% was excreted in the third 24 hr. These excreted fractions correspond with the loss of activity from the blood.

F. Clearance of Antibody from the Tumour

In 18 patients the percentage of the injected dose of ^{131}I-labelled 791T/36 present per gram of tumour was calculated after correction for the decay of ^{131}I between injection and resection of the tumour. The results are shown plotted against the number of days between injection and resection of the tumour in Fig. 6. There is a significant correlation between these two variables ($p < 0.003$); the mean percentage of the injected dose per gram of tumour resected within 48 hr of injection was 0.0065 ± 0.002 and the half-life of the ^{131}I-labelled 791T/36 within the tumour was 4 days.

The T : NT ratio for counts per minute per gram, on the other hand, bears no relationship to the interval between injection and resection of the tumour.

G. Development of Anti-mouse Antibody

In the four patients tested for the presence of anti-mouse antibodies, these were detected after the single injection of 791T/36 between 7 and 90 days after injection (Pimm *et al.*, 1983).

H. Site of Antibody Localization

Samples of tumour and normal tissue from seven resected colorectal cancers, after injection of ^{131}I-labelled 791T/36, were minced and forced through a 60-mesh grid (Snary *et al.*, 1976). It was found that in all seven the vast majority of the radioactivity (83.6%) was in the fibrous portion

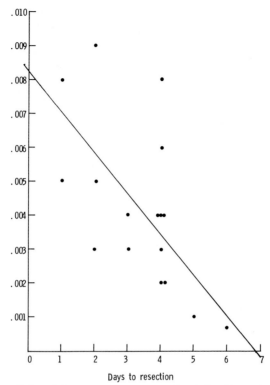

Fig. 6. Percentage of injected dose per gram tumour with relationship to days after injection.

of the tumour. Chromatography and antigen extraction showed that this antibody was in the form of complexes with a 72,000-MW protein (Price *et al.*, 1984), identical in terms of molecular weight to that found on the cell surface of 791T osteogenic sarcoma cells (Price *et al.*, 1983), and a cultured colon carcinoma cell line (Campbell *et al.*, 1984).

In addition, autoradiographs were made from tissue derived from freshly resected tumours of patients injected pre-operatively with ^{131}I-labelled 791T/36. These show that the silver grains are to be found within the lumina of the pseudoacini and stroma of the tumour rather than overlying the tumour cells (Armitage *et al.*, 1984) (Fig. 7).

This corresponds with the findings of immunohistology using 791T/36 on sections of colorectal cancer, where the antibody has been shown to bind to the gland contents of the tumour pseudoacini and in the tumour stroma (Armitage *et al.*, 1984).

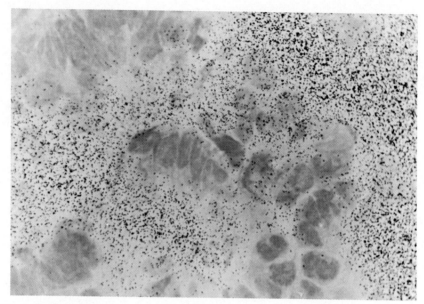

Fig. 7. Autoradiograph of a tumour from a patient injected with ^{131}I-labelled 791T/36 showing deposition of silver grains (antibody) in stroma and pseudoacini. (From Armitage *et al.*, 1984.)

VI. DISCUSSION

A. 791T/36

These studies have shown that the anti-tumour monoclonal antibody 791T/36 consistently localizes in colorectal cancer. This localization has allowed external imaging by γ camera of patients with colorectal cancers who were injected with radiolabelled antibody. Positive imaging was achieved in 8 of 11 (73%) patients with lesions outside the pelvis but in only 5 of 12 (42%) patients with intrapelvic lesions (rectosigmoid and rectal lesions). The lower detection rate of the latter group is due to the urinary excretion of ^{131}I with accumulation of radionuclide in the bladder. Even when the bladder was completely emptied prior to imaging, sufficient activity remained to mask effectively many intrapelvic lesions. The use of a different radionuclide such as ^{111}In, which is not excreted in the urine, may overcme this problem and has been used successfully by other workers (Fairweather *et al.*, 1984).

All 31 resected specimens of colorectal cancer showed positive local-ization of the tumour on γ-camera imaging with good congruity to the size and contours of the tumour.

This increased uptake in the tumour was clearly shown in the counting of the resected specimen samples. Only 1 of the 31 resected specimens had a T : NT tissue ratio of less than 1 : 1. Patient 30 had a huge, poorly differentiated cancer of the rectum, invading the bladder; whilst there was a positive specimen image due to the bulk of the tumour, the T : NT was 0.7 : 1 when samples were counted for radioactivity. For the re-mainder, however, there was consistent preferential localization of an-tibody in the tumour, with an overall mean T : NT ratio of 2.5 : 1 (range 0.7–5.8 : 1). Whilst with a specific antibody one might have expected a greater than two and one-half times uptake in tumour over normal colon, this ratio is of the same order of uptake as in other published series. Mach, using a paired label technique with a monoclonal anti-CEA an-tibody, found a mean T : NT ratio of 3.2 : 1 between colorectal tumour and normal mucosa (Mach *et al.*, 1981). The same team found a mean T : NT ratio of 1.7 : 1 between colorectal tumour and normal mucosa, but 4.3 : 1 between tumour and normal serosa using a specific anti-co-lorectal cancer monoclonal antibody 17-1A (Mach *et al.*, 1983).

The double labelling study, with a T : NT ratio of 3.3 : 1 for 791T/36 and 1.1 : 1 for NMI, indicates that the preferential uptake of 791T/36 is a specific antibody–antigen reaction. This was further investigated with the biochemical studies into the antibody–antigen complexes within the tumour. It was established that the injected 791T/36 was complexed with a 72,000-MW protein, this being identical in molecular weight to the791T/36-determined antigen on the cell surface of 791T osteogenic sarcoma cells (Price *et al.*, 1983).

Although there is preferential uptake of antibody in colorectal cancer, the absolute quantity of antibody localized is small. From specimens re-sected during the first 48 hr, only 0.0065% of the injected dose was pres-ent per gram of tumour. This represents a tissue level of 65 ng/g from an injected dose of 1 mg antibody.

The patients with disseminated colorectal cancer had good correlation between clinical/radiological and laparotomy findings and the result of immunoscintigraphy. The mean image T : NT ratios after subtraction is 4.3 : 1. This is very similar to the result in those patients with positive *in vivo* images of primary colorectal cancers, where the mean T : NT ratio after subtraction was 4.4 : 1. These T : NT ratios are somewhat higher than those for resected specimens. Quantitation of the tumour uptake of antibody from patient images is affected by the geometry of the source of activity and the detector. The T : NT ratio is measured from images of a concentration of activity in a tumour at a depth within a patient with overlying and underlying activity in the circulation, unlike those images of resected specimens. These data, however, imply that a similar preferential localization of antibody is occurring in metastases as in primary colorectal cancers.

As far as the benign lesions are concerned, none of the adenomas showed any significant uptake over normal colon. This is a little surprising, since two of the benign tumours were large villous adenomas which carry a high potential for malignant change. It may be that an increase in the 791T/36-defined antigen within tumour is associated with frank invasion rather than just neoplasia.

Of the non-colonic gastrointestinal malignant tumours studied, only 2 of the 13 showed sufficiently increased uptake in the tumour to give positive *in vivo* images. The rest were not identified by external imaging and, in the limited number of resected specimens—two stomach cancers and two small bowel tumours—no significantly increased uptake could be demonstrated in the tumour on counting of samples from these specimens.

B. 791T/36 Fab Fragments

It has been suggested from animal studies using human tumour xenografts that fragments of monoclonal antibody may be as good as, if not better than, intact antibody for localizing in tumours (Wahl *et al.*, 1983). The theoretical advantage is that antibody fragments are cleared rapidly from the circulation, thus allowing earlier imaging and giving greater contrast between tumour and background.

Using this approach, Mach used Fab fragments of 17-1A colorectal cancer-specific antibody and achieved successful localization in a higher percentage of patients than when intact antibody was used (Mach *et al.*, 1983).

The studies using Fab fragments of 791T/36 on the other hand, did not achieve specific tumour localization on external imaging in any of the patients studied. Analysis of the resected specimens showed increased uptake in tumour in one patient only (patient 69). In the other two patients there was no increased tumour uptake and the absolute counts per gram of tumour were low. It would seem, therefore, that for 791T/36 the monovalent Fab fragment offers little, either for imaging or targeting. The bivalent $F(ab)_2$ fragment may hold more promise and requires further research.

C. Antibody Kinetics

It can be seen that the clearance of 791T/36 is initially rapid during which time the circulating antibody is probably equilibrating with the extravascular compartment. Later there is a slower clearance with a half-life of approximately 2 days. As might be expected, Fab fragments of 791T/36 are more rapidly cleared.

In all the patients tested, a single dose of 791T/36 has resulted in significant production of anti-mouse antibodies. This is similar to the findings of Larson *et al.* (1982) and Miller *et al.* (1981). This anti-mouse antibody may limit furthr administration of monoclonal antibody in two ways. First, circulating anti-mouse antibody may form complexes with injected antibody rendering it ineffective; second, the anti-mouse antibody/monoclonal antibody complexes may produce allergic effects—this was encountered in one patient who developed a skin reaction to the subcutaneous test dose for a second scan.

VII. IMPROVEMENTS IN PATIENT IMAGING

Immunoscintigraphy presents problems both in the production of images and in the quantitation of the relative uptake of antibody within the tumour.

Whichever antibody is employed, the majority of the administered dose remains in the bloodstream, giving increased emission of radiation from the large blood vessels and from particularly vascular organs such as liver, spleen and heart. Since the emission from these 'hot' organs and vessels will obscure the emission from the tumour, it has been necessary to develop methods to overcome this. The most common of these is by computerized blood pool subtraction (DeLand *et al.*, 1980). This technique does, however, assume that the distribution of unbound radiolabelled antibody is identical to the distribution of the subtracting radionuclide. In addition, the differences in energies of the usual label ^{131}I and ^{99m}Tc may cause problems (Mach *et al.*, 1981; Perkins *et al.*, 1984).

Several manoeuvres are available to improve the quality of the patient images and achieve more reliable quantitation of the antibody uptake in the tumour. First, different radionuclides may be used as labels. ^{131}I has a number of disadvantages, which include a fairly long half-life of 8.0 days, high energy of γ emission (364 keV) which has a low efficiency of detection by the γ camera, β particle emission, urinary excretion and thyroid uptake even after blocking with potassium iodide. [123]I has a more suitable energy of γ emission (159 keV); however, its short half life (13 hr), limited availability and relative inefficiency of labelling mean that it is difficult to work with. Nevertheless, Epenetos *et al.* (1982) achieved successful patient imaging using this radionuclide. [99m]Tc also has a suitable energy of γ emission (140 keV) but its half-life of only 6 hr would not permit delayed imaging to allow for antibody accumulation in the tumour and clearance from the blood pool. [111]In, which has a half-life of 2.8 days, γ energies of 247 and 150 keV, lack of β particle emission and is not excreted in the urine, is presently considered the most suitable radionuclide to employ as a label. On the other hand, the labelling of antibodies with metals such as indium requires attachment via a chelating agent which is more difficult that iodination. A number of workers have used ^{111}In-labelled antibodies for imaging (Rainsbury *et al.*, 1983; Fairweather *et al.*, 1984). There is, however, intense hepatic uptake of radiolabelled antibody which will limit the use for imaging liver metastases. Another advantage of ^{111}In is that it is more suitable for emission tomography. Tomographic reconstruction gives the opportunity to visualise the distribution of radiolabelled antibody slice by slice. The emitted radiation by activity overlying or underlying a tumour would be reduced and may obviate the need for blood pool subtraction, thus more accurately reflecting tumour uptake. The technique has been applied to patient imaging, with some success, by Mach *et al.* (1981) and Berche *et al.* (1982). In the latter study, rectilinear scanning visualised 9 of 21 tumour sites whilst emission tomography identified 16 of 17 sites in the same patients using a monoclonal anti-CEA antibody.

Apart from changing the radiolabel, the injected antibody may be altered. The removal of the Fc portion of the antibody to leave the Fab or F(ab)$_2$ fragments should remove non-specific reactions of this portion of the antibody with Fc receptor-bearing cells. In addition, these antibody fragments are more rapidly cleared from the blood than intact antibody, thus giving greater contrast between the fragment fixed in the tumour and that in the circulation. Fab and F(ab)$_2$ fragments of monoclonal antibodies have been successfully used to image patients with colorectal cancer (Mach *et al.*, 1983) and malignant melanoma (Larson *et al.*, 1983).

A further means of achieving rapid clearance of circulating antibody is to follow the initial injection of radiolabelled antibody with an injection of further antibody directed against the first antibody. The second antibody 'mops up' the non-localized first antibody, thus ensuring its rapid removal. Begent *et al.* (1982) used this technique with liposomally-entrapped horse anti-goat immunoglobulin to remove circulating ^{131}I goat anti-CEA. The clearance of the radiolabel was increased and allowed visualisation of three of four gastrointestinal tumours.

Finally, the technique which may allow the most accurate quantiation of antibody localization may be a modification of the 'paired label' technique (Pressman *et al.*, 1957). Radioactive antibody and normal immunoglobulin are injected simultaneously, labelled with different radionuclides. The distribution of normal immunoglobulin in the circulation and non-specifically in the interstitial fluid will correspond exactly to that of active antibody, thus allowing accurate subtraction. Ballou *et al.* (1979) labelled active antibody with ^{131}I and normal immunoglobulin with ^{123}I to image experimental tumours successfully. Mach has used a paired label technique to demonstrate antibody localization in resected tumours, though not for external imaging (Mach *et al.*, 1981, 1983). With the development of ^{111}In- and ^{67}Ga-labelled antibodies, which are similar in characteristics, these two radionuclides may offer the possibility of using a paired label technique for patient imaging.

ACKNOWLEDGEMENTS

This work was supported by a grant from the Cancer Research Campaign. We are grateful to Mrs. C. Mangham for expert and willing secretarial assistance.

REFERENCES

Armitage, N. C., Perkins, A. C., Pimm, M. V., Farrands, P. A., Baldwin, R. W., and Hardcastle, J. D. (1984). *Br. J. Surg.* **71**, 407–412.

Baldwin, R. W., Pimm, M. V., Embleton, M. J., Armitage, N. C., Farrands, P. A., Hardcastle, J. D., and Perkins, A. C. (1984). *In* "Cancer Invasion and Metastasis, Biologic and Therapeutic Aspects" (G. L. Nicholson, and L. Milas, eds.), pp. 437–455. Raven Press, New York.

Ballou, B., Levine, G., Hakala, T., and Souter, D. (1979). *Science* **206**, 844–847.

Begent, R. H. J., Green, A. J., Bagshawe, K. D., Jones, B. E., Keep, P. A., Searle, F., Jewew, R. F., Barratt, G. M., and Ryman, B. E. (1982). *Lancet* **2**, 739–742.

Begent, R. H., Green, A. J., Searle, F., Keep, P. A., Bagshawe, K. D., Jones, B. E., and Jewkes, R. F. (1983). *Proc. Am. Assoc. Cancer Res.* **23**, 801 (abstr.).

Berche, C.,Mach, J. P., Lumbroso, J. D., Langlais, C., Aubry, F., Bucheggar, F., Carrel, S., Rougier, P., Parmentier, C., and Tubiana, M. (1982). *Br. Med. J.* **285**, 1447–1451.

Campbell, D. G., Price, M. R., and Baldwin, R. W. (1984). *Int. J. Cancer* **34**, 31–37.

DeLand, F. H., Kim, E. E., Simmons, G., and Goldenberg, D. M. (1980). *Cancer Res.* **40,** 3046–3049.

Dykes, P. W., Hine, K. R., Bradwell, A. R., Blackburn, J. C., Reeder, T. A., Drolc, Z., and Booth, S. N. (1980). *Br. Med. J.,* 220–222.

Embleton, M. J., Gunn, B., Byers, V. S., and Baldwin, R. W. (1981). *Br. J. Cancer* **43,** 582–587.

Epenetos, A. A., Mather, S., Granowska, M., Nimmon, C. C., Hawkins, L. R., Britton, K. E., Shepherd, J., Taylor-Papdimitrou, J., Durbin, H., Malpas, J. S., and Bodmer, W. T. (1982). *Lancet* **2,** 999–1004.

Fairweather, D. S., Bradwell, A. R., Chandler, S., Baggett, N., and Dykes, P. W. (1984). *Protides Biol. Fluids* **31,** 289–292.

Farrands, P. A., Perkins, A. C., Pimm, M. V., Embleton, M. J., Hardy, J., Baldwin, R. W., and Hardcastle, J. D. (1982). *Lancet* **2,** 397–400.

Finan, P. J., Grant, R. M., DeMattos, C., Takei, F., Berry, P. J., Lennox, E. S., and Bleehen, N. M. (1982). *Br. J. Cancer* **46,** 9–17.

Fraker, P. J., and Speck, J. C. (1978). *Biochem. Biophys. Res. Commun.* **80,** 849–857.

Gold, P., and Freedman, S. O. (1965). *J. Exp. Med.* **122,** 467.

Goldenberg, D. M., DeLand, F. H., Kim, E., Bennett, S., Primus, F. J., van Negell, J. R., Estes, N., DeSimone, P., and Rayburn, P. (1978). *N. Engl. J. Med.* **298,** 1384–1388.

Goldenberg, D. M., Kim, E., DeLand, F. H., Bennett, S., and Primus, J. (1980). *Cancer Res.* **40,** 2984–2992.

Herlyn, M., Steplewski, Z., Herlyn, D., and Koprowski, H. (1979). *Proc. Natl. Acad. Sci. U.S.A.* **76,** 1438–1442.

Kaplan, E., Ben-Porath, M., Fink, S., Clayton, G. D., and Jacobsen, B. (1966). *J. Nucl. Med.* **7,** 807–816.

Larson, S. M., Brown, J. P., Wright, P. W., Carrasquillo, J. A., Hellström, I., and Hellström, K. E. (1983). *J. Nucl. Med.* **24,** 123–129.

Mach, J. P., Buchegger, F., Forni, M., Ritschard, J., Berche, C., Lumbroso, J. D., Schreyer, M., Giradet, C., Accolla, R. S., and Carrel, S. (1981). *Immunol. Today* **2**(12), 239–249.

Mach, J. P., Chatal, J. F., Lumbroso, J. D., Buchegger, F., Forni, M., Ritschard, J., Berche, C., Douillard, J. Y., Carrel, S., Herlyn, M., Steplewski, Z., and Koprowski, H. (1983). *Cancer Res.* **43,** 5593–5600.

Miller, R. A., Maloney, D. G., McKillop, J., and Levy, R. (1981). *Blood* **58,** 78–86.

Pavel, D. G., Zimmer, A. M., and Patterson, V. N. (1977). *J. Nucl. Med.* **18,** 305–308.

Perkins, A. C., Whalley, D. C., and Hardy, J. G. (1984). *Nucl. Med. Commun.* **5,** 501–512.

Pimm, M. V., Armitage, N. C., Perkins, A. C., Hardcastle, J. D., and Baldwin, R. W. (1984). *Behring Inst. Mitt.* **74,** 80–86.

Pressman, D., and Keighley, G. (1948). *J. Immunol.* **59,** 141–146.

Pressman, D., Day, E. D., and Blau, M. (1957). *Cancer Res.* **17,** 845–850.

Price, M. R., Campbell, D. G., Robins, R. A., and Baldwin, R. W. (1983). *Eur. J. Cancer Clin. Oncol.* **19,** 81.

Price, M. R., Pimm, M. V., Page, C. M., Armitage, N. C., Hardcastle, J. D., and Baldwin, R. W. (1984). *Br. J. Cancer* **49,** 809–812.

Rainsbury, R. M., Westwood, J. H., Coombes, R. C., Neville, A. M., Ott, R. J., Kalirai, T. S., McCready, V. R., and Gazet, J. C. (1983). *Lancet* **2,** 934–938.

Smedley, H. M., Finan, P., Lennox, E. S., Ritson, A., Takei, F., Wraight, P., and Sikora, K. (1983). *Br. J. Cancer* **47,** 253–259.

Snary, D., Woods, F. R., and Crumpton, M. J. (1976). *Anal. Biochem.* **74,** 457.

Wahl, R. L., Parker, C. W., and Philpott, G. W. (1983). *J. Nucl. Med.* **24,** 316–325.

Wochner, R. D., Adoptepe, M., Van Amborg, A., and Potchen, E. J. (1970). *J. Lab. Clin. Med.* **75,** 711–720.

CHAPTER 8

Clinical Prospective Study with Radioiodinated Monoclonal Antibodies Directed against Colorectal Cancer

J. F. Chatal,*,† J. Y. Douillard,*,†
Jean Claude Saccavini,‡ M. Kremer,*,†
C. Curtet,*,† C. Maurel,* J. Aubry*
and B. Le Mevel*,†

*Unité 211 INSERM
Nantes, France
†Centre René Gauducheau
Nantes, France
‡Office des Rayonnements Ionisants
Gif-sur-Yvette, France

I. INTRODUCTION

After apparently total excision of a colorectal cancer, there is great likelihood of recurrence during the following 2 yr for stages B and C

MONOCLONAL ANTIBODIES FOR CANCER
DETECTION AND THERAPY

(Cass *et al.*, 1976; Hojo and Koyama, 1982; Rich *et al.*, 1983). The development of tumour markers, particularly of the carcinoembryonic antigen (CEA), has made it possible to detect recurrences before the appearance of clinical signs, so that second-look surgery was considered feasible. This procedure was determined by a significant elevation in serum CEA concentration. Encouraging results were obtained with this method since isolated recurrences were resected in a percentage of cases ranging between 7 and 72% (Ellis, 1975; Evans *et al.*, 1978; Minton and Martin, 1978; Welch and Donaldson, 1978; Steele *et al.*, 1980; Wanebo, 1981). Appreciable improvements in survival time were thus obtained. However, this approach had certain inconveniences occasioned by negative laparotomies or the discovery of benign lesions causing transient or non-specific elevations in serum CEA level (Rittgers *et al.*, 1978;). Moreover, in certain cases of recurrence, particularly local recurrences, serum CEA concentration rose only slightly or late, so that the tumours were inextirpable (Moertel *et al.*, 1978; Finlay and McArdle, 1983). A new marker associated with gastrointestinal carcinomas, the CA 19-9 antigen, has been isolated and seems to be complementary to CEA (Sears *et al.*, 1982). The follow-up of high-risk patients by serum assays involving both markers simultaneously may increase the percentage of early detection of recurrences. Yet, although such early biological detection is certainly of value, it does not allow localization which is very important to the surgeon. When a recurrence is suspected on the basis of the serum level of markers (CEA and CA 19-9), it must be visualized to provide grounds for a possible indication of surgery. Among the conventional diagnostic methods used, computed tomography and ultrasonography can help in diagnosing localization, but they lack specificity and have certain limits, especially in the exploration of the pelvis, a frequent site of recurrences (Baker and Way, 1978; Husband *et al.*, 1980; Lee *et al.*, 1981; Moss *et al.*, 1981; Kelvin *et al.*, 1983; Reznek *et al.*, 1983; Temple *et al.*, 1983). Immunoscintigraphy, introduced more recently (Dykes *et al.*, 1980; Kim *et al.*, 1980; Mach *et al.*, 1981), has the advantage of providing better specificity. The clinical results, obtained at first with radioiodinated polyclonal antibodies and then with monoclonal antibodies (Mach *et al.*, 1983; Baldwin *et al.*, 1983; Chatal *et al.*, 1984), have concerned mainly retrospective studies intended to define the diagnostic sensitivity of the method as a function of the nature of the antibody injected.

The present study concerns the diagnostic application of three monoclonal antibodies: an anti-CEA antibody designated as 202, kindly provided by Dr. J. P. Mach, Institut du Cancer, Lausanne, Switzerland; and

two monoclonal antibodies, designated as 17-1A and 19-9, which recognize different antigens associated with gastrointestinal carcinomas,
kindly provided by H. Koprowski, Wistar Institute, Philadelphia, Pennsylvania. The characteristics of these antibodies have been previously
reported (Koprowski *et al.*, 1979; Herlyn *et al.*, 1980; Magnani *et al.*, 1981;
Haskell *et al.*, 1983). After determination of the complementary specificity
of these antibodies by an immunohistochemical study, and of the scintigraphic detection parameters by a radiopharmacokinetic study in colic-
tumour-bearing nude mice, the purpose of the work was to define, on
the basis of a prospective study, the value of immunoscintigraphy in
comparison with conventional methods for localization of recurrences
of colorectal cancers.

II. IMMUNOHISTOCHEMICAL STUDIES

To determine the specificity of the anti-CEA and 19-9 antibodies, an
immunohistochemical study was performed using the immunoperoxidase technique in the avidin–biotin complex (Kremer *et al.*, 1983).

A. Primary Tumours

The frequency of CEA and CA 19-9 antigen expression was determined
in 122 cases of primary tumours. Out of 36 colorectal adenocarcinomas,
results were positive in 29 cases with the 19-9 antibody (81%) and in 34
cases with the anti-CEA antibody (94%). The two antibodies appeared
to be complementary as some tumours which were negative with the
19-9 antibody were positive with the anti-CEA antibody, and vice versa.

For the other gastrointestinal adenocarcinomas tested (pancreas,
stomach, biliary tract), the frequency of positivity was 100% (23 of 23)
with the 19-9 antibody and 78% (18 of 23) with the anti-CEA antibody.
For non-gastrointestinal adenocarcinomas (breast, parotid, ovary, bron-
choalveolar), results were positive in 38% of cases (24 of 63) with the
19-9 antibody and in 30% (19 of 63) with the anti-CEA antibody. The
staining was not very intense in these cases and concerned only a low
percentage of cells.

TABLE I

PATTERNS OF CEA AND CA 19-9 EXPRESSION IN PRIMARY COLORECTAL
CARCINOMA AND RECURRENCE[a]

	Primary tumour	Recurrence	Number
CEA	+ +	+ +	7
	+ +	+	3
	+ +	FR or −	2
CA 19-9	+ +	+ +	3
	+ +	+	3
	+ + or +	FR or −	4
	−	−	2

[a] + +, Strong staining and more than 50% stained cells; +, weak staining and less than 50% stained cells; FR, focal reaction (only a few groups of stained cells); −, no staining.

B. Primary Tumours and Recurrences

In 12 cases the immunohistochemical study was performed on the primary tumour and the recurrence (Table I) to determine whether the antigenic expression of the recurrence was the same as that of the primary tumour and would thus indicate the nature of the radiolabelled antibody to be injected to localize the recurrence.

With the anti-CEA antibody, the antigenic expression of the recurrence was positive in 7 cases and identical with that of the primary tumour. In 3 cases the staining of the recurrence was less positive than that of the primary tumour, and in 2 cases it was negative when that of the primary tumour was positive. In these last 2 cases the staining of the recurrence was positive with the 19-9 antibody.

With the 19-9 antibody results were positive at the same intensity in 3 cases for both the primary tumour and the recurrence. In 3 cases the staining of the recurrence was less intense than that of the primary tumour. In 4 cases it was negative when that of the primary tumour was positive. In the 2 remaining cases results were negative for both the primary tumour and the recurrence. In the 6 cases in which the recurrence did not express CA 19-9, staining was positive 3 times with anti-CEA.

Admittedly, these results concern a short series, yet they show that it is sometimes not possible to predict the antigenic expression of the recurrence searched for on the basis of that of the primary tumour, and that the expression of the two antigens would appear to be complementary. It is thus advisable to inject both radiolabelled antibodies systematically to increase the chances of covering the antigenic spectrum of the recurrence.

III. EXPERIMENTAL STUDIES

In order to define the parameters to be considered when using radiolabelled monoclonal antibodies for diagnosis of cancer patients, a pharmacokinetic study was carried out in nude mice engrafted with human tumours. The aim of this work was, first, to assess the conservation of the antibody immune function after labelling and to define the optimal specific activity and, second, to determine the biodistribution of the labelled antibody at the tumour site and in the normal tissues and blood of the human-tumour-bearing nude mice. Two monoclonal antibodies with specificity for human colorectal carcinoma were tested, including 19-9 and 17-1A antibodies. Intact immunoglobulins and F(ab')$_2$ fragments were used and compared. Three human tumours (two colorectal carcinomas and one melanoma) grown as cell lines were engrafted in nude mice by infusion of $1–2.10^7$ live cells subcutaneously in the flank.

A. Immunoreactivity

Iodination of the antibodies was performed comparatively using two conventional labelling methods. Chloramine T-mediated iodination was compared with the iodogen method. The labelled proteins were then purified in a Biogel 2 (Biorad) glass column chromatograph.

An *in vitro* binding assay to the cell lines mentioned previously was performed using 5.10^5 cells in 50 μl PBS incubated for 4 hr with the labelled monoclonal antibodies at the desired specific activity. Comparison of the chloramine T and iodogen methods relative to conservation of antibody immune function showed a clear advantage for the iodogen method which provides a higher binding percentage than the chloramine T method, probably because of its milder conditions.

The influence of the specific activity on monoclonal antibody reactivity was determined by using the same *in vitro* binding assay with varying specific activities ranging from 40 to 5 μCi/μg for intact immunoglobulin and from 40 to 1 μCi/μg for F(ab')$_2$ fragments. Optimum binding under the described experimental conditions occurred for a specific activity of 10 μCi/μg or less for intact antibody and 1 to 2 μCi/μg for F(ab')$_2$ fragments when using the iodogen method.

B. Biodistribution

Based on the results obtained *in vitro*, a biodistribution study was performed in tumour-bearing nude mice to determine the kinetics of uptake and clearance of the radiolabelled antibody at the tumour site and in normal tissues and blood (Douillard *et al.*, 1983). This experimental approach provided information about the accumulation of antibodies in tumour and tissues, the ratios between tumour and normal tissue antibody concentrations and the specificity of antibody binding by a paired labelling method.

Biodistribution was first studied with the 17-1A monoclonal antibody. Increasing values for binding were observed at the colorectal tumour site up to 5 days (12.3% injected dose/g) and remained stable at this level up to 9 days, the end point of the experiment. In blood, normal tissues and melanoma tumour, the kinetics were quite different, with an early maximum uptake between 2 and 24 hr and then decreasing values. The differences in antibody-binding kinetics to colorectal tumour and other tissues resulted in increasing tumour : blood (0.4–2.2) and tumour : organ ratios with the passage of time. The localization index as defined by Moshakis *et al.* (1981) and reflecting the specificity of binding, rose from 1.05 at 2 hr to 5.7 at 9 days, but never exceeded 1.1 during the experiment for all organs and melanoma tumours. A similar experiment conducted with 17-1A F(ab')$_2$ fragments gave a different kinetics, with early maximum uptake at 24 hr in tumours and normal tissues and values decreasing to very low percentages at 5 days. As noted for 17-1A intact antibodies, differential kinetics occurred at the colorectal tumour site and in normal tissues, blood or melanoma tumours, resulting in increasing colorectal carcinoma tumour : organ ratios, with higher values for F(ab')$_2$ fragments than for intact antibodies. The localization index was comparable for F(ab')$_2$ fragments and intact 17-1A antibodies.

The biodistribution of the 19-9 monoclonal antibody was analyzed under similar experimental conditions. Maximum uptake occurred at 24 hr at the colorectal tumour site (5.1%), the blood (5.4%) and all organs. Faster antibody clearance in normal tissues and melanoma resulted in increasing colorectal tumour : tissues ratios during the entire experimental course. The localization index confirmed the specificity of binding at the colorectal tumour site (4.1 at 9 days). Similar experiments were performed with $F(ab')_2$ fragments. Faster clearance in normal tissues and melanoma tumours led to high colorectal tumour : organ ratios (80 at 7 days for tumour:blood). Much lower uptake was observed in the spleen and liver than with intact antibody.

Based on the experimental results obtained in the animal, 4 to 5 days after infusion would appear to be the optimal time for scanning since antibody accumulation at the tumour site is still high enough to allow external detection, whereas non-specific binding to normal tissues and blood is low due to faster clearance, which leads to higher tumour : organ ratios that should provide better contrasted images. Moreover, $F(ab')_2$ fragments should be preferred to intact antibodies since they result in higher tumour : tissue ratios due to faster clearance and less non-specific binding to Fc receptor positive cells than in normal tissues.

These experimental data were further confirmed by scintigraphy (Fig.1). Colorectal tumour detection was possible 2 days after injection of ^{131}I 19-9 $F(ab')_2$ despite the low tumour : background ratio. Rescanning at day 5 provided a better contrasted image with no accumulation at the melanoma site.

IV. CLINICAL STUDIES

A. Retrospective Studies

Before comparing a new diagnostic technique with conventional methods, it is advisable to define its performances first, i.e., its sensitivity and specificity as based on retrospective studies. With radioiodinated anti-CEA antibodies, whether polyclonal or monoclonal, Mach et al. (1981) found a sensitivity of 50% as compared with the more optimistic value of 75% reported by Dykes et al. (1980), and especially that of 90% reported by Kim et al. (1980). For these works the scintiscans were recorded within the 3 days following injection, and interpretation of images was often subjected to the questionable procedure of computerized subtraction (Rankin and McVie, 1983).

With the 17-1A antibody, diagnostic sensitivity was 54% (Mach et al., 1983); with the 19-9 antibody, sensitivity was 66% (Chatal et al., 1984). In the latter study, the scintiscans were recorded more than 4 days following injection and without computerized subtraction. In addition, this study demonstrated the potential value of injecting a combination of two antibodies of different specificities in order to increase tumour de-

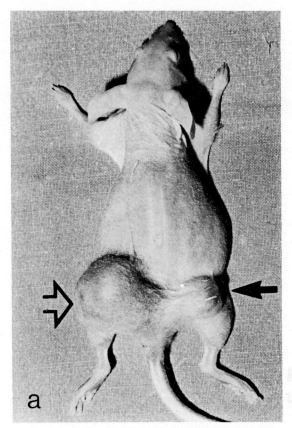

Fig. 1. Immunoscintigraphy of a human-tumour-bearing nude mouse. (a) Nude mouse bearing a colon carcinoma on right side (closed arrow) and a melanoma on left side (open arrow).

tection sensitivity. This association of antibodies is even of greater interest within the scope of a prospective study in which the antigenic expression of the tumour searched for is obviously unknown a priori.

B. Prospective Study

1. Patients

This study involved 25 patients who raised the problem of recurrence of a colorectal carcinoma (rectosigmoid, 20; descending colon, 3; caecum,

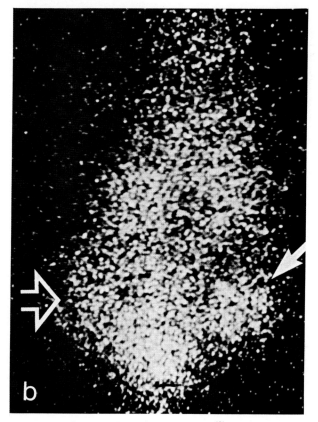

Fig. 1. (b) Immunoscan performed 2 days after injection of ^{131}I 19-9 F(ab')$_2$. Poorly contrasted colorectal tumour visualization.

1; transverse, 1). On the basis of Dukes' staging system, all the patients were initially at Stage B$_2$ (13 cases) or C (12 cases). The criteria suggestive of recurrence were clinical and/or biological. They were entirely clinical in 4 cases (pelvic pains in 2 cases, pelvic heaviness and oedema of the lower left member in 1 case, and associated fatigue and weight loss in 1 case). They were clinical and biological in 6 cases and entirely biological in 15 cases. The biological follow-up of the patients consisted in serial assays of CEA and CA 19-9 antigen. A recurrence was suspected when there was significant and persistent elevation of a least one of the two markers.

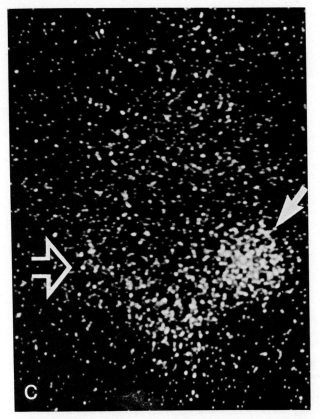

Fig. 1. (c) Immunoscan performed at 5 days. Well contrasted colorectal tumour uptake (closed arrow). No visualization of melanoma (open arrow).

2. Methodology

For the 25 patients, who all gave their informed consent, the first examination performed prospectively was immunoscintigraphy. First, thyroid uptake of ^{131}I was blocked by oral administration of Lugol's solution which was begun 3 days before injection and continued for 10 days. A combination of intact anti-CEA 202 antibodies and of $F(ab')_2$ fragments of antibody 19-9 were injected into 22 patients and a combination of $F(ab')_2$ fragments of antibodies 17-1A and 19-9 were injected into 3 patients. The antibodies, which were in equal proportions when combined, were labelled with ^{131}I using the iodogen method, with a specific activity of 5–10 $\mu Ci/\mu g$ for the intact antibody and 1–2 $\mu Ci/\mu g$ for the fragments. An activity ranging between 74 and 129.5 MBq (2–3.5 mCi) was diluted in 100 ml of saline solution and then injected slowly into each patient during a 10- to 15-min period. A total of 32 scintigraphic examinations were performed on the 25 patients, 7 of whom had repeated examinations at 1- to 2-month intervals. In 23 out of the 32 examinations, a single recording was performed on day 5. In 3 cases the recordings were repeated at days 3 and 6, and in 6 cases at days 5 and 7. The intention in these repeated recordings was to determine the specific or non-specific nature of a doubtful focus (Chatal *et al.*, 1984). Prior to each recording the patients received an injection of ^{99m}Tc in the form of albumin, sulfur colloid and diethylenetriamine pentaacetic acid (DTPA), to visualize the blood pool of the heart and great vessels, the liver, the kidneys and the bladder, and thus to facilitate anatomical localization of the foci imaged with ^{131}I. On average, four views were recorded: two inferior abdominal (anterior and lateral) and two liver (anterior and right lateral). Computerized subtraction was never used in the interpretation of the scintiscans and was only occasionally performed for iconographic reasons after the images had been interpreted. The results were noted as positive or negative, with doubtful images considered as negative results.

After scintigraphy, the diagnostic assessment involved ultrasonography for 19 patients and computed tomography for 18. The interval between scintigraphy and ultrasonography or computed tomography was never greater than 2 weeks.

Computed tomography and ultrasonography were performed routinely in several institutions. The only common feature was the use of a real-time scanning technique for ultrasonography and of third-generation scanners for computed tomography.

3. Results

A recurrence was confirmed in 16 patients. In 8 cases confirmation was the result of second-look surgery enabling localization of 10 tumour sites; in 7 others it resulted from the concordance of the results of immunoscintigraphy with those of ultrasonography and/or computed tomography. For the remaining patient, who had an oedema of the left leg, recurrence was confirmed 6 weeks after immunoscintigraphy by palpation of a mass on the left side corresponding to the previous scintigraphic image. A total of 18 recurrence sites were thus confirmed in 16 patients. In 6 of the other patients, the absence of recurrence was confirmed by surgery (1 patient) or as a result of negative follow-up over

TABLE II

RESULTS OF IMMUNOSCINTIGRAPHY IN 22 PATIENTS WITH A SUSPECTED RECURRENCE

Scan results	Documented recurrence[a]	No recurrence
Positive	13 (72%)	1
Negative	5	5
Total	18	6

[a]Number of tumour sites.

more than 6 months (5 patients). For the 3 remaining patients in this study, a recurrence was quite probable due to the persistent elevation of the serum concentration of both markers, but no diagnostic method has as yet permitted localization.

a. Results of Immunoscintigraphy (Table II). Immunoscintigraphy was positive in 13 out of 18 confirmed sites, or 72% of cases: 5 local pelvic

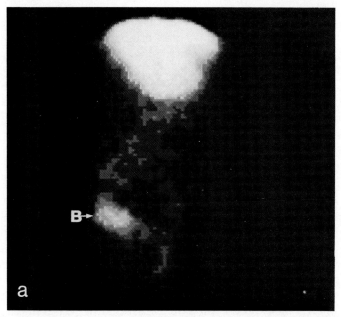

Fig. 2. Visualization of a local recurrence of a rectum carcinoma. Ultrasonography and CT examinations were interpreted as normal. Left lateral view of pelvis. (a) ^{99m}Tc Radioactivity due to ^{99m}Tc-labelled albumin and DTPA. Visualization of bladder (B); (b) ^{131}I Immunoscan showing a focus of abnormal radioactivity behind the bladder (indicated by the arrow). The outline of the bladder has been drawn according to the ^{99m}Tc image.

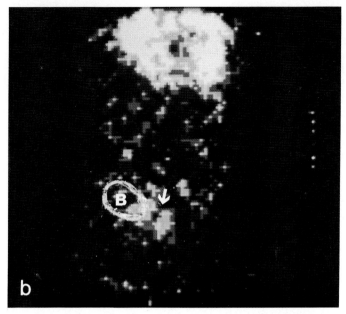

Fig. 2. *(Continued.)*

recurrences (Fig. 2), 4 liver metastases (Fig. 3) and 4 abdominal sites remote from the primary site. Three of the 5 negative cases corresponded to a diffuse pelvic carcinomatosis (accounting for the absence of a scintigraphic focus), a widespread, necrotic pelvic recurrence and small liver metastases approximately 2 cm in diameter. The 2 other negative cases related to a widespread involvement of the left lobe of the liver and to a single liver metastasis, 5 cm in diameter, located in the posterior part of the right lobe, which was surgically removed and in immunohistochemical study expressed CA 19-9 and mainly CEA. In the latter case, a single anterior view of the liver had been recorded, which may well account for the negative result (Fig. 4). For the 6 patients with no confirmed recurrence, scintigraphy was negative in 5 cases and positive in 1 case, that of a patient whose recurrence was searched for in the context of an isolated and persistent elevation of CEA level. At the third and sixth days after injection, scintigraphy showed a small, poorly contrasted spot which, with barium enema, corresponded exactly to the site of anastomosis (Fig. 5). Second-look surgery was performed on the basis of scintigraphic findings and despite normal colonoscopy and computed tomography. The surgeon did not find a tumour recurrence but an inflammatory process with perianastomotic micro-abscesses, which were

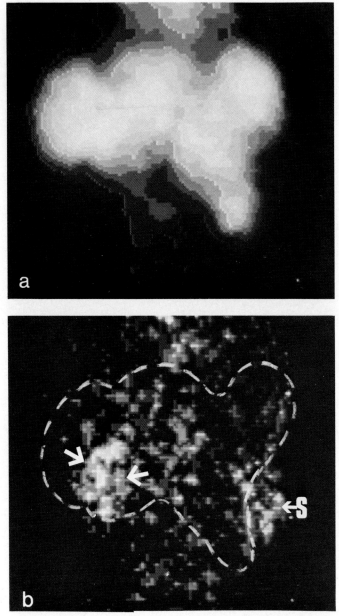

Fig. 3. Isolated liver metastasis of a left colon carcinoma. This patient had a resection of a liver metastasis of the right lobe 8 months before. Ultrasonography and CT examination were interpreted as normal. Anterior view of liver. (a) ^{99m}Tc Radioactivity due to ^{99m}Tc-labelled sulfur colloid. Relative hypertrophy of the left lobe due to previous and partial resection of the right lobe, but no obvious photon-deficient area; (b) ^{131}I Immunoscan showing a focus of abnormal radioactivity in the lower part of the right lobe (arrows). The outline of the liver has been drawn according to the ^{99m}Tc image. S = Radioactivity in stomach.

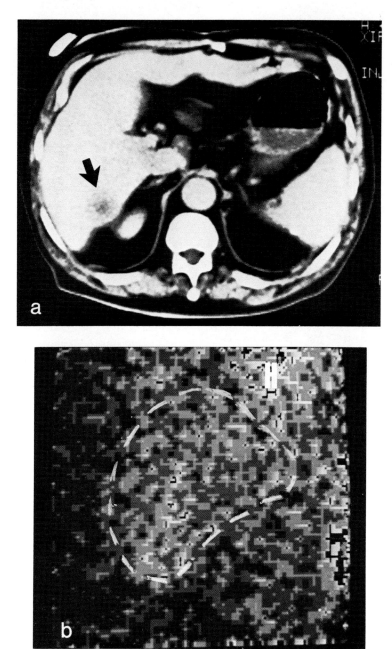

Fig. 4. Isolated liver metastasis of a sigmoid carcinoma. (a) Liver CT scan showing a low-density area in posterior part of right lobe (arrow); (b) anterior view of immunoscan. No abnormal focus. Diffuse and weak liver activity. H = Heart radioactivity.

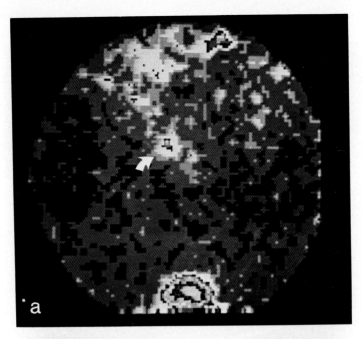

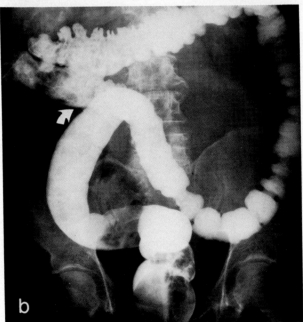

Fig. 5. Suspected recurrence of colon carcinoma due to a persistant elevation of CEA serum level. (a) [131]I Immunoscan. Abdominal anterior view. Small focus of abnormal radioactivity (indicated by the arrow) below the inferior margin of the liver; (b) barium enema showing that the focus of abnormal radioactivity corresponds to the site of anastomosis (arrow).

TABLE III

COMPARATIVE RESULTS OF IMMUNOSCINTIGRAPHY AND ULTRASONOGRAPHY IN DOCUMENTED RECURRENCES

Immunoscintigraphy[a]	Ultrasonography[a]		
	Positive	Negative	Total
Positive	3	5	8
Negative	3	2	5
Total	6	7	13

[a]Number of tumour sites.

removed. One month later another scintigraphic examination proved negative and the CEA level had become normal.

b. Comparative Results of Immunoscintigraphy and Ultrasonography (Table III). Ultrasonography was performed on 19 patients after immunoscintigraphy and when the result of the latter examination was unknown. There were 13 confirmed recurrence sites in 12 of these 19 patients. The results of both techniques were positive for 3 sites of liver metastasis and negative in the case of the small metastases, 2 cm in diameter, of the left lobe of the liver and in that of diffuse pelvic carcinomatosis. Ultrasonography was positive in 3 cases in which immunoscintigraphy had been negative: 2 cases of large liver metastases and 1 of a partially necrotic pelvic recurrence. Finally, ultrasonography was negative in 5 cases in which immunoscintigraphy had been positive: 2 cases of local pelvic recurrence (Fig. 2), 2 of abdominal recurrence remote from the primary site and 1 of liver metastasis (Fig. 3). In this last case, ultrasonography was disturbed by the presence of metal clips from a previous operation. Ultrasonography was negative for the 7 other patients, 4 of whom had no demonstrated recurrence and 3 a probable but not yet confirmed recurrence.

c. Comparative Results of Immunoscintigraphy and Computed Tomography (Table IV). Computed tomography was performed on 13 patients (14 tumour sites) with a demonstrated recurrence in the same conditions as for ultrasonography, i.e., after immunoscintigraphy and when the result of the latter examination was unknown. There was positive correlation of the two techniques for 3 patients, 2 of whom had an abdominal recurrence remote from the primary site and 1 local pelvic recurrence. The correlation was negative for 2 patients, 1 with a local pelvic recurrence and the other a diffuse pelvic carcinomatosis. In 2 cases, com-

TABLE IV

COMPARATIVE RESULTS OF IMMUNOSCINTIGRAPHY AND COMPUTED TOMOGRAPHY IN DOCUMENTED RECURRENCES

Immunoscintigraphy[a]	Computed tomography[a]		Total
	Positive	Negative	
Positive	3	7[b]	10
Negative	2	2	4
Total	5	9	14

[a]Number of tumour sites.
[b]Three out of seven (CT results) were interpreted as doubtful and considered as negative.

puted tomography corrected a false negative result of immunoscintigraphy: that of a widespread, partially necrotic pelvic recurrence and that of an isolated liver metastasis 5 cm in diameter (Fig. 4). Finally, computed tomography was negative or doubtful in 7 cases in which immunoscintigraphy had been positive (as for scintigraphy, a doubtful result of computed tomography was considered negative). The results were interpreted as normal in 1 case of local pelvic recurrence (Fig. 2), 1 case of left abdominal recurrence and 1 case of liver metastasis. The result was also considered normal in another case of liver metastasis, but the examination had been hampered by the presence of metal clips from a previous operation (Fig. 3). The results were interpreted as doubtful in 3 cases of local pelvic recurrence. Each of these 3 cases involved the problem of discriminating between a normal anatomical structure or a post operative fibrosis and a tumour recurrence. Such problems of interpretation have been reported and discussed by several authors. Some have proposed to solve them by applying morphological criteria of differentiation (Husband *et al.*, 1980; Lee *et al.*, 1981), whereas others insist on the necessity of repeating the examinations and of comparing changes in the images with reference to a baseline examination performed during the post-operative period (Kelvin *et al.*, 1983; Reznek *et al.*, 1983).

Finally, computed tomography was normal in 5 other patients: in 2 cases in which the patient's course confirmed the absence of recurrence, in 1 case in which surgery showed no recurrence (whereas scintigraphy had been positive) and in 2 of the 3 cases in which recurrence was considered very likely because of an elevation in marker levels, but not yet confirmed.

d. The Advantages of Immunoscintigraphy in Comparison with the Other Methods. The positive result of immunoscintigraphy was the determining factor in 4 cases in the decision to reoperate. For 3 of these patients the results of ultrasonography and computed tomography were negative or doubtful (1 case). For the fourth patient the result of computed tomography was doubtful and that of the pelvic ultrasonographic examination was technically impossible to interpret. Surgery confirmed recurrence in these 4 patients and excision was apparently total in 3 cases: 2 local pelvic recurrences (Fig. 2) and 1 isolated liver metastasis (Fig. 3). In the remaining case, a pelvic recurrence was associated with small liver metastases, 2 cm in diameter, which were not visualized by any of the methods.

Two other studies have demonstrated the prospective value of immunoscintigraphy. Goldenberg *et al.* (1983) have reported 11 cases in which immunoscintigraphy localized recurrence whereas the results of other methods were negative; however, the other methods included computed tomography and/or ultrasonography for only 5 patients. Begent *et al.* (1981) have reported 9 positive immunoscintigraphic results in 10 patients with an isolated rise in CEA level. Recurrence was confirmed in only 4 patients (once by surgery).

In comparison with ultrasonography and computed tomography, which are methods with a morphological approach, immunoscintigraphy has the advantage of being more specific. A rather well-contrasted scintigraphic focus is highly suggestive of recurrence. As noted previously, on the basis of cases in this study or in the literature, there may be difficulty with ultrasonography or computed tomography in relating an abnormal or doubtful image to a recurrence or to a non-specific structure. The differential diagnosis must then be based on criteria of changes during repeated examinations, which may delay the diagnosis. When a recurrence is suspected because of a rise in the level of one or more antigens associated with tumours, it would seem logical first of all to try to confirm the recurrence by injecting the radiolabelled antibody(s) specifically recognizing the antigen(s).

e. Present Limitations of Immunoscintigraphy. Immunoscintigraphy has different sorts of limitation. First of all, it has immunological limitations due to an absence of close oncological specificity in the antibodies used. It is for this reason that in one case a perianastomotic focus suggested a tumour recurrence (Fig. 5), whereas in fact only a non-specific inflammatory reaction was involved. Immunoscintigraphy also has limitations related to the method of detection. In one case it was negative for a posteriorly located single liver metastasis which in immunoperoxidase study after excision expressed both CEA and CA 19-9 antigens. However, a single anterior view was recorded for this patient (Fig. 4), and it is possible that the metastasis would have been visualized by additional posterior and lateral views.

Immunoscintigraphy, in which positive results are indicated by radioactive uptake areas contrasting with adjacent background, is also limited in cases of diffuse recurrence without clearly defined foci, such as that of diffuse pelvic carcinomatosis in the present study. It is possible that the 3 patients who had a persistent elevation in marker levels but no recurrence as yet demonstrated correspond to this situation of diffuse peritoneal carcinosis, which would account for the negative results of immunoscintigraphy, ultrasonography and computed tomography. The strict follow-up of these patients will determine whether this hypothesis is confirmed or not.

Rockoff *et al.* (1980) demonstrated the limitations of conventional planar scintigraphy by calling attention on the one hand to the ratios between the size and depth of the tumour to be detected, and on the other to its scintigraphic contrast as expressed by the tumour : background ratio. An effort must thus be made to improve the methodological performances.

4. Future Prospects

The application of single photon emission computed tomography should contribute to the improvement of diagnostic sensitivity (Chatal, 1983). Mach *et al.* (1983) already confirmed this tendency by visualizing 13 out of 14 tumours tested, but interpretation was hindered by the existence of many non-specific foci. It will be necessary to overcome these inconveniences by recording images as late as possible after injection of the radiolabelled antibody or antibodies, while maintaining satisfactory count levels and injecting the greatest quantity of radioactive substance compatible with an acceptable radiation dose for the patient. [131]I must also be replaced by a radionuclide better adapted to scintigraphic detection. [123]I may be a good substitute, though it has too short a half-life, in view of the pharmacokinetic characteristics (Epenetos *et al.*, 1982). [111]In is also well adapted to scintigraphic detection and can label an antibody conjugated with a bifunctional agent such as DTPA without altering immunoreactivity (Halpern *et al.*, 1983). However, its clinical application is limited because the high liver and colon activity greatly hinders image interpretation (J. F. Chatal, unpublished personal data).

V. CONCLUSION

The first clinical applications of immunoscintigraphy in the diagnosis of colorectal cancers are of relatively recent date. As the results of retrospective studies obtained with anti-CEA antibodies were conflicting and raised questions as to the clinical value of this new diagnostic method, it proved important to integrate immunoscintigraphy into a prospective study comparing its results with those of the most effective conventional methods such as ultrasonography and computed tomography. This was the purpose of the present study. In view of the results, it may be concluded with due caution that immunoscintigraphy is of real clinical value and that in diagnostic strategy its role is complementary to that of the other methods.

ACKNOWLEDGEMENTS

The authors thank Marie-Antoinette de Cussé for her precious secretarial assistance in preparing this manuscript.

REFERENCES

Baker, C., and Way, L. W. (1978). *Am. J. Surg.* **136**, 37–44.

Baldwin, R. W., Embleton, M. J., and Pimm, M. V. (1983). *Bull. Cancer* **70**, 132–136.

Begent, R. H. J., Keep, P. A., Searle, F., Dent, J., Bagshawe, K. D., Jones, B. E., Jewkes, R. F., and Vernon, P. (1981). *Oncodev. Biol. Med.* **2**, 61.

Cass, A. W., Million, R. R., and Pfaff, W. W. (1976). *Cancer* **37**, 2861–2865.

Chatal, J. F. (1983). *Nouv. Presse Med.* **12**, 2361–2363.

Chatal, J. F., Saccavini, J. C., Fumoleau, P., Douillard J. Y., Curtet, C., Kremer, M., Le Mevel, B., and Koprowski, H. (1984). *J. Nucl. Med.* **25**, 307–314.

Douillard, J. Y., Chatal, J. F., and Saccavini, J. C. (1983). *Bull. Cancer* **70**, 169–171.

Dykes, P. W., Hine, K. R., Bradwell, A. R., Blackburn, J. C., Reeder, T. A., Droll, Z., and Booth, S. N. (1980). *Br. Med. J.* **28**, 220–222.

Ellis, H. (1975). *Br. J. Surg.* **62**, 830–832.

Epenetos, A. A., Mather, S., Granowska, M., Nimmon, C. C., Hawkins, L. R., Britton, K. E., Shepherd, J., Taylor-Papadimitriou, J., Durbin, H., and Malpas, J. S. (1982). *Lancet* **6**, 999–1004.

Evans, J. T., Mittleman, A., Chu, M., and Holyoke, E. D. (1978). *Cancer* **42**, 1419–1422.

Finlay, I. G., and McArdle, C. S. (1983). *Br. Med. J.* **286**, 1242–1244.

Goldenberg, D. M., Kim, E. E., Bennett, S. J., Nelson, M. O., and Deland, F. H. (1983). *Gastroenterology* **84**, 524–532.

Halpern, S. E., Hagen, P. L., Gawer, P. R., Koziol, J. A., Chen, A. W. N., Frincke, J. M., Bartholomew, R. M., David, G. S., and Adams, T. H. (1983). *Cancer Res.* **43**, 5347–5355.

Haskell, L. M., Buchegger, F., Schreyer, M., Carrel, S., and Mach, J. P. (1983). *Cancer Res.* **43**, 3857–3862.

Herlyn, D. M., Steplewski, Z., Herlyn, M. F., and Koprowski, H. (1980). *Cancer Res.* **40**, 717–721.

Hojo, K., and Koyama, Y. (1982). *Am. J. Surg.* **143**, 293–295.

Husband, J. E., Hodson, N. J., and Parsons, C. A. (1980). *Radiology* **134**, 677–682.

Kelvin, F. M., Korobkin, M., Heaston, D. K., Grant, J. P., and Akwari, O. (1983). *AJR, Am. J., Roentgenol.* **141**, 959–964.

Kim, E. E., DeLand, F. H., Casper, S., Corgan, R. L., Primus, F. J., and Goldenberg, D. M. (1980). *Cancer* **45**, 1243–1247.

Koprowski, H., Steplewski, Z., Mitchell, K., Herlyn, M., Herlyn, D., and Fuhrer, P. (1979). *Somatic Cell Genet.* **5**, 957–972.

Kremer, M., Curtet, C., Douillard, J. Y., and Chatal, J. F. (1983). *Bull. Cancer* **70**, 172–173.

Lee, J. K. T., Stanley, R. J., Sagel, S. S., Levitt, R. G., and McClennan, B. L. (1981). *Radiology* **141**, 737–741.

Mach, J. P., Buchegger, F., Forni, M., Ritschard, J., Berche, C., Lumbroso, J. D., Schreyer, M., Girardet, C., Accolla, R. S., and Carrel, S. (1981). *Immunol. Today* **2**, 239–249.

Mach, J. P., Chatal, J. F., Lumbroso, J. D., Buchegger, F., Forni, M., Ritschard, J., Berche, C., Douillard, J. Y., Carrel, S., Herlyn, M., Steplewski, Z., and Koprowski, H. (1983). *Cancer Res.* **43**, 5593–5600.

Magnani, J. L., Brockhaus, M., Smith, D. F., Ginsburg, V., Blaszczyk, M., Mitchell, K. F., Steplewski, Z., and Koprowski, H. (1981). *Science* **212**, 55–56.

Minton, J. P., and Martin, E. W. (1978). *Cancer* **42**, 1422–1427.

Moertel, L. G., Schutt, A. J., and Go, V. L. W. (1978). *JAMA, J. Am. Med. Assoc.* **239**, 1065–1066.

Moshakis, V., McIlhinney, R. A. J., Raghavan, D., and Neville, A. M. (1981). *Br. J. Cancer* **44**, 91–99.

Moss, A. A., Thoeni, R. F., Schnyder, P., and Margulis, A. R. (1981). *J. Comput. Assist. Tomogr.* **5**, 870–874.

Rankin, E. M., and McVie, J. G. (1983). *Br. Med. J.* **287**, 1402–1404.

Reznek, R. H., White, F. E., Young, J. W. R., Kelsey, I., and Nicholis, R. J. (1983). *Br. J. Radiol.* **56**, 237–240.

Rich, T., Gunderson, L. L., Lew, R., Galdibini, J. J., Cohen, A. M., and Donaldson, G. (1983). *Cancer* **52**, 1317–1329.

Rittgers, R. A., Steele, G., Zamcheck, N., Loewenstein, M. S., Sugarbaker, P. H., Mayer, R. J., Lokich, J. J., Mattz, J., and Wilson, R. E. (1978). *JNCI, J. Natl. Cancer. Inst.* **61**, 315–318.

Rockoff, S. D., Goodenough, D. J., and McIntire, K. R. (19800. *Cancer Res.* **40**, 3054–3058.

Sears, H. F., Herlyn, M., Del Villano, B., Steplewski, Z., and Koprowski, H. (1982). *J. Clin. Immunol.* **2**, 141–149.

Steele, G., Zamcheck, N., Wilson, R. E., Mayer, R., Lokich, J., Rao, P., and Mattz, J. (1980). *Am. J. Surg.* **139**, 544–548.

Temple, D. F., Parthasarathy, K. L., Bakshi, S. P., and Mittelman, A. E. (1983). *Surg., Gynecol. Obstet.* **156**, 205–208.

Wanebo, H. J. (1981). *Surgery (St. Louis)* **89**, 290–295.

Welch, J. P., and Donaldson, G. A. (1978). *Am. J. Surg.* **135**, 505–511.

CHAPTER 9

Clinical Applications of Radioimmunolocalisation

R. H. J. Begent and K. D. Bagshawe

Cancer Research Campaign Laboratories
Department of Medical Oncology
Charing Cross Hospital
London, United Kingdom

I. INTRODUCTION

Localization of tumours by external scintigraphy after intravenous administration of radiolabelled antibody directed against a tumour-associated antigen [radioimmunolocalisation (RIL)] might be expected to solve many of the problems of conventional tumour imaging. Although no truly specific tumour antigen is known, there are many tumour-associated antigens which are present in much higher concentrations in certain tumours than in tissues which are normal or affected by other diseases. This feature has the potential to endow RIL with a degree of

MONOCLONAL ANTIBODIES FOR CANCER
DETECTION AND THERAPY

specificity not exhibited by imaging methods such as computerised tomography (CT), ultrasound (US) or nuclear magnetic resonance (NMR) which reflect the physical characteristics of tissues.

The clinical application of new imaging methods depends partly on their comparative performance in terms of sensitivity and specificity and also on ways in which the unique features of each can be exploited to optimize the management of individual patients. There are significant deficiencies with all the existing imaging methods; this chapter discusses the extent to which RIL may fill some of the gaps. Particular attention will be paid to situations where the result has consequences for patient management. Much of the work cited was carried out in experimental systems and on more than 300 patients at Charing Cross Hospital between 1979 and 1984.

II. FACTORS AFFECTING SPECIFICITY AND SENSITIVITY OF RIL

The model provided by human tumours grown as xenografts in immune-deprived animals or at immunoprivileged sites in immunologically normal animals gives some insight into the problems. Specificity depends on localisation of a (specific) anti-tumour antibody by comparison with a non-specific one (Pressman, 1957). A high specificity ratio implies a high value for the ratio of specific antibody in tumour to that in normal tissues divided by the ratio of non-specific antibody in tumour to that in normal tissues. This establishes a basic concept of specificity but does not give the complete picture. It is also necessary to examine the total amount of specific antibody per unit weight of tumour tissue as it is important for a strong signal to be obtained from the tumour by external scintigraphy. The tumour-to-blood or normal tissue ratio for the specific antibody is also important as this will give an indication of the degree of discrimination between tumour and background which can be expected.

Autoradiography on excised tumours makes it possible to define the microscopic site of localisation of antibody administered *in vivo* (Lewis *et al.*, 1982). Some antibodies such as those directed against structural antigens of the cell membrane localise principally on the cell membrane. Others such as those directed against secreted antigens are found largely in extracellular tissue spaces within the tumour. It is not obvious that this difference influences the imaging characteristics of an antibody in the clinical studies which we have performed.

The dwell-time for antibody retained by tumour in comparison with other tissues is also of particular importance. Studies with xenografts show that specific antibody is retained in tumour for longer than non-specific antibody and that the rate of clearance of a specific antibody from tumour is slower than that from blood or other normal tissues (Searle *et al.*, 1981; Goldenberg *et al.*, 1981). The effect of this is to increase the specificity ratio with time after administration of antibody and to increase the tumour : blood ratio with time. Counts per gram of tumour, however, steadily diminish.

The proportion of administered antibody which localises in the tumour is very small. This is not surprising when it is considered that specific localisaton probably depends on passive diffusion of antibody out of the vascular compartment and into the proximity of a concentration of tumour antigen. It appears that the proportion is greater in xenograft systems, being commonly in the region of 2%, whereas 0.1% appears to be a good result in man (Mach *et al.*, 1980). The effect of this problem on tumour imaging is twofold. First, the background radioactivity in normal tissues readily obscures small tumours and, second, the total number of counts in the tumour is very low. These unfavourable circumstances for tumour imaging are further increased by the problem of isotopic decay. In spite of these disadvantages, large tumours which are readily palpable or detectable by simple radiology can sometimes be imaged simply by external scintigraphy particularly if they are away from areas with high physiological blood flow. Imaging of nearly all smaller tumours calls for some attempt to reduce the effect of background radioactivity in normal tissues. There are a number of ways of doing this.

III. REDUCTION OF BACKGROUND RADIOACTIVITY

A. Late Imaging

The longer the time interval between injection of antibody and imaging, the greater will be the tumour concentration relative to background. Therefore, imaging several days after administration of antibody is attractive. This has not proved popular for a number of reasons.

First, the absolute count rate in the tumour declines with time and if it was low initially, levels may become too low for imaging with contemporary γ cameras. This problem is greatest with short half-life radionuclides such as ^{123}I (half-life 13 hr) but is less of a problem with ^{111}In (half-life 2.8 days). ^{131}I with a half-life of 8 days is best from this point of view. This does not, however, make ^{131}I the automatic choice because the lower energies of emission of ^{123}I and ^{111}In mean that they are more efficiently imaged by γ cameras.

B. Subtraction

The fact that clinically useful tumour images were not obtained until Goldenberg *et al.* (1978) introduced the subtraction method establishes their technique as the standard against which others should be judged. The empirical finding that injection of ^{99m}Tc and labelled human serum albumin and ^{99m}TcO$_4$ gives an image of normal tissues similar to that of ^{131}I-labelled antibody given 24 hr previously is generally valid. After equalisation of counts between the ^{99m}Tc and ^{131}I, images and subtraction of the ^{99m}Tc image from that of ^{131}I, localisation of antibody in tumour is shown by residual activity in areas where ^{131}I antibody was relatively more concentrated than ^{99m}Tc subtraction medium. The method has been used to show the presence of tumour when conventional radiology has been negative (Begent *et al.*, 1980; Begent and Bagshawe, 1983; Goldenberg *et al.*, 1983; Halsall *et al.*, 1981; van Nagell *et al.*, 1980). The method suffers from a number of disadvantages as follows.

1. Different Energies of ^{131}I and ^{99m}Tc

It is necessary that radionuclides of different energies be used in a subtraction procedure so that they can be distinguished by the γ camera. The higher energy radionuclide (^{131}I) gives a slightly larger image than ^{99m}Tc. This tends to produce haloes around the outside of the body and of organs in which radioactivity is present in the highest concentrations. The heart and liver are the most striking of these (for review, see Begent and Bagshawe, 1983).

2. Different Distribution of Antibody and Subtraction Medium in Different Organs

When inspecting images generated by the subtraction technique, it is important to see that the distribution of the two radionuclides is similar in organs which would be expected to be normal. Frequently, the dis-

TABLE I

ARTEFACTS ASSOCIATED WITH SUBTRACTION

Site of artefact	Putative explanation
Thyroid	Uptake of iodide in spite of blocking
Cardiac	Different distribution of ^{131}I and ^{99m}Tc in the circulation
Right and inferior cardiac borders	'Halo effect' due to different energies of ^{131}I and ^{99m}Tc in the circulation
Inferior hepatic border	'Halo effect' due to different energies of ^{131}I and ^{99m}Tc
Hepatic (diffuse)	Immune complex deposition
Stomach	Uptake of iodine in the mucosa
Renal and bladder	Different distribution of ^{131}I and ^{99m}Tc in the urinary tract
Right colon	Excretion of iodide in the gut
Compensatory (possible at many different sites)	Excess of ^{99m}Tc over ^{131}I in one area giving non-specific excess of ^{131}I over Tc in another

tribution is very similar but if, for instance, there is a greater concentration of ^{99m}Tc than ^{131}I in the circulation, subtraction will give apparently negative amounts of radioactivity in the heart and major vessels and relatively positive appearances in other organs. Thus, these organs would appear misleadingly positive. Other organs in which discrepancies due to different handling of the two media occur include the thyroid gland, where some free iodide is taken up in spite of blocking of the thyroid; the stomach where free iodide or ^{99m}Tc may accumulate; the urinary tract in which either isotope may be predominantly excreted at the time of imaging; and the gastrointestinal tract into which some free iodide is probably secreted. In our experience the latter is most commonly seen in the region of the caecum or ascending colon. Views on subsequent days sometimes show this to have moved around the colon. Administration of potassium perchlorate can diminish uptake of iodide in the stomach but does not appear to have any effect on other parts of the bowel. The artefacts produced in these various ways are listed in Table I. Unilateral hydronephrosis is particularly prone to lead to misinterpretation due to retention of iodide in the dilated renal pelvis. A feature of these artefacts is that they frequently produce very impressive positive results with higher count rates than those found when antibody localises specifically in tumours. Ironically this sometimes gives a clue to their nature. One should not be too surprised by this observation when considering the very small percentage of administered antibody which localises specifically in tumours.

It is arguable that the subtraction method can also give false negative results by non-specific localisation of ^{99m}Tc-labelled human serum albumin in tumours. This hypothesis is supported by animal experiments to determine specificity of antibody localisation which show that there is some tendency for proteins to localise non-specifically in tumours. Also, radiolabelled albumin has a tendency to localise in tumours (Bauer et al., 1955). In the subtraction method, human serum albumin is given only a few minutes before imaging and it is possible that false negative results are generated by subtraction of this non-specific accumulation from the image produced by specific retention of antibody.

False negative images with tumours of more than 2 cm may also result from limited antigen expression within the tumour, from poor tumour vasculature or from binding of antibody to circulating antigen to form immune complexes. In the limited number of patients we have studied, such immune complexes stay in the circulation, having a half-life similar to that of monomeric IgG (Begent and Bagshawe, 1983). This is probably not always the case, however, since diffuse liver images are obtained occasionally in the absence of tumour in that organ. This is consistent with accumulation of immune complexes in the Kuppfer cells of the liver.

3. Tumour Images Obtained by Subtraction

Provided that the considerations described previously are taken into account, the subtraction method can provide data of relevance to the management of patients with cancer. Goldenberg et al. first reported this in 1978, using radiolabelled polyclonal antibody directed against carcinoembryonic antigen (CEA). Images were obtained with carcinomas of the colon, rectum, uterine cervix, ovary and other organs. The method was soon applied to a wider range of CEA-producing tumours and to other well-characterised tumour antigens such as human chorionic gonadotrophin (HCG) (Begent et al., 1980; Goldenberg et al., 1980a; Searle et al., 1984) and α-fetoprotein (AFP) (Goldenberg et al., 1980b; Halsall et al., 1981).

4. Interpretation of Results

As described previously, the amount of radioactivity bound specifically by the tumour will be very low in relation to the total dose given. This is a problem in statistical manipulation of data. The administered dose is limited by safety requirements to about 2 mCi of [131]I. The specific count rates in tumours are so low that those remaining after subtraction may not be amenable to useful statistical manipulation. Not surprisingly, subjective interpretation of such data is hazardous when trying to locate a small tumour in order to make an important decision about a patient's management. Objective assessments of the results are therefore highly desirable. The raw data from ^{131}I and ^{99m}Tc images are the most suitable for statistical manipulation and the method we have developed depends on this approach (Green *et al.*, 1984).

Images are created by subtracting pixel by pixel a percentage of the ^{99m}Tc images from those of ^{131}I until total counts are equalised. The subtracted images are assessed visually and areas which appear positive are defined as regions of interest (ROI). These are outlined and the number of counts of ^{131}I and ^{99m}Tc in the ROI are measured. For comparison, similar areas within the same organ or tissue, which do not appear positive, are also selected. These are designated ROI 1 and ROI 2 respectively. The ratio of ^{131}I in ROI 1 to that in ROI 2 is calculated and known as RI. Similarly the ratio for ^{99}Tc^m (RT) in these two areas is calculated. If a result is positive, RI will be higher than RT. The factor *Fx* is derived as follows:

$$Fx = \frac{RI - RT}{Ex}$$

where *Ex* is the sum of the standard deviations of RI and RT.

Thus, if no tumour is found, an *Fx* value of zero would be expected and one standard deviation away from this would give an *Fx* value of 1. Figure 1 shows the results of such an analysis of patients with colorectal cancer with raised serum CEA but no palpable tumour. It can be seen that those areas with tumour give higher *Fx* values than those without and that there is some overlap. In practice it has been found that *Fx* values in excess of +4 give a 93% chance of true positivity in patients with subclinical recurrence of colorectal cancer using antibody to CEA. *Fx* values between +2 and +4 are an indication for further investigation at the site concerned. This numerical analysis gives a basis for interpretation of results in a way that is useful in clinical decision making and also in comparison of different antibodies or imaging techniques. It may also be used with other radionuclides such as ^{111}In-labelled antibody and ^{99m}Tc subtraction medium.

C. Acceleration of Clearance of Background

This may be achieved in a variety of ways which are potentially of great interest because they avoid many of the artefacts associated with subtraction.

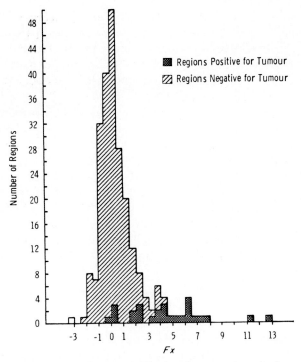

Fig. 1. *Fx* values in patients after apparently complete resection of colorectal cancer who had a raised serum CEA but no palpable tumour recurrence. High values are seen in many of those subsequently found to have tumour at the site concerned but false negatives occur. An *Fx* value of 4 gives a useful point for discrimination between positive and negative for the purposes of clinical decision making.

1. Second Antibodies

Non-tumour-bound antibody can be actively removed from the circulation and tissue spaces using a second antibody directed against the anti-tumour (first) antibody. The immune complex thus formed is cleared from the circulation by the reticuloendothelial system either directly or through clearance of a liposome to which the second antibody is attached before administration.

It was shown by Keep *et al.* (1983) that antibody could be cleared from the circulation of animals bearing xenografts of human colorectal carcinoma by liposome-entrapped second antibody (LESA) without a corresponding removal of antibody from the tumour. Improved tumour imaging was achieved with LESA directed against goat antibody to CEA in patients with gastrointestinal cancer (Begent *et al.*, 1982). It was suggested by Bradwell et al. (1983) that second antibody without the liposome would achieve the same result. Comparative experiments were performed at Charing Cross Hospital which showed that with one antibody–antigen system in mice that there was no improvement in efficiency using LESA but that either method gave an eightfold improvement in tumour : blood ratio of radioactivity. Satsifactory tumour images have been obtained in man with second antibody alone with some monoclonal anti-tumour antibodies but, in our experience, the method has failed to produce clearance with others of the same species and subclass. Possible reasons for this have been discussed (Begent et al,, 1983a). Although results are preliminary, tumour imaging in patients appears more satisfactory with second antibody, either liposome entrapped or not, than with the subtraction method. An example of the improvement achieved with LESA in man is given in Fig. 2.

2. Immunoglobulin Fragments

The use of F(ab)$_2$ fragments of immunoglobulin G antibodies has been suggested as a means of improving images. They will not be taken up non-specifically by Fc receptors in normal tissues. It has been shown by Buchegger et al. (1983) and Herlyn et al. (1983) that superior tumour : blood ratios are achieved with F(ab)$_2$ fragments than with intact immunoglobulin in animals. Imaging data, although not quantitative, support this hypothesis but the advantage is less striking than in the animal studies (Mach et al., 1983; Larson et al., 1983).

3. ^{111}Indium

When this radionuclide is chelated to an antibody (Buckley and Searle, 1984), it is cleared from the circulation more rapidly than iodine-labelled antibodies being taken up preferentially in the liver (Rainsbury et al., 1983; Fairweather et al., 1983). The mechanism of this uptake which persists for several days is not clear but it does have the effect of reducing background. Also it appears that the linkage of indium to antibody is relatively stable so that the proportion of administered radionuclide persisting in the tumour is higher. The result of these two factors is an enhanced tumour : blood ratios which has to be offset against the accumulation of the radionuclide in the liver. The importance of the latter will depend on the clinical circumstances but since so many tumours metastasize to the liver it is likely to be a considerable problem for staging of patients or for selecting those for resection of drug-resistant disease on the assumption that tumour is localised exclusively in some other

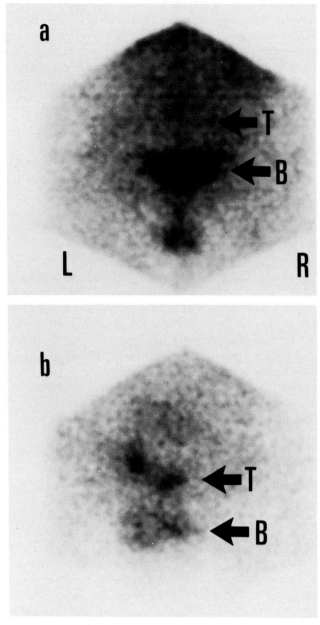

Fig. 2. Images of the pelvis with the patient sitting above the γ camera (a) immediately before LESA; (b) 24 hr after LESA. B = Bladder containing free ^{131}I; some free ^{131}I is seen below this in the urethra. T = Tumour behind the bladder. (From Begent *et al.*, 1982.)

site. When subtraction studies are done using ^{99m}Tc as the subtraction medium, high Fx values are achieved and it seems likely that improved sensitivity in tumour detection will be achieved.

IV. MEANS OF INCREASING RADIOACTIVITY PER GRAM OF TUMOUR

Provided that antigen in the tumour mass is not saturated with diagnostic doses of antibody, increasing the amount of antibody given should increase radioactivity per gram of tumour. This topic has not been much explored because the total dose of radiation which can be given is limited by doses acceptable for safety in a diagnostic procedure (Begent, 1984). This need not prevent administration of increased amounts of antibody for therapy (Pimm and Baldwin, 1984). The main hope of achieving better results in imaging, however, is with antibodies which are more efficiently localised in tumour. Antibodies can be compared in terms of affinity constant or of the proportion localising in each gram of tumour in animal tumour models. The most promising antibodies can then be compared in imaging studies. The Fx system for analysis of results (Green *et al.*, 1984) enables this to be done in a quantitative way; an example of comparison of the monoclonal and polyclonal antibodies directed against CEA is shown in Fig. 3. In this example there is little difference between the two antibodies investigated. No striking differences have been seen, in our experience, between antibodies which have performed in a comparable way in animal tumour models. If saturation of tumour-associated antigen is achieved with some antibodies then a combination of antibodies may be beneficial. Experience to date, however, does not suggest that saturation occurs in the context of imaging. Combinations of monoclonal antibodies may have other advantages (see below).

Relevance of Specificity Ratios in Clinical Imaging

Monoclonal antibodies with specificity for a single epitope are in a sense more specific than conventional antisera which contain antibodies with specificities for a number of different epitopes on the same antigen. There is, however, no reason why a single monoclonal antibody should give better results in RIL than a polyclonal antibody. Indeed, some mon-

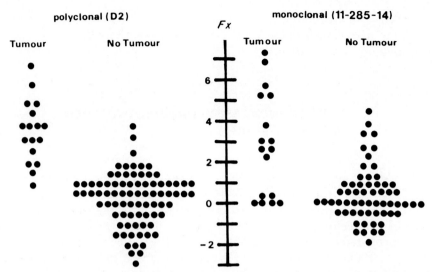

Fig. 3. *Fx* values in patients with recurrent or metastatic colorectal cancer obtained with two different antibodies directed against CEA. High positive values are more frequent in sites of known tumour. There is little apparent difference between the affinity-purified goat polyclonal antibody (D2) and the monoclonal (11-285-14) which originated from Dr. C. H. Ford and was kindly donated by Eli Lilly and Co.

oclonal antibodies which first appeared specific for a particular antigen have been shown to have cross-reacting sites on molecules in which conventional serology has failed to demonstrate homology. This appears to be because the same amino acid sequence or pattern of glycosylation occurs on sites other than the tumour antigen. The conventional polyclonal antibody can overcome this problem by having several different clones of antibody reacting with different or overlapping epitopes on the molecule. Any cross reactions which these antibodies have with otherwise unrelated molecules are thus diluted out (for review, see Lane and Koprowski, 1982). Theoretically, this objection can be overcome by using a mixture of monoclonal antibodies directed against different epitopes.

Monoclonal antibodies which would react with different epitopes on the same molecule are now being generated in quite large numbers. It seems only a matter of time before favourable combinations can be characterised or possibly even selected for individual patients on the basis of reactivity of a panel of antibodies with the patient's tumour in tissue sections.

V. CLINICAL APPLICATIONS OF RIL

The value of an investigation in clinical practice depends on its ability to provide information not available by other means, to do so at significantly lower cost or with less disturbance to the patient. Radioimmunolocalisation must be compared with CT, US and NMR. It will take several years to make good comparisons and since the competing investigations are simultaneously being improved, any superiority of RIL may soon be challenged. It should be remembered that there are now more methods of investigation relevant to a particular disease process than it is economically practical to apply and that each test applies cumulative emotional stress to the patient.

A. Spatial Resolution

Radioimmunolocalisation has been widely reported to locate tumours of 2 cm or above (Goldenberg et al., 1980c) but lesions of 0.5 cm have been located (Begent et al., 1980). The concentration of radioactivity in a tumour and its relationship to background will affect sensitivity as discussed previously. These factors will depend on accessibility and concentration of antigen in the tumour as well as the characteristics of the antibody. It follows that below a certain size the dimensions of a tumour are unlikely to bear a direct relationship to the ability of RIL to detect it even if it is known to express the relevant antigen. On the other hand, CT, US and NMR do have relatively well-defined limits of sensitivity in particular tissues. For example, CT can locate tumours of 2–3 mm in diameter in the lungs but may not show a much larger tumour lying between loops of bowel, particularly if the tumour is diffuse as is common in ovarian carcinoma. The abdomen, therefore, is a site where RIL may compare well with other methods in terms of spatial resolution and as the method improves it may compete more successfully in the thorax and brain.

B. Biochemical Information

The ability to locate the site of production of a tumour-associated antigen is a unique feature of RIL and theoretically enables it to discriminate between viable and necrotic masses of tumour or between tumour and masses of other pathogenesis. However, such distinctions are so important in clinical practice that biopsy or excision and histological examination are likely to remain the usual practice. The sensitivity of careful histological examination is unlikely to be matched by RIL; however, the latter sometimes finds a place where, for various reasons, biopsy or excision of a suspected tumour is not appropriate.

Nuclear magnetic resonance spectroscopy (Evanochko *et al.*, 1983; Ross *et al.*, 1984) is a competing, non-invasive method of obtaining biochemical information about tumours. Whether these data for metabolism of phosphorus or other substances will discriminate between tumours and other tissues remains to be seen.

C. Anatomical Assessments

While CT, US or NMR show the tumour and normal structures around it, this is not true of RIL. Bone scanning and colloid isotope liver scanning have been used simultaneously with RIL to try to resolve the problem but the approach is complicated and rather limited in application. It should be noted that a small tumour with a high count rate will appear larger than it really is by RIL. Therefore, other investigations are likely to be preferable to RIL if the purpose of imaging is to determine the local extent or dimensions of a known tumour for staging, planning of surgery or monitoring the course of disease.

D. A Unique Role for RIL

A major strength of RIL is that it gives both localising and biochemical information. This combination can be used to advantage when a tumour is known to produce a serum tumour marker which can also be a target for RIL. Where the serum tumour marker can predict clinically evident relapse, location of the recurrent tumour becomes urgent in case it can be resected or successfully treated at an early stage by other means. Radioimmunolocalisation with antibody directed against the serum tumour marker concerned is the logical investigation for this task and has been found valuable in colorectal cancer, gestational choriocarcinoma and anaplastic germ cell tumours of the ovary and testis.

1. Colorectal Cancer

A rise in serum CEA after apparently curative resection of cancer of the colon or rectum frequently predicts clinically evident relapse by several months (N. I. H. Consensus Statement, 1981; Tate, 1982). Radioimmunolocalisation with antibody to CEA was performed in 31 patients in the Charing Cross Hospital series who had raised serum CEA but no physical signs of recurrence. Using the Fx method for analysis of results and excluding false positive sites, it was evident that an Fx of 4 gave good discrimination between positive and negative when sites of known artefacts were excluded (Fig. 1). Tumour was later confirmed by surgery or conventional imaging methods such as CT or US in 93% of the sites giving Fx values greater than 4. A negative result was less useful, 47% of patients having false negative RIL (Begent et al., 1985). The most frequent sites of recurrence were in the liver and pelvis. Eight patients were consider for resection of tumour. Three had tumour resected, one was a metachronous carcinoma (see Fig. 4), one a benign polyp and one a recurrence in the laparotomy scar. Four patients were found to have unresectable tumour at laparotomy but one achieved a complete response after chemotherapy and radiotherapy and remains apparently tumour-free 2 yr after finishing treatment. One patient was considered unfit for surgery because of chronic obstructive airways disease. In four patients, CT of the abdomen failed to show tumour at sites where it was correctly identified by RIL.

In the context of early recurrence of colorectal cancer, RIL was sometimes able to provide unique information. It was capable of locating tumours in the lumen of the bowel, on peritoneal surfaces and in the liver and other viscera. This repertoire is beyond the scope of any other single investigation and there is no doubt that some patients have enjoyed prolonged disease-free survival as a result of the information provided.

The numerical values given by the Fx method provide an important means for determining whether a result is sufficiently positive for decisions about a patient's management to be based on it. This well-defined clinical situation provides an opportunity for comparison of different antibodies and imaging technologies.

2. Gestational Choriocarcinoma

A small proportion of the young women who develop this tumour still die of drug-resistant disease. Location of deposits of tumour confined to sites from which they can be surgically resected can sometimes lead

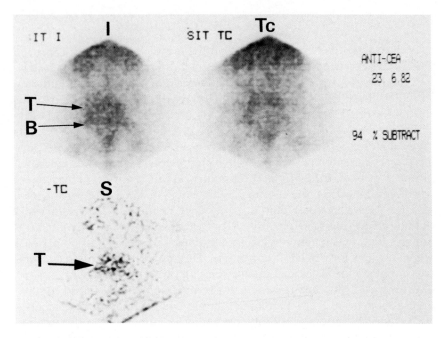

Fig. 4. Radioimmunolocalisation showing a metachronous tumour in the sigmoid colon. Views with the patient sitting above the γ camera showing distribution of (I) [131]I antibody; (Tc) ^{99m}Tc subtraction medium; (S) residual activity behind the bladder after subtraction. Fx was 6.4; B = bladder; T = tumour deposit.

to a cure when this cannot be achieved with drugs alone. Serum human chorionic gonadotrophin levels are a very sensitive marker of the progress of such tumours; rising values whilst a patient is receiving chemotherapy can give a clear indication of drug resistance before enlarging masses are detectable by the most sensitive imaging methods. (Begent *et al.*, 1980; Begent and Bagshawe, 1983). Radioimmunolocalisation with antibody directed against HCG can identify the sites of disease in these patients though positive results are rarely achieved with serum HCG below 50 IU/litre. In some, the tumour is too disseminated for resection but in six patients at Charing Cross Hospital tumours located by RIL have been resected and this has contributed to the achievement of sustained complete remission. An example is shown in Fig. 5.

3. Anaplastic Germ Cell Tumours

These tumours may contain malignant or differentiated tissues originating from any of the three germ cell layers. Their components are

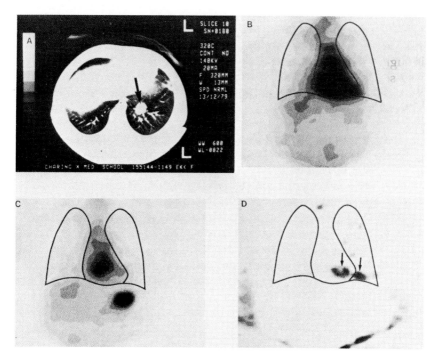

Fig. 5. Computerised tomography and RIL of pulmonary tumour in a patient with cho-riocarcinoma. (A) CT of the lower thorax showing an opacity in the left lower lobe (arrowed). (B) [131]I γ-camera image of anterior chest and upper abdomen after administration of ^{131}I anti-HCG. The radionuclide is concentrated principally in the heart. (C) [99m]Tc γ-Camera image of anterior chest and upper abdomen. The radionuclide is concentrated principally in the heart and stomach. (D) Image produced by computer subtraction of C and B. The increased uptake in the left lower zone suggests the presence of two deposits of chorio-carcinoma (arrowed). At thoracotomy, two deposits were found and removed, the smaller being 5 mm in diameter. (From Begent *et al.*, 1980.)

often mixed and numerous different tumour-associated antigens may be expressed in the same tumour. Therefore, RIL with one antibody is unlikely to give complete information about the status of a tumour. Images of HCG- and AFP-producing germ cell tumours have been obtained (Begent *et al.*, 1980, 1983b; Javadpour *et al.*, 1981; Halsall *et al.*, 1981; Goldenberg *et al.*, 1980a) and there are examples in which drug-resistant deposits of these germ cell tumours have been localised and successfully resected as a result.

The presence of drug-resistant tumours can be predicted by raised values of AFP or HCG and RIL with the appropriate antibody performed.

There are instances in which tumours located in this way have been successfully resected at Charing Cross Hospital and other institutions (Javadpour et al., 1981).

E. Patients without Raised Serum Tumour Markers

There are many malignancies in which relapse is common but there is no good serum tumour marker system. In these diseases RIL can be used to monitor patients who are potentially at risk of recurrence, although the yield may be lower than that achieved when there is a rise in a serum tumour marker. Nevertheless we have used RIL to locate recurrence of colorectal cancer in two patients with no increase in serum CEA. In both cases the recurrence was completely resected.

It is likely that other applications of RIL will emerge in which the result influences management. These may include staging and monitoring of the course of disease. Also, if antibody-directed therapy of cancer becomes effective, RIL will be useful in confirming that the antibody does bind to the tumour in vivo before therapy is undertaken.

VI. CONCLUSION

Radioimmunolocalisation can give information about human malignancy which is not obtainable by the best conventional methods. In some instances this has been used to provide prolonged tumour-free survival. There are many technological advances to be made with the method and it is likely that its performance will improve. Imaging methods which demonstrate high concentrations of antibody in tumour relative to normal tissue establish the principle necessary for successful antibody-directed therapy of cancer. This may ultimately be the most important consequence of RIL.

ACKNOWLEDGEMENTS

We are indebted to our colleagues in the Cancer Research Campaign Laboratories at Charing Cross Hospital Medical School whose work made this review possible. We are also grateful to all those in the several other departments at Charing Cross Hospital who have helped in these studies.

This work was supported by the Cancer Research Campaign and the Medical Research Council.

REFERENCES

Bauer, F. K., Tubis, M., and Thomas, H. B. (1955). *Proc. Soc. Exp. Biol. Med.* **90,** 140–142.

Begent, R. H. J. (1984). *Immunol. Today* **5** (4), 98.

Begent, R. H. J., and Bagshawe, K. D. (1983). *In* "Oncodevelopmental Markers" (W. H. Fishman, ed.), pp. 167–188. Academic Press, New York.

Begent, R. H. J., Stanway, G., Jones, B. E., Bagshawe, K. D., Searle, F., Jewkes, R. F., and Vernon, P. (1980). *J. R. Soc. Med.* **73,** 624–630.

Begent, R. H. J., Keep, P. A., Green, A. J., Searle, F., Bagshawe, K. D., Jewkes, R. F., Jones, B. E., Barratt, G. M., and Ryman, B. E. (1982). *Lancet* **2,** 739–742.

Begent, R. H. J., Green, A. J., Keep, P. A., Bagshawe, K. D., Searle, F., Jones, B. E., Jewkes, R. F., Ryman, B. E., and Barrett, G. M. (1983a). *Lancet* **1,** 1047–1048 (letter).

Begent, R. H. J., Boultbee, J., Jewkes, R., Katz, D., and McIvor, J. (1983b). *Clin. Oncol.* **2** (1), 117–157.

Begent, R. H. J., Keep, P. A., Searle, F., Green, A. J., Mitchell, H. D. C., Jones, B. E., Dent, J., Pendower, J. E. H., Poskins, R. A., Reynolds, K. W., Cooke, T. G., Allen-Mensch, T., and Bagshawe, K. D. (1985). *Br. J. Surg.* (in press).

Bradwell, A. R., Vaughan, A., Fairweather, D. S., and Dykes, P. W. (1983). *Lancet* **1,** 247 (letter).

Buchegger, F., Haskell, C. M., Schreyer, M., Bianca, R., Scazziga, R., Randin, S., Carrel, S., and Mach, J. P. (1983). *J. Exp. Med.* **158,** 413–427.

Buckley, R. G., and Searle, F. (1984). *FEBS Lett.* **166,** 202–204.

Evanochko, W. T., No, T. C., Lilly, M. B., Lawson, A. J., Corbett, T. B., Durant, J. R., and Glickson, J. D. (1983). *Proc. Natl. Acad. Sci. U.S.A.* **50,** 1–5.

Fairweather, D. S., Bradwell, A. R., Dykes, P. W., Vaughan, A. T., Watson-James, S. F., and Chandler, S. (1983). *Br. Med. J.* **287,** 167–170.

Goldenberg, D. M., DeLand, F. H., Kim, E. E., Bennett, S., Primus, F. J., van Nagell, J. R., Estes, N., DeSimone, P., and Rayburn, P. (1978). *N. Engl. J. Med.* **298,** 1384–1388.

Goldenberg, D. M., Kim, E. E., DeLand, F. H., van Nagell, J. R., and Javadpour, N. (1980a). *Science* **208,** 1284–1286.

Goldenberg, D. M., Kim, E. E., DeLand, F. H., Spremulli, E., Nelson, M. O., Gockerman, J. P., Primus, F. J., Corgan, R. L., and Alpert, E. (1980b). *Cancer* **45,** 2500–2505.

Goldenberg, D. M., Kim, E. E., DeLand, F. H., Bennett, S., and Primus, F. J. (1980c). *Cancer Res.* **40,** 2984–2992.

Goldenberg, D. M., Gaffar, S. A., Bennett, S. J., and Beach, J. L. (1981). *Cancer Res.* **41,** 4354–4360.

Goldenberg, D. M., Kim, E. E., Bennett, S. J., Nelson, M. O., and DeLand, F. H. (1983). *Gastroenterology* **84,** 524–532.

Green, A. J., Begent, R. H. J., Keep, P. A., and Bagshawe, K. D. (1984). *J. Nucl. Med.* **25,** 96–100.

Halsall, A. K., Fairweather, D. S., Bradwell, A. R., Blackburn, J. C., Dykes, P. W., Howell, A., Reeder, A., and Hine, K. R. (1981). *Br. Med. J.* **283**, 942–944.

Herlyn, D., Powe, J., Alavi, A., Mattis, J. A., Herlyn, M., Ernst, C., Vaum, R., and Koprowski, H. (1983). *Cancer Res.* **43**, 2731–2735.

Javadpour, N., Kim, E. E., DeLand, F. H., Salyer, J. R., Shah, U., and Goldenberg, D. M. (1981). *JAMA, J. Am. Med. Assoc.* **246**, 45–49.

Keep, P. A., Searle, F., Begent, R. H. J., Barratt, G. M., Boden, J., Bagshawe, K. D., and Ryman, B. E. (1983). *Oncodev. Biol. Med.* **4**, 273–280.

Lane, D., and Koprowski, H. (1982). *Nature (London)* **296**, 200–202.

Larson, S. M., Brown, J. P., Wright, P. W., Carrasquillo, A., Hellström, I., and Hellström, K. E. (1983). *J. Nucl. Med.* **24**, 123–129.

Lewis, J. C. M., Bagshawe, K. D., and Keep, P. A. (1982). *Oncodev. Biol. Med.* **3**, 161–168.

Mach, J. P., Carrel, S., Forni, M., Ritschard, J., Donath, A., and Alberto, P. (1980). *N. Engl. J. Med.* **303**, 5–10.

Mach, J. P., Chatal, J. F., Lumbroso, J. D., Buchegger, F., Forni, M., Ritschard, J., Berche, C., Douillard, J. Y., Carrel, S., Herlyn, M., Steplewski, Z., and Koprowski, H. (1983). *Cancer Res.* **43**, 5593–5600.

N.I.H. Consensus Statement (1981). *Br. Med. J.* **282**, 373–375.

Pimm, M. V., and Baldwin, R. W. (1984). *Eur. J. Cancer Clin. Oncol.* **20**, 515–524.

Pressman, D. (1957). *Ann. N. Y. Acad. Sci.* **69**, 644–650.

Rainsbury, R. M., Ott, R. J., Westwood, J. H., Coombes, R. C., Neville, A. M., Ott, R. J., Kalirai, T. S., McCready, V. R., and Gazet, J.-C. (1983). *Lancet* **2**, 934–938.

Ross, B., Marshall, V., Smith, M., Bartlett, S., and Freeman, D. (1984). *Lancet* **1**, 641–646.

Searle, F., Boden, J., Lewis, J. C. M., and Bagshawe, K. D. (1981). *Br. J. Cancer* **44**, 137–144.

Searle, F., Partridge, C. S., Kardana, A., Green, A. J., Buckley, R. G., Begent, R. H. J., and Rawlins, G. A. (1984). *Int. J. Cancer* **33**, 429–434.

Tate, H. (1982). *Br. J. Cancer* **46**, 323–330.

van Nagell, J. R., Kim, E. E., Casper, S., Primus, F. J., Bennett, D., DeLand, F. H., and Goldenberg, D. M. (1980). *Cancer Res.* **40**, 502–506.

CHAPTER 10

Localisation of Cancer of the Ovary and Metastases Using ^{123}I-labelled Monoclonal Antibody HMFG-2 Compared to Surgical Findings

K. E. Britton,* M. Granowska* and J. Shepherd*,†

*Department of Nuclear Medicine
† Department of Gynaecological Surgery
St. Bartholomew's Hospital
London, United Kingdom

Ovarian cancer is the second most common cause of death due to cancer in women. It often presents late and then requires radical surgery and repeated courses of chemotherapy. Because the deposits are often in the form of peritoneal seedlings or matted to bowel or omentum, the use of ultrasound and X-ray computed tomography is not very successful in staging or in judging response to chemotherapy or recurrence. Therefore a 'second-look' or even 'third-look' operation with, if necessary, further debulking surgery is performed. The clinical requirements are for, first, an imaging technique that would diagnose whether or not any pelvic mass is due to ovarian cancer before surgery; and second, an imaging technique that would help to demonstrate the distribution of metastases and their response to chemotherapy and their recurrence or not,

201

so as to avoid the need for the 'second-look' operation. This chapter summarises the use of radioimmunoscintigraphy in this context.

I. ANTIBODY

The monoclonal antibody HMFG-2 is an epithelial-specific, tumour-associated antibody. The hybridoma-producing HMFG-2 was derived from the fusion of the mouse myeloma cell line NSI with the spleen cells of a mouse which had received an initial injection of human milk fat globule (HMFG) followed by a boost with cultured normal milk epithelial cells (Taylor-Papadimitriou *et al.*, 1981). By immunoperoxidase staining of formalin-fixed, paraffin-embedded sections, the spectrum of reactivity of the antibody has been determined (Arklie *et al.*, 1981). It reacts with primary and metastatic breast tumour, ovarian cancer and colonic cancer and weakly with some normal epithelial cells.

HMFG-2 reacts with an antigenic determinant carried on a high molecular weight (>300K) glycoprotein (Burchell *et al.*, 1983) found in the HMFG. This component has been shown to consist of at least 50% carbohydrate (Shimizu and Yamauchi, 1982) and seems to be a mucin-like molecule with a high serine, threonine and proline content and O-linked sugars. The site recognised by HMFG-2 is present in only low numbers on the extracellular mucin-like molecule excreted by the lactating (and other secretory) epithelial cells, but it is present in higher numbers in the cell membrane of many tumours, particularly those of breast and ovarian origin (Burchell *et al.*, 1983; Taylor-Papadimitriou *et al.*, 1983). This is perhaps not unexpected in view of the fact that the mouse which provided the spleen for the fusion producing HMFG-2 was injected both with a product of the differentiated cell (the milk fat globule) and with a growing mammary epithelial cell. The binding of HMGF-2 to HMFG can be inhibited by peanut agglutinin, wheat germ agglutinin and Limumus polyhemus, lectins that are specific for Galβ1—3GalNAc, $\beta(1\rightarrow4)$ GlcNAc and sialic acid, respectively. These results indicate that the antigen is carbohydrate in nature. The antibody is of the IGg1 class.

II. THE RADIONUCLIDE LABEL

In order to demonstrate the localisation of the antibody *in vivo*, an appropriate radioactive label is required. The choice of label depends on the physical properties of available radionuclides and their suitability for labelling antibodies.

^{131}I has the disadvantage of producing β rays which give 80% of the radiation due to this radionuclide. The long half-life of 8 days means also that only a relatively small amount of activity can be given since the radiation dose is related to the product of the activity given and the half-life. The high γ-ray energy of 364 keV penetrates the thin crystal of the modern γ camera so the efficiency of count collection is poor. However, the ready availability, low expense and ease of labelling with ^{131}I commend it as the label with which new studies are undertaken.

^{123}I has a γ-ray energy ideal for the γ camera (159 keV) and short half-life of 13.2 hr which allows a count rate to be obtained which is about 100 times that obtained with ^{131}I for the same administered activity. Its availability, however, is limited, usually once weekly, and in lower activity than ^{131}I, it is also costly. For labelling, added carrier stable iodine is necessary to push the reaction to completion; thus synthesis of the labelled antibody is a little more difficult than with ^{131}I.

The labelling of antibody with iodine has been a standard procedure for decades since ^{125}I- labelled antibody is the cornerstone of the *in vitro* radioimmunoassay procedures for the measurement of hormones, etc. The chloramine T and iodogen techniques are the most frequently used, the latter being the milder of the two methods. The essential requirement is to label the antibody at a site away from the active centre so as not to affect its immunospecificity. To this end a 1 : 1 iodine to antibody molar ratio is recommended.

The use of iodine-labelled antibody has some disadvantages. The patient requires loading with stable iodine usually in the form of potassium iodide 60 mg b.d. from the day before and for 3 days after the study for ^{123}I and for 2 weeks after ^{131}I. The *in vivo* metabolism of iodine-labelled antibody is relatively rapid and about 20% free iodine is liberated in 24 hr. However, it is evident from animal studies that the iodine label attached to antibody bound to tumour does not come off and it is the unbound labelled antibody that is metabolised. Thus, it does matter whether the iodine is bound or free in blood or tissues other than the cancer; it all contributes to the background 'noise' against which the signal from the cancer target is to be determined.

^{111}In has an excellent γ-ray energy for the γ camera (171 keV) but its abundance of γ rays is considerably less than ^{123}I and the presence of a second γ-ray energy of 267 keV means that a medium-energy collimator which has reduced resolution has to be used. Its longer half-life of 67 hr has the potential commercial advantage that there would be time for a manufacturer to label, undertake quality control, package and distribute ready labelled antibody to centres undertaking radioimmunoscintigraphy. The labelling procedure is more complex and requires the use of bifunctional chelate, one end of which binds the indium and the other binds the protein. The cyclic anhydride of diethylenetriamine pentaacetic acid (DTPA) is a satisfactory chelate for this purpose. ^{111}In-labelled antibody is less rapidly metabolised in the body, circa 5% per 24 hr, than radioiodine-labelled antibody. However, a higher than expected liver uptake of the ^{111}In-labelled antibody may be seen, giving an absorbed radiation dose to the liver of about 3 rad/mCi administered (Fairweather *et al.*, 1983). Free ^{111}In is bound to plasma transferrin and [^{111}In]DTPA is excreted in the urine.

^{99m}Tc is the standard radionuclide of nuclear medicine being generator produced on site (γ-ray energy 140 keV), but it has two major disadvantages in this context. It is particularly difficult to label biologically active proteins in a way so that they remain stable *in vivo* for 24 hr and its short half-life of 6 hr means that too little activity is present at the time of maximum antibody uptake which is between 12 and 24 hr.

III. LABELLING WITH ^{123}I

^{123}I has a half-life of 13 hr, no β rays and a γ ray energy of 0.159 MeV, which is ideal for the γ camera. ^{123}I is produced by the Atomic Energy Research Establishment, Harwell, using a cyclotron. By means of a 55 MeV-proton beam using diiodomethane as the target, the ^{127}I is converted to ^{123}Xe which decays to ^{123}I.

$$^{127}\text{I (p, 5n)} \, ^{123}\text{Xe} \rightarrow \, ^{123}\text{I}$$

This reaction produces ^{123}I totally free of ^{124}I and with less than 0.5% ^{125}I. ^{123}I is produced on the sides of the flask containing the ^{123}Xe as it decays. ^{123}I is dissolved in sodium hydroxide and dispensed into sterile vials and dried.

The iodogen reaction is used with ^{123}I to label the monoclonal antibody. The iodogen is dissolved in dichloromethane to make iodogen solution and evaporated to dryness at 37°C in sterile propylene tubes. Iodogen reagent is then coating the inside of the tube and these tubes can be stored at 5°C for 6 months without loss of reactivity.

Once the iodogen tubes are prepared and the HMFG antibodies have been made available, the following technique is used for labelling. Pure ^{123}I, the mouse monoclonal antibody, 1–2 mg/ml in 10^{-5} M, Tris buffer, pH 7.4 and potassium iodide, 4×10^{-4} M in water are mixed in the iodogen tube. Potassium iodide is added because it is necessary to increase the ionic stength of the iodine for the labelling reaction to proceed to completion.

The mixture is left at room temperature for 10 min with gentle shaking. The mixture is decanted on to a Sephadex G-50 filtration column in a 20-ml syringe pre-washed with 1% human serum albumin in phosphate-buffered saline. After a 5-ml void volume, the eluate is collected in 2-ml aliquots, activity assayed and passed through a micropore filter into sterile vials.

Quality control is undertaken using 10-μl samples from before and after gel filtration. They are spotted at an origin of 10-cm absorbent strips. These are developed in an ascending manner with 85% methanol and the radioactivity of the strips is determined. The labelling efficiency is typically over 70%. Iodinated protein is precipitated at origin and free ^{123}I is at solvent front. Reactivity of iodinated antibody with breast cancer cells is tested using enzyme-linked immunosorbent assay (ELISA). It is shown that this iodogen method leaves the active centre of the antibody intact with its avidity unaltered. This is also confirmed by direct radioimmunoassay.

IV. PATIENTS

Patients with suspected or known ovarian cancer, between 30 and 75 yr of age, were under the care of the gynaecologist (J. S.). The procedure was explained and each gave signed consent. Potassium iodide 60 mg b.d. was given orally the day before and for 3 days after the study. A skin test with the antibody was performed prior to the study to test for allergy. The patients were divided into four groups.

Group 1. Patients with a mass in the abdomen or pelvis of undiagnosed cause but for which there was a reasonable clinical suspicion that it was due to ovarian cancer.

Group 2. Patients with clinically obvious ovarian cancer in order to determine the extent of the disease before operation. The extent of the disease was determined at surgery in order to 'stage' the ovarian cancer, which assessment forms the basis of therapy.

Group 3. Patients who had been operated on for ovarian cancer elsewhere having histological proof of the disease but who had been referred for specialist treatment at the gynaecology/oncology unit at St. Bartholomew's Hospital. The extent of the disease determined by imaging was compared with that determined by other techniques, untrasound and X-ray computed tomography.

Group 4. Patients with ovarian cancer who had already undergone complete or incomplete surgical resection of disease and had had chemotherapy. In some of these a 'second-look' operation was necessary to determine presence of any or the extent of residual disease as a guide to further treatment and in others chemotherapy had failed and re-operation was indicated.

V. PROCEDURE

The patient lies supine on the scanning couch and a γ camera is placed over the pelvis anteriorly. The injection of 2–3 mCi of ^{123}I-labelled monoclonal antibody containing 0.5 mg of antibody is given intravenously to the patient. Dynamic studies are recorded for the first 10 min directly into the computer. Static images are then taken, anteriorly and posteriorly of the whole of the abdomen together with marker scans. These are transferred directly into the computer. Similar procedures occur at 4 and 22 hr. Then the patient goes for surgery later that morning.

One of the problems with this sort of imaging is that the detail of tumour may not be clear and than a technique of background correction may be required. The method employed in this study is to subtract the 10 min image from the 4-hr and from the 22-hr image, using radioactive markers placed on the patient to co-ordinate the two pictures. Transparent films of the marker positions on the persistance scope are made at the early visit, and the patient's skin marked. At each subsequent visit, the markers are repositioned on the patient and the patient is repositioned until the image of the marker on the persistance scope fits that on the previously recorded film positioned over the scope. The computer is also programmed so that the recorded images can be moved and fixed one pixel at a time, vertically, horizontally or by rotation so that an exact superimposition of the later image over the earlier image may be made. Although many primary ovarian tumours and their metastases may be seen without background subtraction, the use of the subtraction technique has resulted in the unequivocal identification of metastases with relatively low uptake (Granowska *et al.*, 1983, 1984).

VI. CLINICAL EXAMPLES

A 64-yr-old woman had a laparatomy at another hospital showing extensive serious adenocarcinoma and was referred for specialist treatment (Group 3, Stage III). Radioimmunoscintigraphy showed uptake in the right side of the pelvis (Fig. 1) and inferior to the spleen (Fig. 2) which was confirmed at re-operation (Fig. 3).

A 58-yr-old woman presented with a left pelvic mass (Group 1). A local area of increased uptake was shown there on radioimmunoscintigraphy (Fig. 4). At operation it was shown to be a Krukenberg tumour—a metastasis from occult carcinoma stomach.

A 40-yr-old woman presented with an abdominal mass thought to be an ovarian cyst (Group 1). Radioimmunoscintigraphy showed marked uptake (Fig. 5). The mass was confirmed at operation (Fig. 6) and shown to be benign teratoma on histology.

A 55-yr-old woman completed her courses of chemotherapy (Group 4b, Stage III) for ovarian serous cystadenocarcinoma and radioimmunoscintigraphy was performed (Fig. 7), before the second-look operation.

A 44-yr-old woman presented with a pelvic mass with clinical evidence of abdominal spread (Group 2, Stage IV). Radioimmunoscintigraphy showed evidence of tumour and metastases and this was confirmed at operation (Fig. 8). Histology showed a poorly differentiated adenocarcinoma. She then received five full courses of chemotherapy and further imaging was undertaken. The imaging findings before the first operation and before the second operation are shown in Fig. 9 for posterior views of the pelvis, and Fig. 10 for anterior views of the pelvis. These views taken together show the rather faint distribution of labelled antibody corresponding to the findings at the first operation (Fig. 8). A second-look operation showed large areas of necrotic tissue but multiple biopsies showed viable cancer which confirmed the findings at imaging.

VII. RESULTS

For patients with known ovarian cancer in Groups 2, 3 and 4, the correlation between the findings at radioimmunoscintigraphy and the findings at subsequent surgery are summarised in Table I. One poor correlation and one equivocal result was found but the other 37 studies showed good correlation between the imaging and surgical findings (Figs.

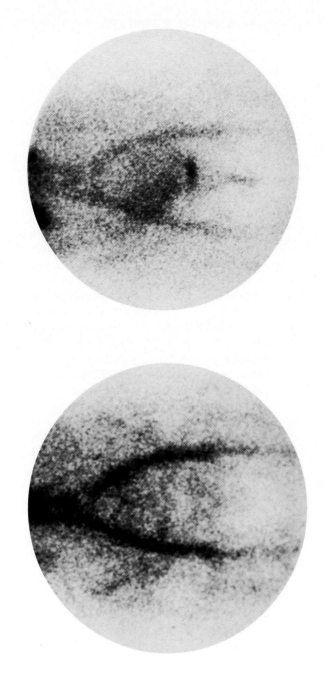

Fig. 1. Anterior view of the pelvis (left) 10-min image; (right) 21-hr image. Increased uptake with time is seen in the right side of the pelvis.

208

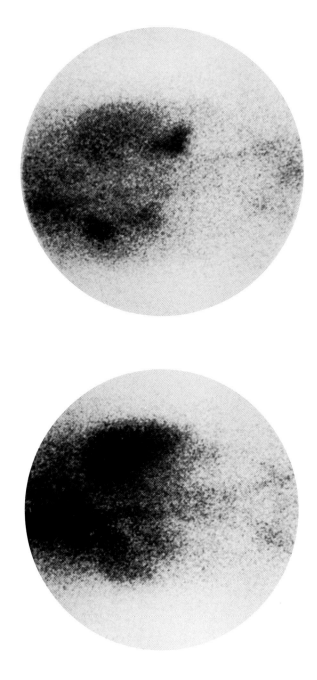

Fig. 2. Posterior view of the abdomen (left) 10-min image; (right) 21-hr image. Increased uptake is seen just inferior to the spleen on the late image. Some retention of free iodine is noted in the right renal pelvis.

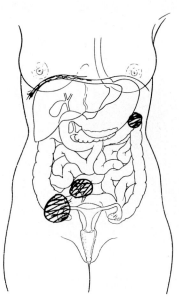

Fig. 3. Surgical findings show masses in the right pelvis, the site of uptake in Fig. 1, and a mass in the splenic flexure noted as a site of uptake on the posterior view in Fig. 2.

1, 3, 8 and 9). It so happened that no patient in Group 1 had ovarian cancer. Poor correlations between imaging and the surgical findings were found in patients with fibroids, two benign ovarian tumours and a tubo-ovarian abscess. Equivocal results were found with lymphoma and a metastasis from alveolar cell carcinoma of the lung. Good correlations were found in the patients with metastases from colon carcinoma and stomach carcinoma, known to take up HMFG-2 (Table II). Uptake in the benign teratoma is shown in Fig. 5 and in the pelvic secondary tumour from carcinoma of the stomach in Fig. 4. Seven patients showed the typical pattern of ovarian cancer—that of low early uptake which increases to a high value by 22 hr. Two were the large benign tumours, four were carcinoma of the gastrointestinal tract known to react with HMFG-2 and one was a vaginal secondary from hepatoma. High early uptake in fibroids and tubo-ovarian abscess decreasing with time characterises a dominantly vascular lesion. This pattern of change with time may now be distinguished using computer analysis. The results summarised in Table II emphasise that the HMFG-2 imaging is good in staging and determining the results of chemotherapy in known ovarian cancer but poor in screening patients presenting with a pelvic mass or those who are suffering from carcinoma or the ovary.

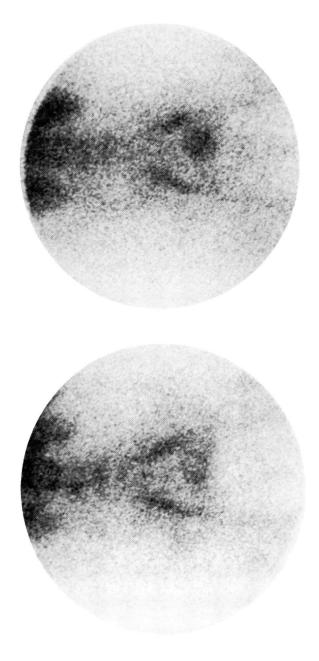

Fig. 4. Posterior views of the pelvis (left) 10-min image; (right) 4-hr image. Increasing uptake with time is seen focally in the left side of the pelvis, found to be due to a pelvic metastasis from carcinoma of the stomach.

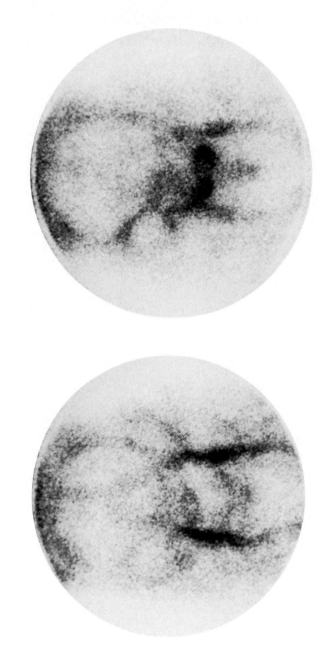

Fig. 5. Anterior views of the pelvis (left) 10-min image; (right) 22-hr image. There is increasing uptake with time in the rims of two circular lesions, small on the right side, large centrally and to the left with an area of increased uptake inferior to these lesions.

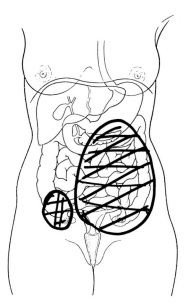

Fig. 6. Surgical findings corresponding to Fig. 5. Histology was a benign teratoma.

VIII. DISCUSSION

The results show that there was a good (95%) correlation between the findings at radioimmunoscintigraphy and those at surgery in patients with known ovarian carcinoma of all stages (Table I, Figs. 1–3, 7–10). However, patients in Group I with a pelvic mass of uncertain cause were generally not correctly diagnosed (Table II), giving an overall correlation of 77%. On two occasions, histologically benign tumours took up the labelled HMFG-2 antibody (Fig. 5). These findings indicate that with large benign ovarian tumours, there is sufficient uptake of HMFG-2 antibody by normal ovarian tissue to enable imaging. In addition, there may be some architectural change tending to expose normally epithelial surface antigens more directly to the circulation. The uptake of HMFG-2 in gastrointestinal cancer fits in with the known distribution of the HMF-G glycoprotein antigen. Thus, it is clear from these findings that radioimmunoscintigraphy has no place at present in the screening of women with a pelvic mass as to whether or not they have ovarian cancer. A much more specific antibody is required.

By contrast, in the context of known ovarian cancer in all groups of patients and at all stages of the disease, there is a very good correlation

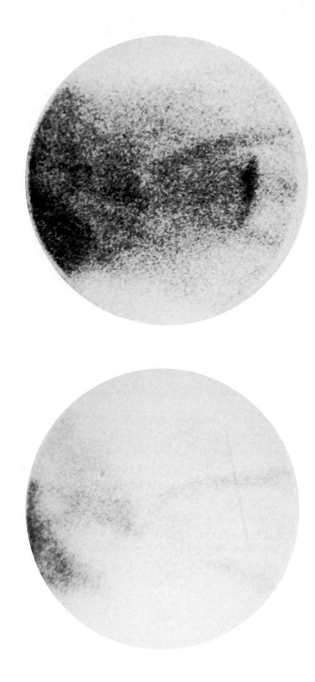

Fig. 7. Anterior view of the abdomen and pelvis (left) 10-min image; (right) 21-hr image. Increased uptake with time is seen in the abdomen and pelvis.

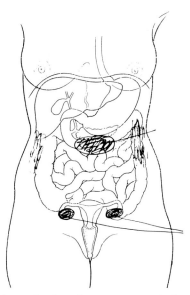

Fig. 8. Surgical drawing shows the sites of tumour masses in the ovaries and in the upper abdomen.

between the results of imaging and the findings at operation. This raises the hope that the determination of the presence or absence of viable cancer cells, particularly seeding the peritoneum or omentum, may be demonstrable without the need for a second- or third-look operation.

It is worth considering the requirements for improvements in radioimmunoscintigraphy. The basic requirement is more labelled antibody on the tumour. The higher the count rate from the tumour, the better the image contrast and resolution for the statistical error depends on the square root of the total counts. Thus, 100 counts per picture element has an error of ± 10, an error of 10%, whereas 10,000 counts per picture element has an error of ± 100, an error of 1%. This error, due to Poisson distribution noise, must be reduced to enhance the signal.

It would be advantageous to increase the number of radionuclides per molecule over the one-to-one relationship. However, the chance of affecting the active centre increases with further labelling. It is essential to confirm that the labelled antibody has the same immunoreactive properties as the unlabelled antibody through direct radioimmunoassay or the ELISA technique.

The rate of specific uptake of the antibody by the tumour will follow Michaelis–Menten kinetics and be more rapid initially, falling off with time. Although there is little specific evidence, calculations based on the

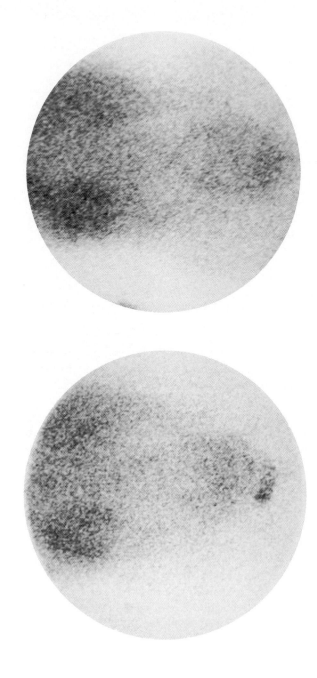

Fig. 9. Posterior views of the pelvis, 21-hr images. Left side before the first operation, uptake in the pelvis is noted superior to the activity in the bladder; right side after chemotherapy, uptake in the pelvis is more prominent.

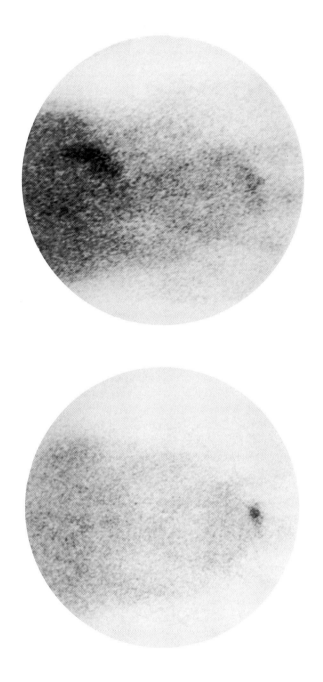

Fig. 10. Anterior views of the pelvis, 21-hr images. Left side before the first operation, uptake in the upper abdomen in the left and right flanks and centrally merging into the liver and spleen is noted; right side after chemotherapy, findings are similar, but there is also free iodine in the stomach.

217

TABLE I

RADIOIMMUNOSCINTIGRAPHY OF KNOWN OVARIAN CANCER; CORRELATION WITH SURGICAL FINDINGS[a]

Group	Poor	Equivocal	Good	Total
2			15	15
3			6	6
4	1	1	16	18
Total	1	1	37	39

[a]Total results: 37 of 39; 95% good correlation.

circulation and re-circulation time suggest that most uptake will be within the first 12 hr after injection. There are thus two imaging strategies: one is to image early using a high-activity, short-lived radionuclide such as ^{123}I or ^{111}In with the advantage of high sensitivity and low statistical error and thus high detectability, but with the disadvantage of higher non-tumour background; and the other is to image late with a long-lived radionuclide such as ^{131}I when the target : background ratio has improved but at the cost of low sensitivity, high noise and reduced discrimination.

In order to improve the uptake of the antibody by the tumour, a number of requirements should be met. The antibody should be more specific, ideally totally cancer specific and should also be very avid. It must not only be able to bind but also to have staying power on the antigen so that the antibody does not disconnect and so that the radiolabel is not metabolised off the bound antibody. It may be that the class of antibody is important because the diffusibility of the antibody may be a limiting factor in getting it from the circulation to the tumour surface. Antibody fragments may be effective in improving access, but fragmentation of the γ-globulin may reduce its avidity.

Another requirement is to reduce the non-tumour distribution of the labelled antibody. Approaches to this problem include the use of Fab_2 fragments which are cleared more quickly from the blood (Mach *et al.*, 1981) and the use of a second antibody injected either free or carried on liposomes to precipitate and clear the labelled antibody (Begent *et al.*, 1982). The antibody not taken up by the tumour is metabolised in the body. For iodine-labelled antibody, about 20% free iodine is liberated per day. This release of iodine in the circulation is not particularly important, for the γ camera, of course, cannot distinguish between free and bound iodine in the circulation. It is all noise that tends to obscure the signal. The crucial requirement is lack of metabolism of the labelled antibody on the cancer cell. However, the slower the uptake of the an-

TABLE II

RADIOIMMUNOSCINTIGRAPHY OF SUSPECTED AND KNOWN OVARIAN CANCER; CORRELATION WITH SURGICAL FINDINGS[a]

Group	Poor	Equivocal	Good	Total
1	5	5	4	14
2			15	15
3			6	6
4	1	1	16	18
Total	6	6	41	53

[a]Total results: 41 of 53; 77% good correlation.

tibody by the tumour, the more important becomes the need for the labelled antibody to remain stable and unmetabolised in the circulation.

The question is often asked as to the smallest detectable size of lesion. Over about 2 cm in diameter there is an approximate correspondence between physical size and apparent image size; below 2 cm the detectability depends primarily on the activity in the lesion. Thus, the head of a pin less than 1 mm across if sufficiently radioactive would appear as an image perhaps 2 cm across. It is, therefore, clear that detectability depends on activity on the target. This is the primary endeavour necessary to improve imaging with radiolabelled antibodies. Counts count in nuclear medicine.

Provided there is specific uptake of the labelled antibody, there are several ways by which the signal may be enhanced in relation to the noise. The standard nuclear medicine technique is to inject a second labelled agent which has no specific uptake by the abnormality of interest but has a similar distribution as that of the first labelled agent that has not been taken up; and to subtract the non-specific image from the specific image. Goldenberg *et al.* (1980) used ^{99m}Tc-labelled albumin and DTPA to mimic the distribution of ^{131}I-labelled anti-carcinoembryonic antigen not taken up by the tumour. This approach, by using two radionuclides of different γ-ray energies, is fraught with physical problems. The attenuations of the γ rays, ^{99m}Tc and ^{131}I, are different as is their scattering. Thus subtraction leads to edge and other artefacts. The most objective approach using this technique is that of Green *et al.* (1984).

The alternative approach is to compare an image taken early after intravenous injection of the labelled antibodies with those taken at later times. The basis for this is that the early image would show mainly the vascular and extravascular distribution of the antibody, whereas the later images would, in addition, show the specific uptake. In order to compare these images, a careful patient-repositioning protocol is undertaken as described earlier. This is followed by a repositioning protocol applied to the series of computer images. Once the images are accurately superimposable, one of a series of Change Detection algorithms may be applied. These show sites of significant positive uptake with time to a predetermined confidence level—95, 99, 99.5% etc., and also the regions of signficantly decreasing uptake with time. This objective method of identifying sites of specific antibody uptake appears very encouraging (Nimmon *et al.*, 1984).

Single photon emission tomography is an alternative approach to improving the contrast resolution of a suspected tumour (Berche *et al.*, 1982). Transverse, cranial or sagittal sections of the radionuclide distribution are obtained using computer analysis of the data accumulated during the rotation of the camera around the patient. The taking of sections acts in effect as a form of contrast enhancement of the lesion. This should enable quantitation of the amount of uptake to be performed. Unfortunately there are a number of problems including data reconstruction artefacts due to enhancement of statistical noise, misalignment and patient and organ movement and the inability to perform accurate corrections for tissue attenuation. Relative quantitation, i.e., in comparison to an appropriate phantom or an adjacent area of 'normal' uptake, may be performed so that, for example, uptake in the tumour may be compared with uptake in the liver. Apparent tumour volumes may be determined for lesions over 2 cm in diameter.

A further requirement is a lack of adverse effects of the labelled antibody on the patient. The immunogenicity of the labelled antibody should be as low as possible. Patients with known sensitivities to foreign proteins or with positive skin tests to the proposed injection should not be studied. Although we have had no reactions in our series in which four patients have been studied twice, the development of anti-HMFG-2 antibodies remains a potential problem especially if therapy with labelled antibody is to be considered. The preparation must be virus and DNA free, and standards of purity for such biological materials are under discussion.

An important clinical requirement is that the labelled antibody is only taken up by viable and not by necrotic cells, since this is essential in the evaluation of chemotherapy. In one patient (Figs. 9 and 10), viable cells were thought to be present on imaging and, although the surgical picture showed areas of necrosis, the multiple biopsies showed viable cells.

In conclusion, screening patients with ovarian cancer is not worthwhile with this technique. Assessing the response to chemotherapy and providing evidence of recurrence of known ovarian cancer are methods usefully undertaken using ^{123}I-labelled HMFG-2 monoclonal antibody. Whether intravenous administration or intraperitoneal instillation of HMFG-2 labelled with ^{131}I for radiation therapy of peritoneal deposits of ovarian cancer will be effective, remains to be determined. It is likely that more specific and more avid antibodies will be required.

ACKNOWLEDGEMENT

This work was supported by the Imperial Cancer Research Fund.

REFERENCES

Arklie, J., Taylor-Papadimitriou, J., Bodmer, W., Egan, M., and Millis, R. (1981). *Int. J.Cancer* **28**, 23–29.

Begent, R. H. J., Keep, P. A., Green, A. J., Searle, F., Bagshawe, K. D., Jewkes, R. F., Jones, B. E., Barratt, G. M., and Ryman, B. E. (1982). *Lancet* **2**, 739–741.

Berche, C., Mach, J. P., Lumbroso, J. D., Langlais, C., Aubry, F., Buchegger, F., Carrel, S., Rougier, P., Parmentier, C., and Tubiana, M. (1982). *Br. Med. J.* **285**, 1447–1451.

Burchell, J., Durbin, H., and Taylor-Papadimitriou, J. (1983). *J. Immunol.* **131**, 508–513.

Fairweather, D. S., Bradwell, A. R., Dykes, P. W., Vaughan, A. T., Watson-James, S. F., and Chandler, S. (1983). *Br. Med. J.* **287**, 167–170.

Goldenberg, D. M., Kim, E. E., Deland, F. H., Bennett, S., and Primus, F. J. (1980). *Cancer Res.* **40**, 2984–2992.

Granowska, M., Shepherd, J., Britton, K. E., Ward, B., Mather, S., Taylor-Papadimitriou, J., Epenetos, A. A., Carroll, M. J., Nimmon, C. C., Hawkins, L. A., and Bodmer, W. F. (1983). *J. Nucl. Med.* **24**, P15.

Granowska, M., Shepherd, J., Britton, K. E., Ward, B., Mather, S., Taylor-Papadimitriou, J., and Bodmer, W. F. (1984). *Nucl. Med. Commun.* **5**, 485–499.

Green, A. J., Begent, R. H. J., Keep, P. A., and Bagshawe, K. E. (1984). *J. Nucl. Med.* **25**, 96–100.

Mach, J.-P., Buchegger, F., Farni, M., Ritschard, J., Berche, C., Lumbroso, J.-D., Schreyer, M., Girandet, C., Accolla, R. S., and Carrel, S. (1981). *Immunol. Today* **2**, 239–249.

Nimmon, C. C., Carroll, M. J., Flatman, W. D., Marsden, P., Granowska, M., Horne, T., and Britton, K. E. (1984). *Nucl. Med. Commun.* **5**, 231.

Shimizu, M., and Yamauchi, K. (1982). *J. Biochem. (Tokyo)* **91**, 515–524.

Taylor-Papadimitriou, J., Peterson, J. A., Arklie, J., Burchell, J., Ceriani, R. C., and Bodmer, W. F. (1981). *Int. J. Cancer* **28**, 17–21.

Taylor-Papadimitriou, J., Burchell, J., and Chang, S. E. (1983). *In* "Monoclonal Antibodies and Cancer. Armand Hammer Symposium" (R. Dulbecco and R. Langman, eds.), pp. 227–238. Academic Press, New York.

CHAPTER 11

Efficiency and Tolerance of the Treatment with Immuno-A-chain-toxins in Human Bone Marrow Transplantations

F. K. Jansen,* G. Laurent,* M. C. Liance,*
H. E. Blythman,* J. Berthe,[†] X. Canat,*
P. Carayon,* D. Carriere,[†] P. Casellas,*
J. M. Derocq,* D. Dussossoy,* A. A. Fauser,[‡]
N. C. Gorin,[§] O. Gros,* P. Gros,* J. C. Laurent,*
P. Poncelet,* B. Remandet,[†] G. Richer* and H. Vidal*

*Immunotoxin Project
[†]Department of Toxicology
Centre de Recherches Clin. Midy
Groupe Sanofi
Montpellier, France
[‡]Med. Univ. Klinik
Freiburg, Federal Republic of Germany
[§]Hôpital St. Antoine
Paris, France

MONOCLONAL ANTIBODIES FOR CANCER
DETECTION AND THERAPY

I. INTRODUCTION

Immuno-A-chain-toxins (I-A-chain-Ts) have been described in the literature (Gilliland *et al.*, 1980; Jansen *et al.*, 1980; Krolick *et al.*, 1980; Masuho and Hara, 1980; Miyazaki *et al.*, 1980; Raso and Griffin, 1980) since 1980 (Sanofi *et al.*, 1978). They are conjugates between subunits of very potent toxins, their A-chain or active chain (the toxic moiety), and antibodies specifically directed against target cells, in order to increase the antibody-mediated cytotoxicity. Thus, immunotoxins (ITs) combine the potential of the most powerful toxins with the specificity of selected monoclonal or polyclonal antibodies (Abs).

Another class of ITs described since 1970 (Moolten and Cooperband, 1970; Thorpe *et al.*, 1978; Youle and Neville, 1980), are conjugates between Abs and whole toxins, composed of an A and B chain, i.e., I-ricin-Ts, which share the same principal advantages. But each of these IT classes also has its inconvenience. Whole toxins coupled to antibodies maintain part of their non-specific binding sites, such as ricin for sugar residues, and are able to bind non-specifically to any cell. Under *in vitro* conditions, this non-specific binding can be greatly diminished by high lactose concentrations (Youle and Neville, 1980). In contrast, I-A-chain-Ts show almost no non-specific binding to non-target cells, but their cytotoxic potency is diminished because of the lacking B chain and its helper function. This inconvenience can be overcome *in vitro* in the presence of NH_4Cl at high concentration, which inhibits the neutralization of I-A-chain-Ts in the lysosomes of target cells (Casellas *et al.*, 1982a,b; Jansen *et al.*, 1982).

Both ITs show high potency *in vitro*, while their *in vivo* efficacy is not yet convincing, since the necessary adjuvants, high lactose or NH_4Cl concentrations, respectively, cannot be maintained *in vivo*. Nevertheless, attempts are being made to render I-ricin-Ts more specific *in vivo* by blocking the non-specific binding site of the whole ricin (Thorpe *et al.*, 1984). On the other hand, I-A-chain-Ts may in the future become more potent *in vivo* with the help of free (Youle and Neville, 1982) or bound B chains (Vitetta *et al.*, 1983) or in the presence of drugs with potentiating properties similar to lysosomotropic amines (Casellas *et al.*, 1982a,b; Jansen *et al.*, 1982) or carboxylic ionophores (Casellas *et al.*, 1984a,b).

The high *in vitro* potential of ITs can now be used in the treatment of human bone marrow needed to rescue leukemia patients with autologous or allogeneic marrow when they had been treated with supralethal, bone marrow toxic doses of irradiation and/or conventional drugs. In autologous transplantation marrow, contaminating leukemic cells have to be destroyed, while in allogeneic transplants mature T cells should be eliminated in order to inhibit graft versus host disease (GvHD). Such approaches were realized on human bone marrow with lectins (Reisner *et al.*, 1983), with antibodies alone (Filipovich *et al.*, 1982; Prentice *et al.*, 1982), with antibodies and complement (Prentice *et al.*, 1984; Ritz *et al.*, 1982), with antibodies immobilized on magnetic or other beads (Treleaven *et al.*, 1984) or with I-ricin-Ts (Filipovich *et al.*, 1984).

Immunotoxins assembled with A chains, I-A-chain-Ts, are now under clinical evaluation. They are almost non-toxic *in vivo* and can therefore be directly infused with the whole marrow into the patient. I-A-chain-Ts also show low toxicity to stem cells *in vitro*. A first representative of such new drugs assembled with the T101 antibody directed against a pan T antigen on human lymphocytes is utilized in autologous and allogeneic bone marrow transplantation. As compared with I-ricin-Ts or the other methods for purging of bone marrow, the advantages of I-A-chain-Ts are more of a practical order. Such drugs necessitate much less time-consuming manipulations of the marrow with the danger of infections and may be more potent in specific cytoreduction than the other methods (Casellas *et al.*, 1985).

In the following sections we descibe the general properties of I-A-chain-Ts, their potency in eliminating leukemia cells or normal T cells in human bone marrow, their potential *in vivo* effect when administered with the bone marrow to the patient and the future development of I-A-chain-Ts.

II. GENERAL REMARKS ON I-A-CHAIN-Ts

The main properties of I-A-chain-Ts are specific cytotoxicity against their target cells combined with low non-specific toxicity towards unrelated cells. The general properties of I-A-chain-Ts will only be summarized because of the available literature (Möller, 1982).

A. Activity of I-A-chain-Ts

1. Specificity of Cytotoxicity

The A chains of potent polypeptide toxins are about 10^3–10^5 less toxic than the original whole toxins, since they can no longer bind to cells.

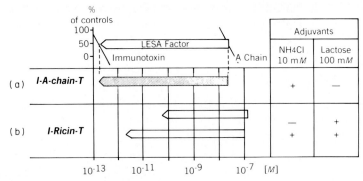

Fig. 1. Specific activity of I-A-chain-Ts versus I-ricin-Ts and corresponding LESA factors. (a) T101 I-A-chain-Ts or free A chain were incubated in increasing concentrations and in the presence of 10 mM NH₄Cl with CEM cells for 20 hr at 37°C. The ratio of the A-chain concentration versus the IT concentration leading to 50% leucine uptake inhibition is called LESA factor (ligand-enhanced specific activity factor). (b) T101 I-ricin-T (from Drs. Leonard and Royston, La Jolla) was incubated with CEM cells for 20 hr in the presence of 100 mM lactose or with lactose plus 10 mM NH₄Cl. The non-specific activity was evaluated on antigen negative Raji cells, showing the same sensitivity to A chain as CEM cells.

By the conjugation to an antibody they acquire the capacity to bind to target cells only, which results in specific cytotoxicity.

By analogy with a therapeutic index *in vivo*, the specific cytotoxicity of ITs can be estimated by the ligand-enhanced specific activity factor (LESA) (Jansen *et al.*, 1982). This factor indicates the relation of the free A-chain concentration versus the antibody bound A-chain concentration leading to the same inhibition of leucine incorporation (50%) into the target cells (Fig. 1). This factor varies considerably for different ITs from low to high specific activities with LESA factors from 10^1 to 10^4. Several reasons may explain this variability. The nature of the antigen and/or the antibody and their respective densities on target cells influence the specific activity (Casellas *et al.*, 1984a). High-affinity antibodies kill target cells in much lower concentrations, e.g., $10^{-14}M$ with the T101 IT, than low-affinity antibodies. LESA factors also depend on the non-specific cytotoxicity of free A chain on the target cells or of unrelated IT on these cells. In both cases, relatively high concentrations, of the order of $5 \times 10^{-7}M$ are needed.

2. Kinetics of Cytotoxicity

The toxic activity of the A chain is based on its capacity to inhibit protein synthesis by an enzymatic modification of ribosomes (about 2000

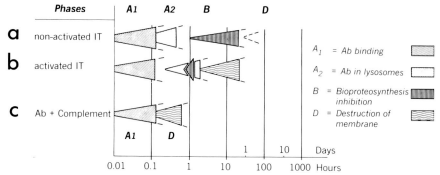

Fig. 2. Kinetics of the non-activated and activated T101 IT in relation to complement lysis in general. (a) The time needed to induce 50% of responses (T50) was evaluated for four different responses: the antibody binding with radioactive antibodies (A1 phase), the entry into secondary lysosomes of IT-coated gold particles examined under the electron microscope (A2 phase), the inhibition of leucine uptake by the cells, indicating protein synthesis inhibition (B phase) and the destruction of the cell membrane, as measured by propidium iodine uptake with cytofluorometry. (b) The same responses were measured with the T101 I-A-chain toxin activated by the presence of NH_4Cl. (c) For comparison the generally expected A1 and D phases of complement lysis are indicated.

ribosomes per minute) (Olsnes and Pihl, 1980). After the binding of the antibody moiety of an IT to the membrane, the A chain must be translocated into the cytoplasm to reach the ribosomes. When complete inhibition of protein synthesis is reached, cells may survive for a limited time with their existing protein equipment, before their membranes become permeable for dye solutions. The kinetics of this sequence of events are of considerable significance for the potency of ITs, since IT treatment only becomes efficient if the inhibition of cell proliferation by IT is more rapid than the proliferation of the target cells themselves.

The whole process until cell death may be subdivided into four different phases: A, Antibody binding and endocytosis; B, Bioproteosynthesis inhibition; C, Colony formation inhibition; D, Destruction of the cell membrane. Phases A and B describe the interaction of the IT with the cell by the antibody in phase A and the A-chain moiety in phase B. Phases C and D indicate the cell reaction in phase C by the inhibition of physiological cell activities, i.e., mixed lymphocyte reaction (MLR) or colony formation, and in phase D by cell membrane destruction.

With an example of an IT with slow kinetics, the T101 IT directed against the T1 antigen (65 kDa of human T lymphocytes), the time points were measured at which 50% of the maximum effect of each phase (T50) was reached on CEM cells (Fig. 2). They were of the order of 10 min for antibody binding (phase A1) and about 30 min for the entry into secondary lysosomes (phase A2). This was studied with the electron microscope by the incorporation of IT-coated gold particles (Carrière *et al.*, 1985). The B phase lasted about 20 hr to obtain 50% inhibition of bioproteosynthesis, while the D phase kinetics were too long to be measurable, since cell proliferation interferes with cell destruction after the 24-hr incubation period.

3. Acceleration of Kinetics

In the presence of 10 mM ammonium chloride, known to increase the pH of secondary lysosomes, the whole process of cell destruction becomes considerably accelerated (Fig. 2b). This may be explained by an inhibition of the neutralization of ITs in secondary lysosomes. The A1 phase of antibody binding remains constant but the A2 phase, concerning the uptake into secondary lysosomes, is prolonged about five times, from 30 min to 2.5 hr. The B phase, which includes the translocation and protein synthesis inhibition, becomes extremely short, 1.6 hr. It is now accomplished before the T50 of the A2 phase is reached, suggesting that the translocation step is enhanced and might be effected in the pre-lysosomal compartment. The D phase kinetics (dye exclusion of 50% of cells) are of the order of 20 hr.

The acceleration of the kinetics results in an important increase of efficiency in the corresponding dose–response curves. The T101 IT can now kill 50% of target cells in concentrations of 5×10^{-13} M (Jansen *et al.*, 1982). This corresponds to less than 40 ITs bound per target cell. A similar increase of efficacy is found in the inhibition of colony formation. The capacity of cytoreduction was increased from 1 to 4 logs.

4. Cytotoxic Capacity

There is a discrepancy between the capacity of ITs to inhibit protein synthesis and colony formation on the one hand, and their capacity to kill cells, as studied by dye uptake, on the other hand. First, the kinetics of the cell destruction (phase D for a CEM clone: T50 = 10 hr) are about seven times longer than those of protein synthesis inhibition (T50 = 1.5 hr). Therefore, in a certain percentage of target cells the membrane remains intact although protein synthesis is completely blocked. These cells seem to survive when measured with the dye exclusion test after 24 hr of incubation with IT.

Second, the kinetics of the destruction phase do not, as expected, follow first-order kinetics over several days but become increasingly longer.

With a CEM clone which possesses only the low amount of 5000 antigens per cell, even after 6-day incubation with IT, about 25% of cells are still excluding the dye. This may be explained by the proliferation of IT-resistant cells. Dye exclusion tests are, therefore, not appropriate to demonstrate the whole cytotoxic capacity of ITs, mainly because of the involved slow cytotoxic kinetics of the destruction phase D.

B. Comparison with Other Methods

1. Lysis by Antibodies Plus Complement

The most efficient complement-dependent lysis is generally obtained with antibodies of the IgM class, while highly potent ITs may be produced with antibodies of every isotype. As published earlier (Jansen et al., 1981), an IgM monoclonal antibody against Thy-1.2 with complement produced 50% cytotoxicity in concentrations of about $10^{-10} M$. The same activity was reached with this antibody as IT. In colony formation assays on a Burkitt lymphoma cell line, a cytoreduction of more than 4 logs after several treatments with a cocktail of Abs and complement was described (Bast et al., 1983a), while the T101 IT alone produced a similar or even better cytoreduction on CEM cells (Casellas et al., 1984a, 1985). The in vitro efficacy of both methods may be similar, if the comparison is made between the best ITs and the most efficient IgM antibodies plus complement against the same antigen. However, an individual complement binding IgG is often much less active with complement than with an A chain as IT, i.e., the T101 antibody is only moderately active in complement-mediated lysis (Royston et al., 1980).

Even if the in vitro efficacy of both methods will be considered to be similar, ITs show some practical advantages for the treatment of human bone marrow. Complement lysis needs a time-consuming manipulation of the marrow, i.e., isolation of nucleated cells, and sometimes multiple incubations and washes (Bast et al., 1983b). Such manipulations run the risk of infection and a loss of stem cells. With I-A-chain-Ts, no manipulation is needed. The whole marrow can be treated without separation of erythrocytes and the I-A-chain-T can be injected together with the marrow into the patient because of its very low toxicity.

Another problem with complement is the difficulty in obtaining standardized preparations without toxicity towards stem cells, and in their large-scale production. With one batch of several grams of I-A-chain-T, however, more than 1000 bone marrows can be treated without risk of stem cell damage.

2. Cytotoxicity of I-ricin-Ts

In collaboration with Drs. J. E. Leonard and I. Royston (La Jolla, California), T101 antibodies coupled to whole ricin or to ricin A chain were compared for their potency and specificity (Gros *et al.*, 1984). When both products are used with their corresponding adjuvants, ammonium chloride for I-A-chain-Ts and lactose plus ammonium chloride for I-ricin-Ts, they revealed a similar efficiency in dose–response curves, showing almost the same LESA factors (Fig. 1). Specific activities were found with both ITs in very low concentrations of $2 \times 10^{-13}M$ (I-A-chain-T) and $2 \times 10^{-12}M$ (I-ricin-T). In stem cell assays, however, this I-A-chain-T seems to be 20 times less toxic than the corresponding I-ricin-T when it was compared with the results published on GEMM colony formation (Vallera *et al.*, 1983) with the corresponding I-ricin-T (Fig. 3) (see Section III,A,2). In colony formation assays with CEM cells, both classes of IT reduced target cells to a similar extent by more than 4 logs.

An inconvenience of I-ricin-Ts is their *in vivo* toxicity, if they are injected with the marrow into the patient, because the high lactose concentration rapidly becomes diluted in the circulation. Therefore, I-ricin-Ts have to be thoroughly eliminated, after treatment of the marrow, by three washes (Filipovich *et al.*, 1984). For the same reason, I-ricin-Ts without definite blockage of the non-specific binding site of the B chain of ricin cannot be envisaged for therapy of residual leukemic cells *in vivo*.

Since I-A-chain-Ts are reinjected with the marrow, they may have a therapeutical effect on residual leukemia cells *in vivo*, although their efficiency is considerably restricted by the absence of ammonium chloride (see Section IV,B).

C. Pharmaceutical Production and Controls

Appropriate quantities of I-A-chain-Ts can now be produced for clinical studies. The aim of pharmaceutical production is a regular and reproducible supply of the active principle under severe controls. The potency and innocuity of such products have to be proven in pre-clinical and clinical studies with stable products presented in a clinically useful form.

1. Production

The purification of the components of I-A-chain-Ts and their conjugation procedures were performed, as described earlier (Jansen *et al.*,

1980, 1982; Sanofi *et al.*, 1978; Blythman *et al.*, 1981), but in pharmaceutically appropriate quantities. The A chain of the plant toxin ricin was obtained from 10 kg of castor beans in quantities of 10 g at a time. As described, (Jansen *et al.*, 1982) whole ricin was extracted and isolated by affinity on Sepharose gels. A chain was obtained by reduction and purified from B-chain contamination by affinity and ion-exchange chromatography and finally by immunoadsorption on anti-B-chain antibodies. Monoclonal antibodies were obtained and purified in quantities of several grams from mouse ascites, so that batches of 1–6 g of ITs could be produced and purified at once. A ratio of about two A chains per antibody and a yield of about 80% with respect to antibodies are reproducibly obtained. These quantities allowed an extensive toxicology study and are sufficient for the treatment of more than 1000 bone marrow grafts with the same batch of this I-A-chain-T.

2. Process Controls

In order to ensure the reproducibility of this IT, the raw materials of biological origin and the final products are extensively controlled by well-defined standard procedures, which have to be accessible to control institutions, such as the FDA. The ricin A chain is checked for its degree of purity by its isoelectric point and molecular weight, and for its activity and absence of slightest B-chain contaminations by methods of acellular and cellular protein synthesis and toxicity in mice. The monoclonal antibodies are also checked for molecular weight, isoelectric point, and especially their binding capacity on target cells. Besides these criteria, the final I-A-chain-T is characterized for the mean A chain per antibody ratio, the disulphide nature of the linkage, the content of free antibody, the antibody and toxin activities mentioned previously, and finally for the specific IT activities, as examined by dose–response, colony formation and kinetics studies. With the T101 IT, all antibody and A-chain activities were maintained after coupling.

3. Sterility Controls

The monoclonal antibodies are a product from animal tumor cells, hybridomas, also known to secret endogenous C-type viruses. Other type viruses may also be present in the animal or the hybridoma. Therefore, extensive controls are effected on the hybridoma cell line, the mouse ascites and the final IT products for 12 murine viruses: LCM virus, Reovirus I and III, polyoma virus, pneumonia virus, adenovirus virus, minute virus, hepatitis virus, ectromelia virus, sendai virus, GDV virus and

K virus. The presence of these viruses is detected by inoculation of the test products in mice and appearance of specific antibodies (MAP), or by specific cytopathic effects on sensitive cell lines. Retroviruses are detected by reverse-transcriptase measurements. Normal sterility controls also include all standard tests on fungi, mycoplasma and bacteria.

4. Stability

The activities of I-A-chain-Ts are very stable over more than 1 yr if the products are maintained at 4° in sterile solutions, although they may have a tendency to form small visible precipitates. This was avoided by lyophilizing ITs under optimal conditions concerning the concentration of the active principle, protein ballast, pH, sugar and ion content. After reconstitution they then remain clear without loss of activity for at least 1 week at 4°C.

III. CLINICAL VALUE OF I-A-CHAIN-Ts FOR THE *EX VIVO* TREATMENT OF HUMAN BONE MARROW

Well-selected I-A-chain-Ts, such as the T101 IT, were shown to be highly potent *in vitro* in the presence of the activator ammonium chloride. In contrast, their *in vivo* efficacy is still reduced since potentiating agents are not yet applicable. It appears, therefore, that to date the most promising clinical use of ITs may be the cleaning up of human bone marrow with respect to leukemia cells for autologous transplantation or of mature T cells for allogeneic transplantation. The optimal *in vitro* conditions for highest efficacy of IT without toxicity for stem cells are briefly mentioned as follows.

A. Toxicity towards Non-target Cells

The absence of toxicity of ITs towards bone marrow stem cells, which are needed to rescue leukemia patients' depleted marrow, is of great importance. However, the destruction of non-stem cells like mature T cells in the marrow with an anti-T cell IT, should have no major consequence, since new T cells can grow out from stem cells. The non-specific toxicity of ITs was determined in two complementary approaches: (1) on antigen negative cell lines; and (2) on bone marrow stem cells.

TABLE I

NON-SPECIFIC TOXICITY ON LEUKEMIA CELL LINES: PERCENTAGE OF COLONIES AFTER TREATMENT WITH T101 IT[a]

Immunotoxine/ target cells	Concentration of IT (A-chain) (M)			
	10^{-9}	10^{-8}	10^{-7}	10^{-6}
Anti-DNP/CEM	100	50	25	2
Anti-CEA/CEM	90	60	25	3
Anti-T-65/DAUDI	150	100	25	1.5
Anti-T-65/RAJI	100	100	70	7
Mean, colony formation	110–27	78–25	36–22	3–2.5

[a]Different ITs were incubated in increasing concentrations with corresponding antigen negative cells for 20 hr at 37°C in presence of 10 mM NH$_4$Cl. Cell colony formation was examined in assays with cloning efficiencies of 30–50%. After about 15 to 20 days of culture, colonies were counted with an automatic colony counter.

1. Toxicity on Unrelated Cell Lines

With three different I-A-chain-Ts potentiated by ammonium chloride (an anti-CEA, an anti-DNP and an anti-human T cell IT), the inhibition of colony formation was studied on different antigen negative cell lines in respect to the antibodies. The incubation was effected under the optimal conditions for IT efficacy on target cells, i.e., in the presence of the potentiator 10 mM ammonium chloride for 20 hr at 37°C and with increasing IT concentrations. An inhibition was only found for high concentrations, a slight toxicity with $10^{-8}M$ and a marked effect with $10^{-7}M$ concentrations (Table I). The similarity of the results with different I-A-chain-Ts indicates that the non-specific toxicity is mainly due to the A chain and much less to the antibody used.

2. Toxicity on Bone Marrow Stem Cells

A similar toxicity as with the cell lines was found on stem cells by Dr. A. A. Fauser, Freiburg, West Germany. Stem cell assays were carried out for colony-forming units, CFU-C and CFU-GEMM, with increasing concentrations of the T101 I-A-chain-T or free A chain on crude bone marrow on the one hand or Ficoll-Hypaque separated mononuclear cells on the other. In the presence of 10 mM NH$_4$Cl and after an incubation of 24 hr at 37°C, no toxicity was found with the T101 I-A-chain-T and only a minor effect with free A chain in concentrations up to $10^{-8}M$

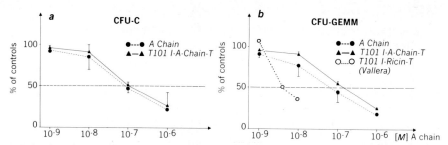

Fig. 3. Toxicity of T101 IT and A chain towards stem cells. CFU-C and CFU-GEMM colonies were determined by Dr. A. A. Fauser, Freiburg, West Germany, after incubation of normal unseparated marrow with increasing concentrations of IT or free A chain for 20 hr at 37°C and in the presence of 10 mM NH₄Cl. The toxicity of a T101-ricin-T in the CFU-GEMM assay is reproduced and adapted from Vallera *et al.* (1983).

(Fig. 3). As with the unrelated cell lines, toxicity only slowly increased with higher concentrations of both products. Complete inhibition of colony formation is only found with 100 times higher A-chain concentrations of more than 10^6 M.

Since the stem cell toxicity of IT is about the same as with free A chain, it depends essentially on the A-chain moiety. The incubation conditions do not increase the inherent A-chain toxicity since a diminution of the NH₄Cl concentration, a lower temperature of 25°C or a shorter incubation time of 8 hr have no influence. It can be concluded that at 10^{-8} M concentrations under the defined optimal conditions, there is no toxicity on stem cells, suggesting that the hematological recovery of patients rescued with an IT-treated marrow should not be diminished.

B. Efficiency against Leukemia Cells in Autologous Bone Marrow

Patients with radiosensitive or chemiosensitive tumors can be more effectively treated, if higher bone marrow toxic doses are employed. Such an aplasia must be rescued by bone marrow transplantation. Autologous bone marrow harvested in complete remission may, nevertheless, be contaminated by less than 5% residual leukemic cells, which should be eliminated before reinfusion in the patient to avoid a leukemia relapse by these cells. Several leukemia patients were treated with the J-5 anti-CALLA monoclonal antibody and rabbit complement, and encouraging results were obtained (Ritz *et al.*, 1982). Immuno-A-chain-toxins offer a promising alternative to this method.

Clinical proof for the efficacy in autologous bone marrow treatment will be difficult to obtain. Survival of treated patients probably depends more on radio- or chemioresistant cells within the high tumor burden in the body than on IT-resistant cells out of the much smaller quantity of contaminating leukemic cells in the bone marrow. Definitive evidence of the interest of *ex vivo* immunodepletion has to be obtained from selective comparative clinical trials. For T cell leukemias, these studies might take a long time because of the very low incidence of T-ALL.

1. Leukemia Cell Lines

The optimal conditions for elimination of a maximum of target cells in normal bone marrow were established with the T101 IT and a colony formation assay of CEM cells showing a cloning efficiency of about 50% (Casellas *et al.*, 1985). The specific activity of IT increased with its concentration up to 10^{-8} M. At higher concentrations, as described in Section III,A, non-specific toxicity was detected on unrelated cells and bone marrow stem cells. The 10 mM concentration of the potentiator ammonium chloride was without toxicity on different cell lines. The efficacy of IT was higher at 37°C than at 25° and slightly better after an incubation of 24 hr when compared to 8 hr. The presence of high concentrations of erythrocytes (hematocrit of 30%) did not influence the IT efficacy at all, while concentrations of 2×10^{11}/liter nucleated bone marrow cells diminished its activity considerably (Casellas *et al.*, 1985). However, normal concentrations of nucleated cells in the bone marrow (up to 2×10^{10}/liter) show no detectable inhibitory effect on the efficacy of IT.

The following optimal conditions were selected for maximum activity of IT without toxicity on bone marrow stem cells and were accepted for clinical pilot studies: an incubation of 24 hr at 37°C with 10^{-8} M IT, 10 mM NH_4Cl and a concentration of nucleated bone marrow cells not exceeding 2×10^{10} cells/liter, which corresponds approximately to a normal bone marrow. Under these conditions, the T101 IT has a cytoreduction capacity of more than 4 logs on uncloned CEM cells (Fig. 4) and more than 6 logs on recloned CEM cells.

In about 1 liter of remission bone marrow with less than 5% of contaminating leukemia cells, a maximum of 10^9 leukemic cells could be expected. Despite the potency of IT, with cytoreduction of about 4 logs, on uncloned cells a maximum of 10^5 cells may potentially escape the IT treatment and become a possible source of recurrence.

The apparent limitation of cytoreduction to about 4 logs on uncloned cells can, however, not be attributed to IT itself but to the heterogeneity of the targets with about 0.01% antigen negative cells. This was proven

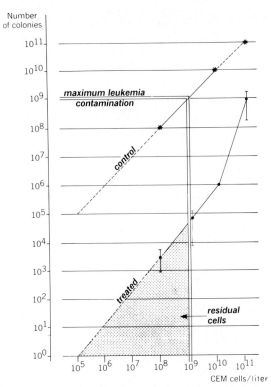

Fig. 4. Cytoreduction of a T leukemia cell line by the T101 I-A-chain-T. After incubation of increasing concentrations of CEM target cells (10^8–10^{11} cells/liter) which were mixed with a constant concentration of 10^{10} nucleated bone marrow cells/liter, the number of clonogenic cells was established in a colony-forming assay of CEM cells. High numbers of colonies were calculated from dilution curves. The maximum contamination of leukemia cells in remission marrows was estimated at 5% and therefore corresponds to about 10^9 cells/liter.

by the fact that escaping clones were insensitive to IT, even after several weeks of culture, and unable to bind it. If the heterogeneity was reduced by repeated cloning of target cells, the same IT achieved a cytoreduction of more than 6 logs, which corresponded to the maximum sensitivity of our method.

In order to circumvent the limitation due to the heterogeneity of the target cells, a cocktail of different ITs was used (the T101 IT and the 3E10 IT anti-HLA-β-microglobulin complex). Thus, on the non-cloned initial cell line, a cytoreduction of more than 6 logs was also achieved. Similar cocktails with ITs specific for different T cell markers are now in preparation for clinical trials.

The feasibility of the elimination of leukemic cells from bone marrow was also shown in animal studies (Thorpe *et al.*, 1982; Krolick *et al.*, 1983).

2. Fresh Leukemia Cells

The activity of I-A-chain-Ts on an individual leukemia is not predictable. The presence of a threshold quantity of antigens is necessary but not sufficient. The heterogeneous distribution of this antigen on individual cells is a second factor beside others (metabolic state . . .). It therefore becomes necessary to measure inidividual leukemias for sensitivity to the various available ITs. By analogy with an antibiogram, this test could be called an "immunotoxogram," and would allow the selection of the most appropriate ITs for each leukemia patient.

The usual test systems for ITs are not appropriate to measure the sensitivity of fresh leukemic cells. Clonogenic assays of fresh cells take a long time to be evaluated and have a very low cloning efficiency. Thus, the selected subclones may no longer be representative of the whole population. Fresh cells are difficult to maintain in culture and in general do not incorporate sufficient leucine to be examined for an inhibition of protein synthesis. Therefore, a short-term cytotoxicity assay was established, which is based on cytofluorometric enumeration of viable (propidium iodine-excluding) cells after a 24-hr incubation with IT and NH_4Cl. This method does not, however, give an absolute evaluation of the cytoreduction but more an estimation of the sensitivity of cells to an IT. Part of the cells inhibited from protein synthesis are still unable to incorporate propidium iodine during the 24-hr assay. However, because of the long kinetics of the membrane destruction phase, a correlation could be established between the percentage of dye-excluding cells and the cytoreduction in a clonogenic assay with several CEM cell lines known to display different sensitivity to the T101 IT (Table II). By comparison with well-characterized established cell lines, this test can indicate a relative sensitivity of fresh leukemia cells to various ITs.

A more simple adaptation of the cytofluorometric method for the use with a fluorescent microscope using the same dyes showed very similar results, so that this assay can now easily be established in a clinical laboratory. First results on eight fresh ALL leukemias showed that the sensitivity to T101 IT is quite variable, ranging from 15 to 92% surviving cells. This is not really unexpected, since the quantity of the T1 (65 kDa) antigen is highly variable from one ALL to another (Royston *et al.*, 1985). It remains hazardous to draw definitive conclusions concerning the re-

TABLE II

COMPARISON OF THE DYE EXCLUSION TEST WITH THE COLONY FORMATION AND THE ASSAY OF PROTEIN SYNTHESIS INHIBITION[a]

Cell lines	Dye exclusion (FACS), (% viable cells)	Clonogenic assay, reduction of clone number (log)	Protein synthesis inhibition, kinetics (T10)
CEM 0.5	66.0	<1	18 H
CEM 5	45.7	~2	8 H
CEM 1	30.0	~4	5 H
CEM 44	18.3	~5	3,5 H

[a] 20 hr after standard treatment (see Section III,B,1 of four different CEM clones, viable cells were measured by propidium iodine exclusion with a FACS cell sorter. Colony formation assays were performed in parallel under standard conditions with the same clones. For the protein synthesis inhibition the time interval was measured at which leucine uptake by intact cells was reduced to 10%. The clones are: CEM 1 with 20,000 antigents per cell and CEM 0.5, CEM 5 and CEM 44 clones bearing 500, 5,000 or 44,000 antigens per cell, respectively.

lationship between sensitivity to various ITs in this test and clinical efficiency, since the dye exclusion is not the best approach for evaluation of IT efficacy. However, this assay might allow the detection of nonreactive leukemias.

C. Efficiency against T Lymphocytes in Allogeneic Bone Marrow

Allogeneic bone marrow transplantation has been found to be a highly promising approach in the curative treatment of high-risk forms of acute leukemia. Nevertheless it is limited by the need for fully matched siblings, only available in about 35% of cases (O'Reilly, 1983). A principal obstacle to this approach is acute GvHD which leads to a morbidity of 30–70% and an indirect mortality in about 25% of affected patients (O'Reilly, 1983). Although the precise mechanism of acute GvHD remains unclear, it is generally accepted that engrafted alloreactive T lymphocytes initiate this process (O'Reilly, 1983). Therefore, different methods have been employed to deplete allogeneic bone marrow of mature T cells in order to prevent GvHD.

1. Present State of T Lymphocyte Depletion

A depletion of T lymphocytes by agglutination with soy bean lectins followed by sheep erythrocyte rosette formation (Reisner *et al.*, 1983) or rosette formation alone (Filipovich *et al.*, 1983) inhibited the appearance of acute GvHD in haploidentical transplants. Coating of T cells with monoclonal antibodies without complement had no effect on the appearance of acute GvHD (Filipovich *et al.*, 1982; Prentice *et al.*, 1982). However, if xenogeneic complement with complement-fixing monoclonal antibodies was used, moderate to severe grades of acute GvHD could be completely inhibited (Prentice *et al.*, 1984).

Immunotoxins against Thy-1.2 on murine lymphocytes assembled with the whole toxin ricin were used for *in vitro* depletion of murine bone marrow and protected about 85% of recipients from lethal GvHD over a major histocompatibility barrier (Vallera *et al.*, 1982). A cocktail of three different I-ricin-toxins was recently employed to eliminate T cells from allogeneic human bone marrow. In two patients treated with the I-ricin-T *in vitro*, the transplants showed prompt peripheral engraftment and no GvHD could be detected (Filipovich *et al.*, 1984). The use of I-A-chain-ITs for T cell depletion is also under clinical study.

2. Efficacy of an I-A-chain-T on T Lymphocytes

We tried to define a precise method of evaluating T101 IT-induced T cell immunodepletion. Functional tests using various mitogens, such as PHA or MLC assays, have been extensively used in several studies (Filipovich *et al.*, 1982; Vallera *et al.*, 1983) and showed a complete inhibition of T cell response after the treatment with a cocktail of I-ricin-Ts against human T cells. Similar results have been found in experiments using the T101 I-A-chain-T (Fig. 5). Nevertheless, these tests do not provide a precise evaluation in terms of cytoreduction. Accurate evaluation of cell-killing efficiency still appears essential to predict a favorable clinical response, since a very low percentage of residual T cells is sufficient to induce a high incidence of GvHD (Korngold and Sprent, 1978). Therefore, a more sensitive T cell growth assay was established to evaluate the IT efficacy. After an incubation with the T101 IT under the defined optimal conditions, normal bone marrow or PBL were cultured in the presence of PHA and T cell growth factor (TCGF) for 3–8 days. The number of viable T cells was evaluated with fluorescent T cell markers by cytofluorometry in comparison to untreated controls (Poncelet *et al.*, 1985). This test system is highly specific and sensitive for T cells, since it com-

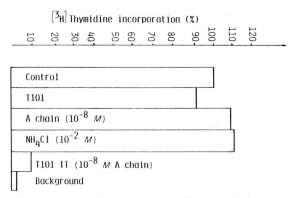

Fig. 5. Inhibition of the PHA response by T101 IT. Peripheral blood lymphocytes were incubated with the T101 IT 24 hr at $10^{-8}M$ and 37°C in presence of 10 mM NH$_4$Cl. After washing they were plated with PHA in microwells. On day 3 they were pulsed overnight with [^{3}H]thymidine and compared for thymidine incorporation with different controls.

bines the specific characterization by T cell markers with the amplification provided by T cell growth induced by specific growth factors (Fig. 6). The T101 IT showed a cytoreduction of almost 99–99.9% in this system. These results were confirmed with a limiting dilution assay after incubation with IT and culture of T cells with TCGF and PHA.

At present, clinical studies are being carried out in several clinics to find out if the cytoreduction of 2 to 3 logs of mature T cells by IT sufficiently inhibits GvHD in fully matched siblings. I-A-chain-Ts showing an efficiency equal to I-ricin-Ts or antibodies with complement, have more practical advantages in clinical use than the other methods, as already described.

IV. POTENTIAL VALUE OF I-A-CHAIN-Ts *IN VIVO*

Since toxicological studies confirmed that I-A-chain-Ts in the doses used (about 2 mg/liter) are completely non-toxic *in vivo*, they are infused with the treated marrow into the patient. It might, therefore, be expected that I-A-chain-Ts have some therapeutic effect *in vivo*, under conditions where the tumor burden is low. Residual leukemia resembles the tumor burden of the experimental conditions in the mouse where ITs showed some effect. In established leukemia, however, an effect could only be expected if I-A-chain-Ts can be potentiated *in vivo* also.

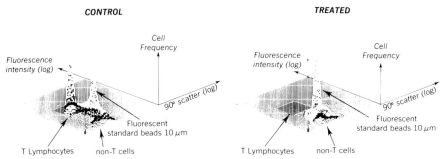

Fig. 6. Growth of T lymphocytes after treatment of normal bone marrow with the T101 I-A-chain-T. After incubation of normal human bone marrow with the IT at $10^{-8}M$ for 20 hr at 37°C in presence of 10 mM NH_4Cl, the marrow was washed and cultured with PHA and TCGF for 6 days. The number of T lymphocytes was analyzed by cytofluorometry and indirect fluorescence with a coctail of anti-T cell monoclonal antibodies directed against T11, T3, T4, T8 and T1. The absolute number of T cells was calculated with respect to non-fluorescent beads introduced for this reason prior to FACS analysis.

A. Toxicity of I-A-chain-Ts

In a first approach, acute and subacute toxicity of the T101 IT was studied in three animal species and thereafter in a clinical phase I pilot study on leukemia patients (Gorin *et al.*, 1984, 1985).

1. Animal Studies

Toxicology studies with the T101 IT were performed on CD1 mice, Sprague-Dawley rats and macaca fascicularis monkeys according to the NCI recommendations for anti-cancer drugs (Report on Anticancer Drugs, 1982). LD_{50} values were obtained with relatively high doses of IT ranging from 20 to 28 mg/kg iv for male and female mice, respectively ($N = 10$ per sex) and more than 44 mg/kg iv for male and female rats ($N = 10$ per sex). In both species renal tubular lesions were a dominant histopathological finding.

In a 1-day toxicity study in rats and macaques, only high doses of 10 mg/kg iv induced transient toxic effects on liver and kidney, which were completely reversible (Table IIIA) A 5-day toxicity study (Table IIIB) of the same IT revealed an accumulative toxicity. Doses of 5 × 2 mg/kg iv induced inconstant and minor focal myocarditis in rats, minor accumulation of lipopigments in hepatocytes and mesentric lymph nodes and early minimal tubulopathy in *Macaca fascicularis*. Dose levels of 5 × 0.2 mg/kg, iv and 5 × 2 mg/kg iv induced minor reaction at the

TABLE III

TOXICOLOGY OF THE T101 IT AFTER SINGLE OR REPEATED (FIVE TIMES) ADMINISTRATION IN RATS AND MONKEYS

Animal species	Dose level (mg/kg iv)			Recovery (weeks)
	0.1	1	10	
1-Day toxicity study				
CD (SR) BR Rats	N.A.D.	N.A.D.	(BUN)	4
Macaca fascicularis			(BUN creatinine) (GOT, LDH, APTT trombine time)	1
	5 × 0.02	5 × 0.02	5 × 2	
5-Day toxicity study				
CD (SR) BR Rats	N.A.D.	Moderate polysynovitis	Moderate polysynovitis Focal myocarditis	6
Macaca fascicularis	N.A.D.	N.A.D.	Minimal tubulopathy Lipid accumulation in hepatocytes and mesenteric lymph nodes	6

injection sites and subacute polysynovitis in rats. All these lesions were reversible.

A single dose of 1 mg/kg iv is safe in rats and macaques. The cumulative safe dose of five daily administrations in the *Macaca fascicularis* is similar to the single dose (5 × 0.2 mg/kg iv). In the rat the cumulative safe dose is inferior to it, but superior to 5 × 0.02 mg/kg iv. The comparison between the non-toxic and the therapeutic doses show a good safety margin.

However, a toxicity due to cross reactivity of the T101 IT with normal T cells could not be evaluated in animals, since this epitope is not expressed on their lymphocytes. In highly irradiated human transplant recipients, no T cells are left for at least 2 weeks, so that this toxicity becomes non-existent. No other cross reactivity of the T101 antibody with other human organs could be detected with a highly sensitive immunoperoxidase staining method assuring the safety of the T101 IT for clinical trials.

2. Clinical Tolerance (Phase I Study)

In a phase I pilot study, the clinical tolerance of the treatment of autologous bone marrow with the T101 IT was studied on four patients with T cell malignancies (Gorin *et al.*, 1985). Three of them had a lymphoblastic lymphoma of stage 3 or 4 and one patient an ALL. Two of the lymphoma patients were in first remission, the third in recurrence under the diaphragm and the ALL patient in a second remission when treated with autologous bone marrow transplantation.

About 1 liter of fresh remission marrow of each patient was distributed in fractions of 100 ml and immediately treated without any cell separation with IT at 37°C under continuous gentle shaking by see-saw movements. The concentration of IT was $10^{-9}M$ (0.2 mg/liter) for the first two and $10^{-8}M$ (2 mg/liter) for the last two patients. The incubation time was increased from 4 hr for the first patient to 20 hr for the others. After treatment the bone marrow fractions were frozen and stored in the standard way (Gorin et al., 1985).

During and after the infusion of the autologous marrow containing up to 2 mg of the I-A-chain-T, no secondary reactions were observed which could be related to the IT treatment. The hematological recovery was also entirely satisfactory, since engraftment in the periphery took place within normal delays: 10^9 leukocytes/liter within 15–31 days; 5×10^8 polynuclear cells/liter within 23–32 days; >0.1 % reticulocytes within 14–26 days; 50×10^9 platelets/liter within 22–47 days and 10^9 lymphocytes/liter within 22–96 days (Gorin et al., 1985).

After complete engraftment two patients underwent viral infections, one of them after a hepatic veno-oclusion. Both died about 4–5 months after the treatment. Another patient, alive 8 months after treatment, showed recurrence under the diaphragm, while the fourth patient is still in complete remission 6 months after transplant.

In conclusion, the T101 IT was not toxic to stem cells in vitro, since there was no inhibition of the hematological reconstitution. The IT is also well tolerated after infusion into the patient, as expected from toxicology. Because of the two infections, however, futher study is needed to determine whether this IT, directed against T cells, has an inhibitory effect on the normal reconstitution of immune functions.

B. *In Vivo* Efficiency

1. Experimental Animals

In two mouse leukemia models, therapeutic effects were obtained with I-A-chain-Ts: WEHI-7 leukemia (2.4×10^5 ip) and an IgM (mouse) anti-Thy-1.2 IT or a virus-induced T2 leukemia (5×10^5 ip) with an IgG_{2a} (rat) anti-Thy-1.2 IT (Blythman et al., 1985). In the latter model, 50% of treated animals definitely survived more than 150 days, while antibody-treated animals showed no long-term survival—only a slight prolongation

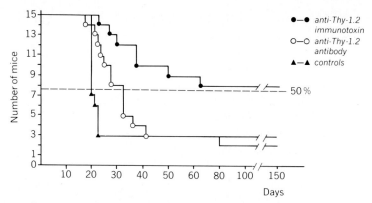

Fig. 7. *In vivo* treatment of a mouse leukemia with an I-A-chain-T. BL.1.1 mice (Thy-1.2 neg.) were injected ip with 5×10^6 T2 leukemia cells and then treated ip during 3 days with a total of 200 μg of an anti-Thy-1.2 IT (IgG from rat, AT 15 E). Survival was established for IT, antibody-treated mice or for untreated controls.

of the median survival time from 20 days in controls to 32 days (Fig. 7). Better results were obtained if the leukemia cells were given intravenously leading to 80% survival on day 72, whereas all controls were dead on day 22 and all antibody-treated mice on day 35.

Significant but less impressive results were obtained with the human T-leukemia cell line Ichikawa in nude mice by ip injection of 2×10^7 leukemia cells and the T101 IT ip during 8 days. A prolongation of the median survival time from 35 days in controls or antibody-treated mice to 50 days in experimental groups was achieved. With the same leukemia model, better results were obtained after iv injection of cells and of the IT 1 day later. In this case about 40% of animals definitely survived until day 220 as compared to only 10% of the antibody-treated animals and none of the controls.

Similar *in vivo* results were also obtained with a mouse mammary carcinoma (Seto *et al.*, 1982) or a murine B cell tumor (Krolick *et al.*, 1982). Immuno-A-chain-toxins therefore showed a significant therapeutic effect, but only if the tumor burden was at the inferior limit, which just allowed tumor take in all animals. With much higher tumor burden comparable to clinical situations, no significant therapeutic effect could be obtained.

2. Clinical Value

To date no results are available to suggest a therapeutic effect of I-A-chain-Ts on residual leukemias. But the small quantity of residual leukemia cells after supralethal treatment resembles the limited tumor burden in the mouse experiments. From the phase I pilot study, no information on IT efficacy can be drawn since the patients were only selected for the presence of T cell markers on their leukemic cells and not for sensitivity to this I-A-chain-T, which varies to some degree in fresh leukemia cells. A phase II study for IT efficacy will be undertaken in the near future with ITs, selected by immunotoxograms for individual leukemias.

V. FUTURE DEVELOPMENTS

The diversification of ITs directed against different antigens of the same target cell is a major objective for the future. Since leukemia cells are heterogeneous, some cells with an insufficient antigen density will escape to a single IT. With a cocktail of ITs with different specificities, no cell clone should escape. A cocktail of three I-ricin-Ts was revealed as superior to the individual ITs for the destruction of T cells (Vallera *et al.*, 1983). Similar cocktails of I-A-chain-Ts are under study for clinical use.

Another tendency of the IT research at present concerns the potentiation of I-A-chain-Ts *in vivo*. The *in vitro* potentiation of the T101 IT with ammonium chloride is already in clinical use (Gorin *et al.*, 1985). Other possibilities of potentiating ITs *in vitro* by B chains are being studied by different groups (Thorpe *et al.*, 1984; Youle and Neville, 1982; Vitetta *et al.*, 1983) but the transposition of the *in vitro* results to *in vivo* experiments remains a major problem to date. Immuno-A-chain-toxins will only become effective on patients with an established tumor, if a clinically useful way of potentiation is found. The most promising clinical model to start an *in vivo* treatment would be the residual leukemia after supralethal treatment and bone marrow transplantation, since the tumor burden is then reduced to a minimum.

VI. CONCLUSIONS

Immuno-A-chain-toxins were pharmaceutically developed and are now being examined in clinical trials for toxicity and efficacy in autologous or allogeneic bone marrow transplantations after supralethal treatment of leukemia or lymphoma patients. Under optimal conditions, I-A-chain-

Ts are highly potent since the T101 IT alone can achieve a cytoreduction of an established leukemia cell line mixed with normal bone marrow of more than 4–6 logs. On mature T cells, cytoreduction achieves 2–3 logs. A combination of several ITs is even more promising. Under defined optimal conditions, bone marrow stem cells are not at all affected, as evaluated by CFU-GEMM assays, and showed prompt peripheral engraftment.

The future will determine whether ITs are more potent than the other methods, i.e., antibodies plus complement, rosette formation or antibodies insolubilized on magnetic or other beads. In any case, they have some practical advantages over these methods since no manipulation of the marrow is needed. The I-A-chain-Ts are injected into the crude marrow, incubated for 20 hr at 37°C and injected with the marrow into the patient. The clinical tolerance to the T101 I-A-chain-T was highly satisfactory, since peripheral engraftment was achieved in normal delays. Besides the practical advantages of the IT treatment, there may be a therapeutic effect on the residual leukemic cells *in vivo*, as suggested by animal experiments. Higher tumor burden, however, would necessitate the potentiation of I-A-chain-Ts *in vivo* in similar ways as already obtained *in vitro*. This might be possible in the near future.

REFERENCES

Bast, R. C., Jr., de Fabristis, P., Maver, C., Lipton, J., Ritz, J., Nadler, L., Sallan, S., Nathan, D. G., and Schlossman, S. F. (1983a). *Cancer Res.* (Abstract) p. 223.

Bast, R. C., Jr., Ritz, J., Maver, P., Lipton, J. M., Feeney, S. E., Sallan, S. E., Nathan, D. G., and Schlossman, S. F. (1983b). *Cancer Res.* **43,** 1389.

Blythman, H. E., Casellas, P., Gros, O., Gros, P., Jansen, F. K., Paolucci, F., Pau, B., and Vidal, H. (1981). *Nature (London)* **290,** 145.

Blythman, H. E., Bord, A., Buisson, I., Jansen, F. K., Richer, G., and Thurneyssen, O. (1984). *Protides Biol. Fluids* **32,** 421–424.

Carrière, D., Casellas, P., Richer, G., Gros, P., and Jansen, F. K. (1985). *Exp. Cell Res.* **156,** 327–340.

Casellas, P., Blythman, H. E., Gros, P., Richer, G., and Jansen, F. K. (1982a). *Protides Biol. Fluids* **30,** 359.

Casellas, P., Brown, J. P., Gros, O., Hellström, I., Jansen, F. K., Poncelet, P., Roncucci, R., Vidal, H., and Hellström, K. E. (1982b). *Int. J. Cancer* **30,** 437.

Casellas, P., Carrière, D., Gros, O., Laurent, J. C., Poncelet, P., and Jansen, F. K. (1984a). *In* "Bacterial Protein Toxins" (J. E. Alouf, F. Fehrenbach, and H. Freer, eds.), pp. 227–234. Academic Press, New York.

Casellas, P., Bourrie, B. J. P., Gros, P., and Jansen, F. K. (1984b). *J. Biol. Chem.* **259,** 9359–9364.

Casellas, P., Canat, X., Gros, O., Poncelet, P., and Jansen, F. K. (1985). *Blood* **65,** 289–297.

Filipovich, A. H., McGlave, P. B., Ramsay, N. K. C., Goldstein, G., Warkentin, P. I., and Kersey, J. H. (1982). *Lancet* **2,** 1266.

Filipovich, A. H., Ramsay, N. K. C., and McGlave, P. (1983). *In* "Recent Advances in Bone Marrow Transplantation" (R. P. Gale, ed.), p. 769. Alan R. Liss, Inc., New York.

Filipovich, A. H., Vallera, D. A., Youle, R. J., Quinones, R. R., Neville, D. M., Jr., and Kersey, J. H. (1984). *Lancet* **1,** 469.

Gilliland, D. G., Steplewski, Z., Collier, R. J., Mitchell, K. F., Chang, T. H., and Koprowski, H. (1980). *Proc. Natl. Acad. Sci. U.S.A.* **77,** 4539.

Gorin, N. C., Douay, L., Laporte, J. P., Zittoum, R., Rio, B, Jansen, F. K., Casellas, P., Poncelet, P., Liance, Voisin, G. A., M. C., Lopez, M., Salmon, C., Le Blanc, G., Deloux, J., David, R., Stachowiak, J., Najma, A., and Duhamel, G. (1985). *Can. Treat. Rep.* (in press).

Gros, O., Casellas, P., Leonard, J., Royston, I., and Jansen, F. K. (1984). *In* "Bacterial Protein Toxins" (J. E. Alouf, F. Fehrenbach, and H. Freer, eds.), p. 269. Academic Press, New York.

Jansen, F. K., Blythman, H. E., Carrière, D., Casellas, P., Diaz, J., Gros, P., Hennequin, J. R., Paolucci, F., Pau, B., Poncelet, P., Richer, G., Salhi, S. L., Vidal, H., and Voisin, G. A. (1980). *Immunol. Lett.* **2,** 97.

Jansen, F. K., Blythman, H. E., Carrière, D., Casellas, P., Gros, P., Paolucci, F., Pau, B., Poncelet, P., Richer, G., Vidal, H., and Voisin, G. A. (1981). *In* "Monoclonal Antibodies and T-Cell Hybridomas" (G. J. Hämmerling, U. Hämmerling and J. F. Kearney, eds.), p. 229. Elsevier/North-Holland, Amsterdam.

Jansen, F. K., Blythman, H. E., Carrière, D., Casellas, P., Gros, O., Laurent, J. C., Paolucci, F., Pau, B., Poncelet, P., Richer, G., Vidal, H., and Voisin, G. A. (1982). *Immunol. Rev.* **62,** 182.

Korngold, R., and Sprent, I. (1978). *J. Exp. Med.* **148,** 1637.

Krolick, K. A., Villemez, C., Isakson, P., Uhr, J. W., and Vitetta, E. S. (1980). *Proc. Natl. Acad. Sci. U.S.A.* **77,** 5419.

Krolick, K. A., Uhr, J. W., Slavin, S., and Vitetta, E. S. (1982). *J. Exp. Med.* **155,** 1797.

Krolick, K. A., Uhr, J. W., and Vitetta, E. S. (1983). *Nature (London)* **295,** 604.

Masuho, Y., and Hara, T. (1980). *Gann* **71,** 759.

Miyazaki, H., Beppu, M., Terao, T., and Osawa, T. (1980). *Gann* **71,** 766.

Möller, G. (1982). *Immunol. Rev.* **62,** 1–216.

Moolten, F. L., and Cooperband, S. R. (1970). *Science* **169,** 68.

Olsnes, S., and Pihl, A. (1980). *In* "The Molecular Actions of Toxins and Viruses" (P. Cohen and S. V. Heyningen, eds.), pp. 51–105. Elsevier/North-Holland, Amsterdam.

O'Reilly, R. J. (1983). *Blood* **62,** 941.

Poncelet, P., and Carayon, P. (1985). *J. Immunol. Methods* (in press).

Prentice, H. G., Blacklock, H. A., Janossy, G., Bradstock, K. F., Skeggs, D., Goldstein, G., and Hoffbrand, A. V. (1982). *Lancet* **1,** 700.

Prentice, H. G., Blacklock, H. A., Janossy, G., Gilmore, M. J. M. L., Price-Jones, L., Tidman, N., Trejdosiewicz, L. K., Skeggs, D. B. L., Panjwani, D., Ball, S., Graphakos, S., Patterson, J., Ivory, K., and Hoffbrand, A. V. (1984). *Lancet* **1,** 472.

Raso, V., and Griffin, T. (1980). *J. Immunol.* **125,** 2610.

Reisner, Y., Kappor, N., Kirkpatrick, P., Pollack, M. S., Cunningham-Rundles, S., Dupont, B., Hodes, M. Z., Good, R. A., O'Reilly, R. J. (1983). *Blood* **61,** 341.

Report on Anticancer Drugs (1982). *Natl. Cancer Inst. Monogr.* **01/82,** 19–30.

Ritz, J., Sallan, S. E., Bast, R. C., Jr., Lipton, J. M., Clavell, L. A., Feeney, M., Hercend, T., Nathan, D. G., Schlossman, S. F. (1982). *Lancet* **2**, 60.

Royston, I., Majda, J. A., Baird, S. M., Meserve, B. L., and Griffiths, J. C. (1980). *J. Immunol.* **125**, 725.

Seto, M., Umemoto, N., Saito, M., Masuho, Y., Hara, T., and Takahashi, T. (1982). *Cancer Res.* **42**, 5209.

Sanofi, S. A., Jansen, F. K., Gros, P., and Voisin, G. A. (1978). French patent no. 2,437,213.

Sobol, R. E., Royston, I., LeBien, T. W., Minowada, J., Anderson, K., Davey, F. R., Cuttner, J., Schiffer, C., Ellison, R. R., and Bloomfield, C. D. (1985). *Blood* **65**, 730–735.

Thorpe, P. E., Ross, W. C. J., Cumber, A. J., Hinson, C. A., Edwards, D. C., and Davies A. J. S. (1978). *Nature (London)* **271**, 752.

Thorpe, P. E., Mason, D. W., Brown, A. N. F., Simmonds, S. J., Ross, W. C. J., Cumber, A. J., and Forrester, J. A. (1982). *Nature (London)* **297**, 594.

Thorpe, P. E., Ross, W. C. J., Brown, A. N. F., Myers, C. D., Cumber, A. J., Foxwell, B. M. J., and Forrester, J. T. (1984). *Eur. J. Biochem.* **140**, 63.

Treleaven, J. G., Ugelstad, J., Philip, T., Gibson, F. M., Rembaum, A., Caine, G. D., and Kemshead, J. R. (1984). *Lancet* **1**, 70.

Vallera, D. A., Youle, R. J., Neville, D. M., and Kersey, J. H. (1982). *J. Exp. Med.* **155**, 949.

Vallera, D. A., Ash, R. C., Zanjani, E. D., Kersey, J. H., Lebien, T. W., Beverley, P. C. L., Neville, D. M., and Youle, R. J. (1983). *Science* **222**, 512.

Vitetta, E. S., Cushley, W., and Uhr, J. W. (1983). *Proc. Natl. Acad. Sci. U.S.A.* **80**, 6332.

Youle, R. J., and Neville, D. M. (1980). *Proc. Natl. Acad. Sci. U.S.A.* **77**, 5483.

Youle, R. J., and Neville, D. M. (1982). *J. Biol. Chem.* **257**, 1598.

CHAPTER 12

The Use of Immunotoxins to Eliminate Tumour Cells from Human Leukaemic Marrow Autografts

Chris Myers[1]

Membrane Immunology Laboratory
Imperial Cancer Research Fund
London, United Kingdom

[1] Present address: Department of Microbiology, University of Texas Health Science Center at Dallas, Dallas, Texas 75235, U.S.A.

I. INTRODUCTION

In a substantial proportion of leukaemia patients, conventional chemotherapy and radiotherapy fail to induce long-term remissions. This has led to a search for new treatments that augment traditional therapy. One such regimen involves increased doses of chemotherapy and radiotherapy followed by bone marrow transplantation. Since the tissue most susceptible to damage by many of the therapeutic agents currently used is the bone marrow, removal and preservation of the marrow before therapy allows higher doses of therapeutic agents to be given to the patient. The increases in drug levels may not be large, but they have proved sufficient to give a major improvement in the survival of patients whose leukaemias can be brought into remission by conventional therapy (Santos and Kaiser, 1982).

There are two approaches to bone marrow transplantation. In autologous transplantation, a patient's marrow is removed and then returned after the treatment. In allogeneic transplantation, the marrow is first ablated with high doses of drugs or irradiation and is then replaced with marrow from a suitable donor.

Most patients do not have an identical twin or immunologically matched sibling to provide bone marrow for transplantation so that partially matched marrow is often used for allogeneic transplantation. This can result in life threatening graft versus host disease (GvHD). Various procedures are currently being tested for the prevention of GvHD in MHC-matched and mismatched transplant recipients. One approach is the use of immunosuppressive drugs, e.g., cyclosporin A (Powles *et al.*, 1980). Another approach is to remove alloreactive T cells from the donor marrow in order to avoid GvHD in the recipient. Removal of T cells can be achieved by rosetting (Filipovitch *et al.*, 1983), complement-mediated cytotoxicity using monoclonal antibodies (Prentice *et al.*, 1984) or monoclonal antibodies coupled to toxins (immunotoxins) (Filipovitch *et al.*, 1984). Each of these methods appears to be very effective at removing T cells from the donor marrow and early clinical trials show a marked reduction in the incidence of acute GvHD. However, it is not yet clear whether the T lymphocytes that emerge from haematopoietic stem cells in the donor marrow will cause chronic GvHD.

Autologous bone marrow transplantation eliminates the problem of GvHD and is the regimen of choice for tumour-bearing patients in which bone marrow involvement is absent or limited (Spitzer *et al.*, 1980). However, its application to leukaemia and lymphoma has been hindered by the need to purge the marrow of infiltrating tumour cells. Any procedure for removing the malignant cells must satisfy two criteria: (1) All clonogenic tumour cells must be removed from the graft; and (2) the reconstituting capacity of the marrow should remain unimpaired. Most procedures which meet these criteria depend upon specific antibodies which recognize antigens present on the tumour cells but not the hae-matopoietic stem cells. They include complement-mediated cytotoxicity (Ritz *et al.*, 1982; LeBien *et al.*, 1983), targeting of drugs (O'Neill, 1979) and toxins (Krolick *et al.*, 1982; Thorpe *et al.*, 1982; Mason *et al.*, 1982; Muirhead *et al.*, 1983) and, most recently, binding of paramagnetic sub-stances to the antibody to enable the tumour cells to be withdrawn in a magnetic field (Poynton *et al.*, 1983; Treleaven *et al.*, 1984). In the present chapter, we describe the experimental use of a conjugate of the mono-clonal antibody, WT-1, and the ribosome-damaging A chain of the plant toxin, ricin, to delete leukaemia cells from bone marrow. Our decision to use an immunotoxin in preference to the other procedures was prompted by their inherent stability, reproducible toxicity and lack of batch-to-batch variability that can occur with complement.

II. THE DISEASE

Thymic acute lymphoblastic leukaemia (T-ALL) has a very poor prog-nosis both in adults and children (Chessells, 1982) although the recent Berlin–Frankfurt–Munster study (Riehm *et al.*, 1983) reports improved prognosis in children subjected to extremely aggressive therapy. T-ALL is thought to originate in the thymus but invariably presents with a high level of peripheral blood infiltration which in itself is a poor prognostic factor (Greaves *et al.*, 1981). The initial response of T-ALL to chemo-therapy is usually very good and remissions are obtained in the majority of cases. With maintenance chemotherapy, initial remissions can last up to 1 yr. Second remissions rarely exceed 6 months. The poor prognosis of this disease combined with the excellent initial responsiveness to chemotherapy make T-ALL a good candidate for early treatment by au-tologous bone marrow transplantation.

III. THE WT-1 ANTIBODY

The monoclonal IgG_{2a} antibody, WT-1, recognizes a human T lineage antigen (M_r 40,000) that is strongly expressed on thymic T blasts and on

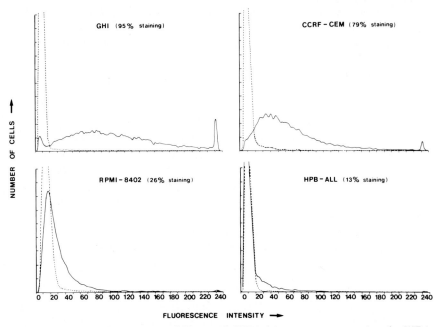

Fig. 1. Reactivity of four T-ALL cell lines with WT-1: histograms representing the WT-1 staining of the four T-ALL cell lines studied. Solid lines represent the WT-1 fluorescence profile and dotted lines the negative control. Figures in parenthesis are the percentages of cells staining more brightly than the control. (From Myers *et al.*, 1984.)

peripheral T cells activated by phytohaemagglutinin, and more weakly on cortical thymocytes and resting peripheral T cells (Tax *et al.*, 1984). WT-1 and other monoclonals with similar specificities (e.g., 3A1, Haynes, 1981; 4A, Morishima *et al.*, 1982) represent the best diagnostic reagents for T-ALL currently available. In a study of 906 miscellaneous fresh leukaemia samples, Vodinelich *et al.* (1983) showed WT-1 to be highly selective for T-ALL. All 80 cases of T-ALL tested were reactive with WT-1, whereas cells from other acute lymphoid leukaemias showed no reactivity. Twenty-four cases of acute lymphoid leukaemia of uncertain phenotype were also tested. Eighteen were reactive with WT-1 and, of these, 14 had at least one other clinical or haematological marker suggestive of T cell leukaemia. None of the six WT-1-unreactive leukaemias in this group displayed other T cell markers. Of the chronic lymphoid leukaemias, only T cell diseases showed reactivity with WT-1. However, in these diseases, not all cases (15 of 19) were reactive and only 30–60% of the leukaemic cells in any individual patient bore the WT-1 antigen. Myeloid leukaemias showed occasional reactivity with WT-1 and staining was seen with 16 of 245 acute myeloid leukaemias, 2 of 7 magakaryoblastic leukaemias, 1 of 16 erythroleukemias, and 6 of 45 myeloid blast crises of CML. Staining in the acute myeloid leukaemias has been shown to be due to biosynthesis of the antigen (Sutherland *et al.*, 1984), suggesting that it may be expressed on a sub-population of normal myeloid cells.

IV. THE IMMUNOTOXIN

Monoclonal antibody WT-1 was provided by Dr. W. Tax (Tax *et al.*, 1982). The WT-1-ricin A conjugate was prepared by Drs. W. C. J. Ross, A. J. Cumber and J. A. Forrester (Chester Beatty Research Institute, London) using the SPDP reagent as described by Myers *et al.* (1984). It contained 0.83 molecules of A chain per antibody molecule. The A-chain moiety of the conjugate was fully active as assessed by inhibition of protein synthesis in a cell-free system and the binding characteristics of the conjugate were indistinguishable from those of native WT-1 antibody as judged by flow cytofluorimetry on the strongly WT-1-positive T-ALL cell line, GH1 (Myers *et al.*, 1984).

V. ANTIBODY-BINDING TO T-ALL LINES

A number of T lymphoblastoid cell lines were screened for reactivity with WT-1; four cell lines giving a wide range of staining intensities were chosen (Fig. 1). GH1 was the most strongly positive line and 95% of the cells were brightly stained. CCRF-CEM was the next brightest cell line and contained 79% positive cells. RPMI-8402 and HPB-ALL were weakly staining lines with only 26% and 13% positive cells, respectively.

VI. CYTOTOXIC EFFECTS OF WT-1-RICIN A ON T-ALL CELLS

A. Effects on Different Cell Lines

The cytotoxic activity of WT-1-ricin A on the four T lymphoblastoid lines chosen was compatible with their levels of staining. Continuous

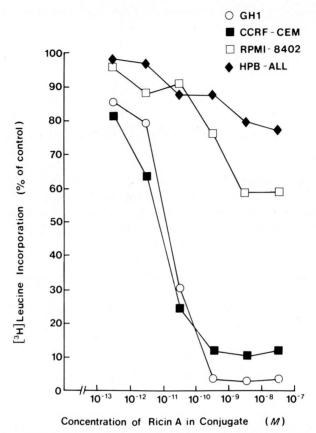

Fig. 2. Effect of WT-1-ricin A on four T-ALL cell lines: [³H]leucine incorporation of four T-ALL cell lines after 24 hr of treatment with various concentrations of immunotoxin. Results are means of triplicate determinations expressed as percentage of uptake of an untreated control. (From Myers *et al.*, 1984.)

incubation of GH1 cells with the immunotoxin at concentrations of 3×10^{-10} M or greater reduced their rate of [³H]leucine incorporation to 2% of that in control cultures, while that of CCRF-CEM cells was reduced to 8% of control. The weakly reactive RPMI-8402 and HPB-ALL lines were less susceptible to the conjugate. They continued to incorporate [³H]leucine to between 60 and 80% of the control levels even after incubation with the immunotoxin at the highest concentration tested, 3×10^{-8} M (Fig. 2).

The poor cytotoxic effect of WT-1-ricin A on HPB-ALL and RPMI-8402 may be due to the fact that a proportion of the cells lack the WT-1 antigen or express it at low levels. There is evidence from the work of Casellas *et al.* (1982) with melanoma cells that there is a threshold level of surface antigen below which immunotoxins are not active.

We attempted to determine whether the cells which were resistant to the immunotoxin differed in antigen expression from those which were susceptible. This was done by treating each of the four cell lines with the immunotoxin for 24 hr, washing them and putting them into culture for a further 24 hr to allow the damaged cells to die. Viable cells were then collected over a single step Ficoll-Hypaque gradient and analyzed for surface expression of the antigen recognized by WT-1. No viable cells were found in the treated GH1 or CCRF-CEM lines. In contrast, in the HPB-ALL and RPMI-8402 lines, the fluorescence profiles of the treated cells were similar to those of the untreated controls. However, it cannot be concluded from this result that the cells that survived were expressing the WT-1 antigen at the time the immunotoxin was added, since, in another experiment, GH1 cells sorted into populations of low and high antigenic expression were found to revert to the staining pattern of the unfractionated cells when cultured for a further 24-hr period. It is possible, therefore, that the HPB-ALL and CCRF-CEM cells that survived exposure to the immunotoxin were transiently deficient in the antigen.

B. Potentiation by Ammonium Chloride

Ammonium chloride had been reported by Casellas *et al.* (1982) to potentiate the cytotoxic action of antibody-ricin A conjugates. The mechanism of the effect is not fully understood but is thought to be due to an increase in lysosomal and endosomal pH caused by the ammonium ion. This inhibits proteolysis of the immunotoxin and gives the A chain a greater chance to traverse the endosomal membrane and enter the cytosol where it can exert its cytotoxic effect. With the cell lines used in the present study, concentrations of up to 6mM ammonium chloride could be included in the cultures without retarding cell growth. When 6mM ammonium chloride was added to GH1 cultures incubated continuously with WT-1-ricin A, there was 100-fold enhancement in the potency of the immunotoxin. 80% reduction in [^{3}H]leucine incorporation was achieved at a $3 \times 10^{-13} M$ concentration of immunotoxin, equivalent to 900 molecules of immunotoxin per cell (Fig. 3).

The mode of action of lysosomotropic agents remains unclear. Fulton *et al.* (1985) describe immunotoxins produced from monoclonal anti-human immunoglobulin and highly purified A or B chains of ricin. The killing of the human B cell line, Daudi, by the A chain immunotoxin was potentiated only 2-fold by ammonium chloride. The same immu-

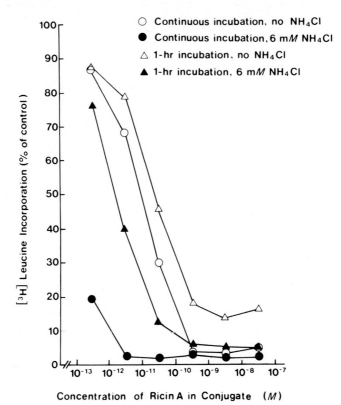

Fig. 3. Effect of ammonium chloride on WT-1-ricin A cytotoxicity. GH1 cells were incubated with immunotoxin in the presence or absence of 6 mM ammonium chloride for 1 or 24 hr. Viability was assayed 24 hr after starting by measuring [^{3}H]leucine incorporation. (From Myers *et al.*, 1984.)

notoxin in the presence of B chain, in the form of B immunotoxin, showed greater than 100-fold potentiation by NH$_4$Cl, suggesting that ammonium chloride action is mainly on the B chain. However, Martin *et al.* (1985) used the same A chain preparation to produce an anti-T cell immunotoxin and showed it to be potentiated about 1000-fold by ammonium chloride in the absence of added B chain, suggesting that the action of lysosomotropic agents may be dependent on a number of parameters.

C. The Influence of Incubation Time on Toxicity

We were concerned that treatment of bone marrow for periods as long as 24 hr *in vitro* before cryopreservation and re-infusion could be detrimental to engraftment. Accordingly, the potentiating effects of am-

TABLE I

CLONAL ASSAY FOR GH1 SURVIVAL AFTER TREATMENT WITH WT-1-RICIN A[a]

	Survival (%)		
Test	1 hr	2 hr	3 hr
1	0.71	0.23	0.11
2	0.48	0.23	0.04

[a] The percentage survival of GH1 cells after treatment with the WT-1 ricin A-chain immunotoxin. GH1 cells were incubated in Iscoves medium at 37°C with 6 mM ammonium
chloride and $3 \times 10^{-9} M$ immunotoxin for 1, 2 or 3 hr prior to washing and culturing in
semi-solid medium. The plating efficiency of the control cells was 17%. Results shown are
the percentage survival of GH1 cells after treatment as compared to this control. (From
Myers *et al.*, 1984.)

monium chloride were also tested in 1-hr incubations. As shown in Fig.
3, the toxicity of WT-1-ricin A to GH1 cells in a 1-hr incubation (followed
by extensive washing and incubation in immunotoxin-free medium for
a further 23 hr) was about 10-fold less than on continuous incubation.
More importantly, the maximal reduction in [^{3}H]leucine uptake that could
be obtained was only 88%, suggesting that a substantial proportion of
cells had survived this short incubation period. However, the addition
of 6mM ammonium to the cells during the 1-hr incubation resulted in
a restoration of the maximum level of toxicity.

D. Clonogenic Assays

A clonal assay was used to determine the percentage of GH1 cells
which survived treatment with WT-1-ricin A under conditions giving
maximal inhibition of protein synthesis. GH1 cells were treated with
$3 \times 10^{-9} M$ immunotoxin in 6mM ammonium chloride for 1, 2 or 3 hr
and were then washed and plated out in a semi-solid growth medium.
The plating efficiency of control cells in this system was 17% and, of
these, less than 1% and 0.1% survived a 1-hr and 3-hr treatment, respectively (Table I).

E. The Lack of Influence of Normal Bone Marrow Cells
   on the Toxicity of WT-1-ricin A to GH1 Cells

Although the foregoing results demonstrate the potent toxicity of WT-
1-ricin A to cell lines to which the antibody binds, the tests do not emulate

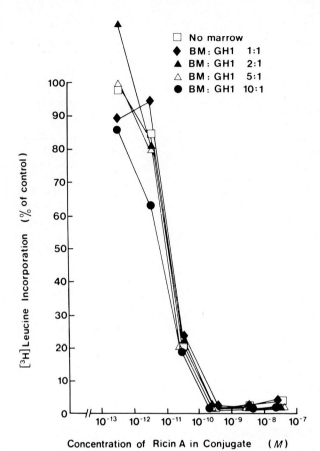

Fig. 4. Effects of excess normal bone marrow on the killing of GH1 cells by WT-1-ricin A. GH1 cells were incubated for 24 hr with immunotoxin and various numbers of normal bone marrow cells. Viability was measured by [³H]leucine incorporation. Bone marrow counts are for mononuclear cells, about 10-fold higher numbers of erythrocytes were also present.

the conditions under which bone marrow would be treated. To approach this situation more closely, high concentrations of normal bone marrow cells were added to GH1 cells to see if any inhibition of toxicity would result from the presence of non-reactive cells. Normal bone marrow cells that had been irradiated (1000 rad) and cryopreserved were found to cause no inhibition of cytotoxicity of the target cells at levels of up to 10 mononuclear cells and 100 erythrocytes per GH1 cell (Fig. 4).

COLLECTED FRACTIONS IN A WT-1 SORT

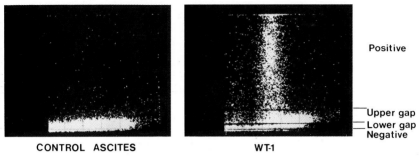

CONTROL ASCITES   WT-1

Fig. 5. Collected fractions in a WT-1 sort. Bone marrow stained with WT-1 and a fluores-ceinated second layer were separated on a FACS I into the four fractions shown. The positive was defined as all cells staining more brightly than with the non-immune mouse ascites control. The remaining fraction was divided into three approximately equal portions as shown. (From Myers *et al.*, 1984.)

VII. THE EFFECT OF WT-1-RICIN A ON NORMAL BONE MARROW CELLS

It was important to show that bone marrow progenitors do not carry the antigen recognized by WT-1. Normal bone marrow cells were stained with WT-1 and then with a FITC-F(ab')$_2$ goat anti-mouse Ig. The cells were then separated on a FACS I (Becton Dickinson) into four fractions as demonstrated in Fig. 5, where the positive fraction contained all those cells with fluorescence greater than that in a non-immune mouse ascites control. The remaining cells were split into three approximately equal groups, labeled in Fig. 5, upper gap, lower gap and negative, respectively. Cells from each of these fractions were analyzed in the CFU-GEMM assay. The positive fraction was found to contain no mixed colony or megakaryocyte colony percursors and less than 1% of the BFU-e and 3% of the CFU-GM in the total marrow. Virtually all the haematopoietic activity was found in the three lower fractions (Table II). This was good circumstantial evidence that normal haematopoietic progenitor cells did not express the WT-1 antigen and so would not bind the immunotoxin.

Next, a series of CFU-GEMM cultures were set up using bone marrow cells that had been pre-treated with immunotoxin. Under the most severe conditions tested (3×10^{-8} M immunotoxin and 6mM ammonium chlo-

TABLE II

COLONY RECOVERY FROM BONE MARROW SORTED BY WT-1 STAINING (%)[a]

	CFU-GM	BFU-e	CFU-Meg	CFU-GEMM
Positive	3	<1	0	0
Upper gap	23	19	12	10
Lower gap	28	19	15	22
Negative	30	23	23	21

[a] Mean percentage recoveries from three sorts with fractions collected as shown in Fig. 5. The percentage positive varied between 15 and 33% and the remaining fractions were adjusted to contain approximately equal fractions of the remainder. (From Myers *et al.*, 1984.)

ride for 24 hr), there was no specific loss of any type of colony-forming cell (Fig. 6).

VIII. THE USE OF MIXTURES OF IMMUNOTOXINS

One possible problem in immunotoxin treatment is that in T-ALL, as in CGL (Greaves, 1982), the truly malignant clonogenic cells (i.e., those with stem cell or self renewal capacity) might represent only a small fraction of the cells in the blood. At present, we can only assume that the clonogenic population bears the same antigens and at similar density to its progeny.

One method for increasing the probability of killing all the tumour cells in an autograft is the use of a cocktail of immunotoxins. Each immunotoxin in such a cocktail must fulfill the criteria listed above and in this light we have begun investigating two other T cell selective monoclonals, RFT-1 (Caligaris-Cappio *et al.*, 1982) and RFT-11, provided by Dr. G. Janossy (Royal Free Hospital, London). These monoclonals are reactive with more mature T cells than WT-1, having specificities similar to OKT-1 and OKT-11A, respectively (Dr. G. Janossy, personal communication). In cell sorter experiments, RFT-1 and RFT-11 showed no reactivity with CFU-GEMM and limited reactivity with other haemopoietic precursors. Likewise, ricin A conjugates of these monoclonals had no specific toxicity on any of the measured precursors.

As can be seen in Fig. 7, the RFT-1 and RFT-11 immunotoxins have different spectra of toxicity on the cell lines tested. These and surface staining data suggest that the three immunotoxins could work in a com-

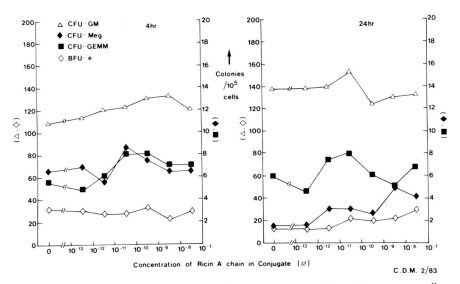

Fig. 6. Effects of WT-1-ricin A on normal bone marrow progenitors. Bone marrow cells were incubated with immunotoxin and 6 mM ammonium chloride for 4 or 24 hr prior to assaying in CFU-GEMM cultures. Each point is the mean of duplicate culture plates. (From Myers *et al.*, 1984.)

plementary fashion. However, until an assay for the clonogenic cell in T-ALL becomes available, it is difficult to judge the clinical potential of an immunotoxin cocktail compared to any of its constituents. Continued examination of the use of cocktails is supported by results obtained using monoclonals and complement. LeBien *et al.* (1983) demonstrate removal of all CALLA-positive cells with a single cycle of treatment using a cocktail of three monoclonals, whilst Bast *et al.* (1983) required three cycles of J5 plus complement. A similar potentiation in the removal of T cells by use of immunotoxin cocktails has also been reported (Vallera *et al.*, 1983).

IX. EVALUATION

The monoclonal antibody WT-1 is reactive with leukaemic cells in all cases of T-ALL tested and WT-1-ricin A is a potent cytotoxic agent for cells carrying its target antigen. Also, WT-1 is unreactive with measurable haemopoietic progenitors and the immunotoxin has no specific deleterious effects on these populations. These properties must be measured against the criteria proposed in the Introduction.

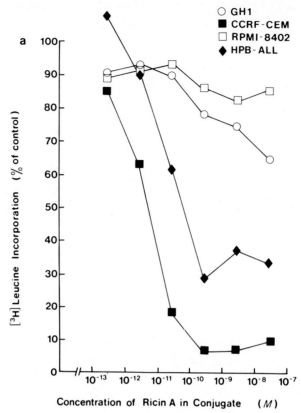

Fig. 7. Effects of RFT-1 and RFT-11 immunotoxins on four T-ALL cell lines. The four T-ALL cell lines were incubated for 24 hr with (a) RFT-1 or (b) RFT-11 before viability was measured by [³H]leucine incorporation. Results are directly comparable with those in Fig. 2.

A. All Clonogenic Tumour Cells Must Be Removed from the Graft

The WT-1-ricin A immunotoxin is a powerful cytotoxic agent for the two human T-ALL cell lines, GH1 and CCRF-CEM, which express the WT-1 antigen at high density, but is relatively ineffective against the more weakly staining cell lines, HPB-ALL and RPMI-8402. In view of this tentative correlation between antigen density and sensitivity to the immunotoxin, any patient considered for therapy would need to have leukaemic cells with high levels of antigen. There is currently no clonal

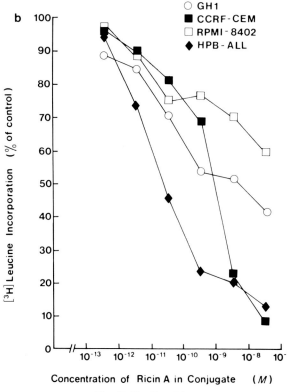

Fig. 7. *(Continued.)*

assay nor animal model by which the effectiveness of the immunotoxin on primary leukaemic cells from a patient can be determined directly: The assumption has to be made that the primary leukaemic cells will behave like a cell line that gives similar density of staining.

The WT-1-binding properties of leukaemic cells from the blood or marrow of 10 patients with T-ALL was determined. As with the cell lines, the tumor cells from each patient displayed a wide variation in the intensity of staining. The median staining in all cases was at least equal to that of CCRF-CEM and in most (6 of 10) was brighter than that of GH1. Also, the primary leukaemic cells tended to be smaller than *in vitro*-adapted cell lines. Thus, these cells expressed surface antigens at a correspondingly higher density for any given level of fluorescence intensity. We do not yet know whether the sensitivity of a cell to an immunotoxin correlates with the total number of antigens per cell, antigen density, or both. In any case, the indications are that the primary leu-kaemic cells will be equally sensitive to the immunotoxin as CCRF-CEM or GH1 cells.

B. The Reconstituting Capacity of the Marrow Should Remain Unimpaired

No reduction in the numbers of committed haematopoietic progenitors (CFU-GM, CFU-meg, BFU-e) or of the multipotential CFU-GEMM was detectable when normal human marrow cells were treated with WT1-ricin A under conditions that give maximal killing of GH1 cells. However, the reliability of these assays as a measure of the reconstituting capacity of bone marrow has been brought into question by the recent findings that rodent (Sharkis *et al.*, 1980) and human (Rowley and Stuart, 1983) marrow treated with 4-hydroperoxycyclophosphamide was fully capable of haematopoietic reconstitution even though all measurable colony types were eliminated. Nevertheless, it is likely that the maintenance of the measurable colony-forming cells in the present study is a good indicator for the retention of reconstituting capacity even though the reverse is not necessarily true. In clinical trials, any doubt over whether or not the pluripotential stem cell is harmed by the immunotoxin will be covered by the standard practice in bone marrow transplantation centres of keeping a reserve of untreated "back up" marrow.

Thus, WT1-ricin A fulfills these criteria for entry into a clinical trial, at least as well as can be demonstrated with the *in vitro* tests currently available. However, there are a number of questions which cannot be answered by these approaches and due caution must be exercised in this respect.

X. POSSIBLE OBSTACLES TO CLINICAL UTILITY

Successful autologous marrow transplantation requires that the patient is reinfused with adequate numbers of bone marrow stem cells. Because most patients considered for autologous marrow transplantation have had extensive chemotherapy, it is important to establish that the numbers of colony-forming cells in the patient's marrow are back within the normal range before instigating transplantation.

One of the biggest obstacles to the treatment of leukaemia by supralethal radiochemotherapy and allogeneic marrow transplantation is the complete elimination of malignant cells from the patient. In leukaemia patients who receive a preparative regimen of high-dose chemotherapy, total body irradiation and an allogeneic marrow graft, typically 40–70% subsequently relapse (Thomas *et al.*, 1979; Barrett *et al.*, 1982; Champlin *et al.*, 1982). Coccia *et al.* (1983) used high-dose cytosine arabinoside (ara-c) with fractionated TBI to treat ALL patients before allogeneic marrow grafting and the early results appear to be better with 6 of 10 patients in remission 1½ yr later. Clearly, this problem applies equally to autologous marrow transplantation but with the additional complication that it will be unclear whether relapse is due to the survival of malignant cells in the patient or to incomplete erradication of malignant cells in the graft.

Finally, it should be noted that a factor which limits the suitability of transplantation is the severity of the treatment itself and the risks associated with it. If the patient to be treated has already received high doses of many commonly used chemotherapeutic drugs, TBI carries an increased risk of myocardial or neural complications (Rubin, 1984). In addition, after transplantation, the patient remains neutropoenic for a period of 2 or 3 weeks. During this time he is highly vulnerable to bacteria and viral infection and strenuous efforts should be made to minimize this risk.

XI. RECENT CLINICAL DEVELOPMENTS

In a study performed in collaboration with Drs. T. A. Lister, A. Z. S. Rohatiner, M. J. Barnett and others at the Medical Oncology Unit, St. Bartholomew's Hospital, London, a patient with T-ALL in second remission received an autologous graft of WT-1-ricin A-treated marrow following intensive radiochemotherapy. The only myeloid or lymphoid marker absent from the marrow after treatment was that recognized by the WT-1 antibody. The patient showed haematopoietic reconstitution indicating that the procedure was not toxic to the bone marrow stem cells in the graft. This study will be reported in detail at a later date.

ACKNOWLEDGEMENT

I gratefully acknowledge all the help in writing this manuscript given to me by Drs. Ellen Vitetta and Phil Thorpe. I thank Ms. Gerry Ann Cheek and Ms. Nicky Coker for their secretarial assistance.

REFERENCES

Barrett, A. J., Kendra, J. R., Lucas, C. F., Joss, D. V., Joshi, R., Desai, M., Hugh-Jones, K., Phillips, R. H., Rogers, T. R., Tabara, Z., Williamson, S., and Hobbs, J. R. (1982). *Br. J. Haematol.* **52,** 181–188.

Bast, R. C., Jr., Ritz, J., Lipton, J. M., Feeney, M., Sallen, S., Nathan, D. G., and Schlossman, S. F. (1983). *Cancer Res.* **43,** 1389–1394.

Caligaris-Cappio, F., Gobby, M., Bofill, M., and Janossy, G. (1982). *J. Exp. Med.* **155,** 623–628.

Casellas, P., Brown, J. P., Gros, O., Gros, P., Hellström, I., Jansen, F. K., Poncelet, P., Roncucci, R., Vidal, H., and Hellström, K. E. (1982). *Int. J. Cancer* **30,** 437–443.

Champlin, R., Ho, W., Arenson, E., and Gale, R. P. (1982). *Blood* **60,** 1038–1041.

Chessells, J. M. (1982). *Semin. Haematol.* **19,** 155–171.

Coccia, P. F., Strandjorg, S. E., Gordon, E. M., Novak, L. J., Shina, D. C., Lazarus, H. M., and Herzig, R. H. (1983) *Proc. Am. Soc. Clin. Oncol.* **2,** 175 (Abstr. C680).

Filipovitch, A. H., Quinones, R., Vallera, D., and Kersey, J. H. (1983). *Erytt. Haematol.* **11,** Suppl. 12, 188 (Abstr. 339).

Filipovitch, A. H., Vallera, D. A., Youle, R. J., Quinones, R. R., Neville, D.M., Jr., and Kersey, J. H. (1984). *Lancet* **1,** 469–471.

Fulton, J. R., Uhr, J. W., and Vitetta, E. S. (1985) Submitted for publication.

Greaves, M. F. (1982). *In* "Chronic Granulocyte Leukaemia" (M. T. Shan, ed.), pp. 15–47. Praeger, New York.

Greaves, M. F., Janossy, G., Peto, J., and Kay, H. (1981). *Br. J. Haematol.* **48,** 179–197.

Haynes, B. F. (1981). *Immunol. Rev.* **57,** 127–161.

Krolick, K. A., Uhr, J. W., Slavin, S., and Vitetta, E. S. (1982). *J. Exp. Med.* **155,** 1797–1809.

LeBien, T. W., Ash, R. C., Zanjani, E. D., and Kersey, J. H. (1983). *Haematol. Bluttransfus.* **28,** 112–116.

Martin, P. J., Hansen, J. A., and Vitetta, E. S. (1985). *Blood* (in press).

Mason, D. W., Thorpe, P. C., and Ross, W.C.J. (1982). *Cancer Surv.* **3,** 189–415.

Morishima, Y., Mashide, K., Yang, S. Y., Collins, N. H., Hoffmann, M. K., and Dupont, B. (1982). *J. Immunol.* **129,** 1091–1098.

Muirhead, M., Martin, P. J., Torok-Storb, B., Uhr, J. W., and Vitetta, E. S. (1983). *Blood* **62,** 327–332.

Myers, C. D., Thorpe, P. E., Ross, W. C. J., Cumber, A. J., Katz, F. E., Tax, W. J. M., and Greaves, M. F. (1984). *Blood* **63,** 1178–1185.

O'Neill, G. J. (1979). *In* "Drug Carriers in Biology and Medicine" (G. Gregoriadis, ed.), pp. 23–41. Academic Press, New York.

Powles, R. L., Clink, H. M., Spence, D., Morgenstern, G., Watson, J. G., Selby, P. J., Woods, M., Barret, A., Jameson, B., Sloane, J., Lawler, S. D., Kay, H. E. M., Lawson, D., McElwain, T. J., and Alexander, P. (1980). *Lancet* **1**, 327–329.

Poynton, C. H., Dicke, K. A., Culbert, S., Frankel, L. S., Jagannath, S., and Reading, G. L. (1983). *Lancet* **1**, 524.

Prentice, H. G., Blacklock, H. A., Janossy, G., Gilmore, M. J. M. L., Price-Jones, L., Tidman, N., Trejdosiewicz, L. K., Skeggs, D. B. L., Panjwani, D., Ball, S., Graphakos, S., Patterson, J., Ivory, K., and Hoffbrand, A. V. (1984). *Lancet* **1**, 472–475.

Riehm, H., Gadner, H., Henze, G., Kornhuber, B., Langermann, H. J., Muller-Weihrich, S., and Schellong, G. (1983). *In* "Leukemia Research: Advances in Cell Biology and Treatment" (S. B. Murphy and J. R. Gilbert, eds.), pp. 251–263. Elsevier, Amsterdam.

Ritz, J. Sallen, S., Bast, R. C., Jr., Lipton, J. M., Clavell, L. A., Feeney, M., Hercend, T., Nathan, D. G., and Schlossman, S. F. (1982). *Lancet*, **2**, 60–63.

Rowley, S. D., and Stuart, R. K. (1983). *Exp. Haematol.* **2**, Suppl. 12, 8 (Abstr. 11).

Rubin, P., (1984). *Int. J. Radiat. Oncol. Biol. Phys.* **10**, 5–34.

Santos, G. W., and Kaiser, H. (1982). *Semin. Haematol.* **19**, 227–239.

Sharkis, S. J., Santos, G. W., and Calvin, M. (1980). *Blood* **55**, 521–523.

Spitzer, G., Dicke, K. A., Litam, J., Verma, D. S., Zander, A., Lanzotti, V., Valdiviesco, M., McCredie, K. B., and Samuels, M. L. (1980). *Cancer (Amsterdam)* **45**, 3075–3085.

Sutherland, D. R., Rudd, C. E., and Greaves, M. F. (1984). *J. Immunol.* **133**, 327–333.

Tax, W. J. M., Willems, H. W., Kibbelaar, M. D. A., de Groot, J., Capel, P. J. A., de Waal, R. M. W., Reekers, P., and Koene, R. A. P. (1982). *Protides Biol. Fluids* **29**, 701–704.

Tax, W. J. M., Tidman, N., Janossy, G., Trejdosiewicz, L., Willems, R., Leevwenberg, J., de Witte, T. J. M., Capel, P. J. A., and Koene, R. A. P. (1984). *Clin. Exp. Immunol.* **55**, 427–436.

Thomas, E. D., Sanders, J. E., Flournoy, N., Johnson, F. L., Buckner, C. D., Clift, R. A., Fefer, A., Goodell, B. W., Storb, R., and Weiden, P. L. (1979). *Blood* **54**, 468–476.

Thorpe, P. E., Mason, D. W., Brown, A. F. N., Simmonds, S. J., Ross, W. C. J., Cumber, A. J., and Forrester, J. A. (1982). *Nature (London)* **297**, 594–596.

Treleaven, J., Gibson, F. M., Vgelstad, J., Rembaum, A., Philipe, T., Caine, G., and Kemshead, J. (1984). *Lancet* **1**, 70–73.

Vallera, D. A., Ash, R. C., Zanjani, E. D., Kersey, J. H., LeBien, T. W., Beverley, P. C. L., Neville, D. M., Jr., and Youle, R. J. (1983). *Science* **222**, 512–515.

Vodinelich, L., Tax, W. J. M., Bai, Y., Pegram, S., Capel, P., and Greaves, M. F. (1983). *Blood* **62**, 1108–1113.

CHAPTER 13

Interest of Globotriaosylceramide Membrane Antigen as Target for Immunotoxins

S. Junqua,* J. Wiels,[†] P. Wils,* T. Tursz[†] and
J. B. Le Pecq*

*Laboratoire de Physico-Chimie Macromoléculaire
[†]Laboratoire d'Immuno-Biologie des Tumeurs
Institut Gustave-Roussy
Villejuif, France

I. INTRODUCTION

The immunotoxins (ITs) were developed in order to specifically kill cells bearing a characteristic membrane antigen. Immunotoxins have generated considerable interest in oncology and this has prompted the search for monoclonal antibodies which could recognize antigens specific for malignant cells. Although many ITs directed against tumor cells were prepared (Jansen *et al.*, 1982; Neville and Youle, 1982; Raso, 1982; Thorpe and Ross, 1982; Vitetta *et al.*, 1982), all of them recognized antigens which were not really specific of malignancy. The monoclonal 38.13 antibody,

MONOCLONAL ANTIBODIES FOR CANCER
DETECTION AND THERAPY

directed against a glycolipid antigen, selectively reacts with target Burk-itt's lymphoma (BL) cells (Wiels *et al.*, 1981). It then appeared that 38.13 antibody could represent an ideal carrier of toxin to selectively kill BL cells. This prompted us to study ITs prepared by linking the 38.13 antibody to gelonin or A chain of ricin.

The ricin toxin consists of two polypeptide chains joined by a disulfide bound. The B chain binds to galactose containing receptors on the cell surface and promotes the internalization and intracellular release of A chain which kills the cell by irreversibly inactivating the 60 S subunit of eukaryotic ribosomes (Olsnes *et al.*, 1974). Gelonin is a single polypeptide chain with properties similar to that of ricin A chain. Therefore gelonin and ricin A chain can only be internalized and kill cells if they are linked to a carrier able to bind to the cell surface.

The 38.13 ITs appeared to possess unusual and unexpected properties. They have cytotoxic potency not only on BL cells but also for several other tumor cells as will be discussed in this chapter.

II. MATERIAL AND METHODS

A. Production of 38.13 Monoclonal Antibody

The production of the 38.13 antibody was achieved by fusing rat splenocytes sensitized *in vivo* with Daudi cells, with murine SP_2O/Ag 14 plasmocytoma cells, according to the method of Kohler and Milstein (1976) and described in detail elsewhere (Wiels *et al.*, 1981). The 38.13 antibody was demonstrated to be a rat IgM.

B. Cell Lines

Detailed reports concerning the origin of the cell lines studied here have been reported (Wiels *et al.*, 1982; Klein *et al.*, 1983). Most of the BL lines were established from BL tumor biopsies in the International Agency for Research on Cancer (IARC, Lyon, France) or kindly provided by Professor G. Klein (Stockholm, Sweden). Lymphoblastoid cell lines (LCL) and other lines originated from various laboratories, including IARC, International Cancer Research Fund (ICRF) (Professor W. Bodmer, London, England) and Uppsala, Sweden (Dr. K. Nilsson). All these lines were routinely cultivated in RPMI medium (Gibco-Biocult, Scotland) supplemented with 10% heat-inactivated fetal calf serum.

C. Preparation of ITs

Ricin was extracted and purified from seeds of *Ricinus communis* and the ricin toxin A chain (RTA) was isolated according to Jansen *et al.* (1982). In order to link RTA to the antibody, activated disulfide groups were introduced on the antibody with the heterobifunctional cross-linker SPDP (Carlsson *et al.*, 1978). The antibody 2-pyridyldisulfide derivatives were mixed with a twofold molar excess of RTA to form 38.13 IgM-RTA IT. An average of 10 molecules of RTA linked per IgM molecule was obtained.

Gelonin (Gel) was isolated from seeds of *Gelonium multiflorum* (Stirpe *et al.*, 1980). As for antibodies, activated disulfide groups have to be introduced into gelonin. An average of 1.5 mole of disulfide groups per mole of gelonin was obtained. After reduction gelonin SH-residues could react with antibody disulfide derivatives to form an IT (38.13 IgM-Gel) as described for 38.13 IgM-RTA.

D. Assays

The assays used here included classical two-step complement-dependent microcytotoxicity, indirect immunofluorescence with fluorescein-conjugated goat anti-rat IgM (Nordic) and fluorescence-activated cell sorter (FACS) analysis.

The protein synthesis inhibition assay in cell culture has been described elsewhere (Wiels *et al.*, 1984b). Briefly 10^5 cells were incubated with various concentrations of ITs or toxin. After various incubation times at 37°C, [^{3}H]leucine was added for 2 hr. Then cells were harvested and the radioactivity incorporated in the cellular proteins was measured in a β counter.

The method of cellular ATP measurement was performed according to the ATP-dependent light emitted by the luciferin–luciferase system (McElroy and Seliger, 1963) after treating the cell membrane with the nucleotide releasing reagent (NRS, Lumac).

TABLE I

REACTIVITY OF 38.13 ANTIBODY WITH VARIOUS CELL LINES AND EXPRESSION OF EBV GENOME[a]

Cell lines	EBV Genome	38.13 Reactivity	
		+	−
Burkitt's lymphoma (BL)	+	25	13
	−	16	3
Lymphoblastoid cell lines (LCL)	+	0	50
T cell lines	−	0	0
Non-lymphoid	−	0	10

[a] The reactivity of various cell lines is tested in complement-dependent microcytotoxicity or indirect immunofluorescence assays. The results are expressed as the number of cell lines showing positive (+) or negative (−) reactivity with 38.13 antibody. EBV-containing cell lines are indicated (+).

III. RESULTS AND DISCUSSION

A. Cellular Reactivity with 38.13 Monoclonal Antibody

Table I shows the reactivity of 38.13 monoclonal antibody with cell lines of lymphoid or non-lymphoid origins. This reactivity has been demonstrated using complement-dependent microcytotoxicity, indirect immunofluorescence and in some cases FACS analysis.

The analysis of a panel of cultured cell lines confirmed the previously suggested anti-BL specificity of 38.13 antibody, since it reacted with 41 out of 57 BL lines so far tested.

None of the 50 EBV-containing LCL studied reacted with 38.13 in complement-dependent microcytotoxicity. In indirect immunofluorescence and FACS analysis, the vast majority of the LCL cells appeared completely unstained. However, occasionally, a low percentage of faintly stained cells could be detected in some lines. As discussed later, this result is consistent with the presence of a small number of antigenic sites on these cells. A complete negativity was observed with two EBV-producer marmoset cell lines, B-95 and M-81, which emphasized the lack of relationship between the expression of the target antigen and the presence of EBV.

Table II shows that in three cases of BL, tumor-derived EBV-negative

TABLE II

**REACTIVITY OF 38.13 MONOCLONAL ANTIBODY WITH BURKITT'S LYMPHOMA
AND LYMPHOBLASTOID CELL LINES OF THE SAME PATIENTS**

Patient number	Cell lines	Origin	EBV-containing cell lines	Chromosomal abnormalities	IF test labeled cells (%)
1	IARC/BL14 A	Burkitt's lymphoma	−	t (8; 14)	62
	IARC/70	Normal B lymphocytes	+	—	0
2	IARC/BL10	Burkitt's lymphoma	−	t (8; 14)	61
	IARC/113	Normal B lymphocytes	+	—	0
3	IARC/BL28	Burkitt's lymphoma	−	t (8; 14)	13
	IARC 139	Normal B lymphocytes	+	—	0

BL cell lines were studied in parallel with EBV-positive LCL obtained from normal peripheral B cells from the same patients. In these three cases, the BL cells reacted with 38.13 antibody, whereas the LCL were negative. These results emphasized further the anti-BL specificity of 38.13 antibody, its lack of relationship with EBV, and showed that BL antigen is not some peculiar histocompatibility antigen shared by BL patients.

Among BL, 16 out of the 57 lines tested did not react with 38.13 (Table I). It is difficult to speculate about the peculiarities of this negative BL subgroup. No difference in either the clinical presentation, the geographical origin or the EBV-content could be found between 38.13 reacting and non-reacting BL. BL antigen expression did not appear either to be restricted to one subtype of the characteristic BL translocations. Indeed, positive BL cases included lines carrying t(8;14), t(8;22) and t(2;8) translocations. Furthermore, IARC/LY65 with a chromosome 8 deletion and BJAB cells in which no specific translocation is observed were also stained with 38.13 antibody.

Finally, 38.13 antibody did not react with normal lymphocytes from peripheral blood, bone marrow and spleen from healthy individuals. Pokeweed mitogen and phytohemagglutinin-activated lymphocytes were also negative (data not shown).

B. Nature of the Target Antigen

Burkitt's lymphoma antigen reacting with 38.13 antibody was shown to be a neutral glycolipid (Lipinski *et al.*, 1982) identified as the globotriaosylceramide (Gb3) or ceramide trihexosyl (CTH) (Nudelman *et al.*, 1983), with the following structure:

$$\text{Gal } \alpha1 \rightarrow 4 \text{ Gal } \beta1 \rightarrow 4 \text{ Glc } \beta1 \rightarrow 1 \text{ ceramide}$$

The substance was previously known as the blood group antigen P^k, a normal intermediate in the P substance synthesis. The P^k antigen has been described on the erythrocytes and the fibroblasts of very rare individuals genetically lacking the *N*-acetylgalactosamine transferase which normally transforms the P^k into the P antigen (Marcus *et al.*, 1976). It must also be pointed out that CTH accumulates in tissues of patients suffering from Fabry's disease (Sweeley *et al.*, 1983).

The 38.13 antibody was shown to react with erythrocytes and fibroblasts of two subjects with the rare P^k phenotype, whereas it was unreactive with erythrocytes or fibroblasts from any other individual tested (Fellous *et al.*, 1985). Recent data obtained in collaboration with S. I. Hakomori (Seattle, Washington) suggested that the accumulation of CTH in Burkitt's cells was not related to an enzymatic defect of *N*-acetylgalactosamine transferase as observed in the subjects with the P^k phenotype. Indeed, Burkitt's cells demonstrated a strikingly high activity in the CTH-synthetizing enzyme, α-galactosyltransferase, when compared with other cell types, such as LCL. (Wiels *et al.*, 1984a). The mechanism of the activation of α-galactosyltransferase observed in Burkitt's cells is currently being investigated.

C. Use of the 38.13 Monoclonal Antibody as Carrier for Toxins

1. Incorporation of [³H]Leucine

As the toxic effects of RTA and Gel are mediated through the inhibition of protein synthesis, incorporation of [³H]leucine by target cells was used *in vitro* to evaluate the biological activity of both ITs.

On Ramos BL cells after 16 hr of incubation, the 38.13 IgM-Gel was about 10^3-fold more active than gelonin alone (Fig. 1). Similar results were obtained with the 38.13 IgM-RTA (Wiels *et al.*, 1984).

Protein synthesis inhibition test gives a relevant evaluation of the primary biological effect of the IT since the two toxin chains act by enzymatically inactivating the ribosomes. However, this test does not provide any information on the actual cellular death induced by IT. After inhibition of protein synthesis, cell membrane integrity is altered much later as seen by trypan blue exclusion. This event can also be followed by the

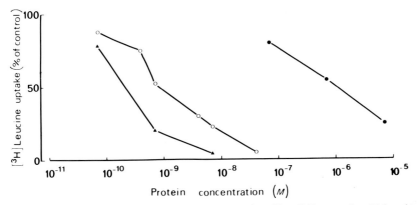

Fig. 1. Inhibition of protein rate synthesis measured in BL cell Ramos after 16 hr of incubation, induced by intact ricin (▲), 38.13 IgM-Gel (○), Gel (●).

determination of the intracellular ATP content which reflects both preservation of cellular energetic metabolism and membrane function.

Whereas the protein synthesis inhibition occurs 2 or 3 hr after treatment with ricin or IT (Wiels *et al.*, 1984b), the decrease of ATP content is only observed after a lag period of about 20 and 30 hr for ricin and 38.13 IgM-Gel, respectively (Fig. 2). Then both ITs give a similar rate of ATP decrease.

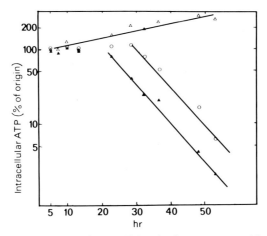

Fig. 2. Intracellular ATP content of BL cell Daudi after treatment with ricin (▲) or 38.13 IgM-Gel (○) as a function of time. Untreated cells (△).

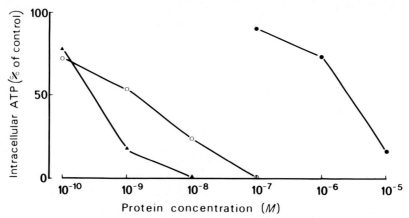

Fig. 3. Intracellular ATP content of BL cell Daudi after treatment with ricin (▲) 38.13 IgM-Gel (○) and Gel (●) as a function of concentration (*M*). Incubation time of 66 hr.

Figure 3 shows the effect of IT on the intracellular ATP content of Daudi BL cells after 66 hr of incubation compared to free Gel and ricin. The results show that a surprisingly long delay separates the primary effect of ricin or IT on protein synthesis and the events which ultimately lead to cell lysis and death.

2. Effect of 38.13 ITs on Various Cell Lines

The 38.13 antibody as discussed previously reacts almost exclusively with Burkitt's cells as seen by indirect immunofluorescence and FACS analysis. Therefore, it was expected that the 38.13 IT activity was limited to these same cells. Surprisingly it was observed that some non-BL cells such as Priess (EBV + LCL), K562 (human granulocyte leukemia) and the murine leukemic L1210 cells were also sensitive to these IT (Fig. 4).

3. Specificity of IT

In order to demonstrate that target cells are not binding any IgM in a non-specific way, an IT containing an irrelevant monoclonal IgM antibody was prepared. Such an obviously irrelevant IgM is the monoclonal IgM antibody directed against the hapten trinitrophenol (TNP). The anti-TNP RTA was obtained by the same procedure as 38.13 IgM-RTA. On TNP-labeled Ramos cells, the anti-TNP RTA was as potent as the intact ricin (Fig. 5). In contrast, the same IT had no effect on unlabeled Ramos cells and behaves almost as free RTA and anti-TNP IgM (Fig. 5). Fur-

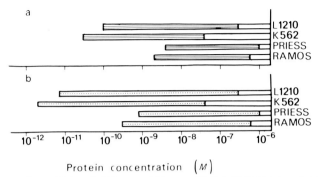

Protein concentration (M)

Fig. 4. Compared sensitivity of different cell lines to 38.13 IgM-RTA (a) and ricin (b). The activity of RTA ▭, ricin ▭ and 38.13 IgM-RTA ▭ is shown by indicating the concentration (M) of protein which causes 50% of protein synthesis inhibition. Ramos is a BL cell line, Priess an EBV-containing lymphoblastoid cell line, L1210 a murine leukemia cell line, K562 a human erythroleukemia cell line.

thermore, an excess of free D-galactose was also shown to inhibit the 38.13 IgM from binding to the reactive glycolipid antigen bearing a terminal galactose (Lipinski *et al.*, 1982). In the same way we demonstrated that addition of 0.1 M galactose in incubation medium was able to protect the target cells significantly against the 38.13 IgM ITs (Wiels *et al.*, 1984b), including the 38.13 Gel. From these studies, it was concluded that a very few number of antigenic sites are probably sufficient to obtain the internalization of the toxins. It is known that a single ricin A chain can cause cell death (Olsnes and Pihl, 1981). Immunotoxins could represent very sensitive reagents to detect antigens present in very small amounts at the cell surface.

Interestingly, the 38.13 IT appeared to be extremely potent on L1210 mouse leukemic cells as shown on Fig. 4. Clearly there is no correlation between the IT activity and the number of membrane antigenic sites, which is high for Ramos cells and quite low for K562, Priess and L1210 cells (since not even detected by conventional immunological methods). Besides, L1210 and K562 cells demonstrated particular sensitivity to ricin (Fig. 4).

Because leukemic L1210 cells, when grafted to DBA/2 mice, are able to multiply and kill the animals, the *in vivo* activity of IT can be examined. In preliminary experiments (Junqua *et al.*, 1985) it was observed that: (1) The IT were not more toxic for the animal than the purified ricin A chain; and (2) intraperitonealy injected 38.13 IgM-Gel increased significantly the life span of mice grafted with L1210 cells. At least 99.99% of the L1210 cells could be killed *in vivo* by treatment with IT.

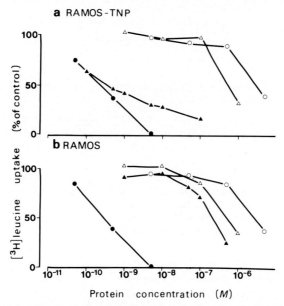

Fig. 5. Effect of anti-TNP IgM-RTA IT on TNP labeled (a) and unlabeled (b) BL cell Ramos. Inhibition of protein synthesis was measured after 16 hr of incubation on cells treated with ricin (●) anti-TNP RTA (▲) anti-TNP IgM alone (△) and RTA (○).

The L1210 experimental system seems to be an interesting model to study *in vivo* the therapeutic properties of ITs. It opens the possibility to test the activity of agents able to potentiate the IT action, such as lysosomotropic compounds and protease inhibitors (Casellas *et al.*, 1982).

IV. CONCLUSIONS

The present work illustrates new perspectives in the use of 38.13 ITs:

1. 38.13 ITs could be used as very sensitive reagents to detect the presence of a small number of antigens at the membrane surface provided that the IT is efficiently internalized and the toxin is released in active form inside the cell. This potential of ITs is also illustrated by the work of Krolick *et al.* (1982) who reported that murine BCL1 leukemic cells were killed by an anti-δ IT, whereas no IgD could be detected on their surface by FACS analysis.

2. 38.13 ITs are active not only on BL cells but also on some other tumor cells which expressed small quantities of antigens otherwise undetected at their surface by usual immunological methods. This observation raises the possibility that these ITs can be used as therapeutic agents for a wide variety of tumor cells. In this respect it was of particular interest to observe that the 38.13 ITs are active *in vivo* against a murine leukemia at doses which do not cause any toxic effect to the animals. This provides a very useful model to test the therapeutic activity of 38.13 ITs for *in vivo* treatment. Finally, the potential use of ITs for the removal of contaminating tumor cells from bone marrow by *in vitro* treatment can also be evaluated in this model.

ACKNOWLEDGEMENTS

We want to thank Drs. A. Balana, B. Ehlin-Henriksson, M. Fellous, S. I. Hakomori, R. Kannagi, G. Klein, G. Lenoir, M. Lipinski and E. D. Nudelman for their contributions in various part of this study and Mrs. M. C. Bouger and C. Tétaud for their expert technical assistance.

This work was supported by grants from CNRS, INSERM, Institut Gustave-Roussy and Association pour la Recherche sur le Cancer.

REFERENCES

Carlsson, J., Drevin, H., and Axén, R. (1978). *Biochem. J.* **173**, 723.

Casellas, P., Brown, J. P., Gros, O., Gros, P., Hellström, I., Jansen, F. K., Poncelet, P., Roncucci, R., Vidal, H., and Hellström, K. E. (1982). *Int. J. Cancer* **30**, 437.

Fellous, M., Cartron, J. P., Wiels, J., and Tursz, T. (1985). *Brit. J. Haematol.* (in press).

Jansen, F. K., Blythman, H. E., Carrière, D., Casellas, P., Gros, O., Gros, P., Laurent, J. C., Paolucci, F., Pau, B., Poncelet, P., Richer, G., Vidal, H., and Voisin, G. A. (1982). *Immunol. Rev.* **62**, 185.

Junqua, S. *et al.* (1985). In preparation.

Klein, G., Manneborg-Sandlund, A., Ehlin-Henriksson, B., Godal, T., Wiels, J., and Tursz, T. (1983). *Int. J. Cancer* **31**, 535.

Kohler, G., and Milstein, C. (1976). *Eur. J. Immunol.* **6**, 511.

Krolick, K. A., Uhr, J. W., Slavin, S., and Vitetta, E. S. (1982). *J. Exp. Med.* **155**, 1797.

Lipinski, M., Nudelman, E. D., Wiels, J., and Parsons, M. (1982). *J. Immunol.* **129**, 2301.

McElroy, W. D., and Seliger, H. H. (1963). *Adv. Enzymol.* **25**, 119.

Marcus, D. M., Naiki, M., and Kundu, S. K. (1976). *Proc. Natl. Acad. Sci. U.S.A.* **73**, 3263.

Neville, D. M., and Youle, R. J. (1982). *Immunol. Rev.* **62**, 75.

Nudelman, E., Kannagi, R., Hakomori, S., Lipinski, M., Wiels, J., Parsons, M., Fellous, M., and Tursz, T. (1983). *Science* **220,** 508.

Olsnes, S., and Pihl, A. (1981). *In* "Pharmacology of Bacterial Toxins" (J. Drews and F. Dorner eds.) p. 355. Pergamon, Oxford.

Olsnes, S., Refsnes, K., and Pihl, A. (1974). *Nature (London)* **249,** 627.

Raso, V. (1982). *Immunol. Rev.* **62,** 93.

Stirpe, F., Olsnes, S., and Pihl, A. (1980). *J. Biol. Chem.* **255,** 6947.

Sweeley, C. C., Klionsky, B., Krivit, W., and Desnick, R. J. (1983). *In* "The Metabolic Basis of Inherited Disease" (J. B. Stanbury, J. B. Wyngaarden, D. S. Frederickson, M. S. Brown, and J. L. Goldstein, ed.), 5th ed., p. 906 McGraw-Hill, New York.

Thorpe, P. E., and Ross, W. C. J. (1982). *Immunol. Rev.* **62,** 119.

Vitetta, E. S., Krolick, K. A., and Uhr, J. W. (1982). *Immunol. Rev.* **62,** 159.

Wiels, J., Fellous, M., and Tursz, T. (1981). *Proc. Natl. Acad. Sci. U.S.A.* **78,** 6485.

Wiels, J., Lenoir, G., Fellous, M., Lipinski, M., Salomon, J. C., Tétaud, C., and Tursz, T. (1982). *Int. J. Cancer* **29,** 653.

Wiels, J., Holmes E. H., Cochran, N., Tursz T. and Hakomori, S. I. (1984a). *J. Biol. Chem.* **259,** 14783.

Wiels, J., Junqua, S., Dujardin, P., Le Pecq, J. B. and Tursz, T. (1984b). *Cancer Res.* **44,** 129.

CHAPTER 14

Monoclonal Antibodies—Their Use in the Diagnosis and Therapy of Paediatric and Adult Tumours Derived from the Neuroectoderm

J. T. Kemshead

Imperial Cancer Research Fund Laboratories
Oncology Laboratory
Institute of Child Health
London, United Kingdom

I. INTRODUCTION

The treatment of malignancies arising in children is becoming increasingly specialised, as it has been found that different tumours respond to different combinations of either drugs and/or radiation therapy. New ways are constantly being sought to improve the differential diagnosis of tumours both *in vivo* (Sweet, 1983) and *in vitro* (Kemshead and Black, 1980). Monoclonal antibodies with their high degree of specificity and availability in almost unlimited amounts have been proposed as being excellent diagnostic and therapeutic tools (Raschke, 1982). This is despite their apparent lack of absolute tumour specificity. Early claims in the literature of antibodies binding exclusively to tumour tissue have not been substantiated (Schnegg *et al.*, 1981; Ashall *et al.*, 1982; Pallensen *et al.*, 1983).

The idea of monoclonal antibodies having operational specificity is more important than the actual distribution of a particular antigen throughout the body. Whilst the search for the 'tumour specific' reagent is by no means over, antibodies that currently exist in the laboratory are being used for *in vitro* diagnosis of tumour type (Kemshead *et al.*, 1983b) and *in vivo* detection of metastatic spread of tumour (Mach *et al.*, 1981). In addition, a variety of attempts have been made to use monoclonal antibodies directly to aid the therapy of patients with malignancy (Schulz *et al.*, 1983). This review will concentrate on these topics with special reference to paediatric solid tumours and tumours derived from the neuroectoderm, arising in both children and adults. The antibodies used for these studies, from our laboratory, have been raised following immunisation of mice with either human foetal brain or human tumour tissue. A list of the antibodies and their derivation is given in Table I.

II. *IN VITRO* DIAGNOSIS OF TUMOUR TYPE

The majority of malignancies can be confidently diagnosed from the clinical picture and the results of conventional histological and cytological investigations. However, two groups of malignancies can be difficult to differentiate, i.e., the small round cell tumours of childhood (neuroblastoma, lymphoblastic leukaemia/lymphoma, rhabdomyosarcoma and Ewing's sarcoma) (Raney *et al.*, 1976; Reynolds *et al.*, 1981) and intracranial neoplasms (Kemshead and Coakham, 1983).

A. The Small Round Cell Tumours of Childhood

Two approaches can be made to using immunohistological procedures for the diagnosis of the small round cell tumours of childhood. Tumour tissue can be acquired either from a biopsy of the primary site or from bone marrow aspirates if there is metastatic spread of the malignancy. In both instances monoclonal antibodies are applied to unfixed tissue; either frozen sections of tumour or suspensions of cells present in the marrow. Binding of antibody is determined indirectly using fluorescein

TABLE I

**MONOCLONAL ANTIBODIES USED FOR DIAGNOSTIC AND
THERAPEUTIC PROGRAMMES**

Monoclonal antibody	Immunogen	Reference
UJ13A	Human foetal brain	Allan *et al.* (1983)
UA1	Human foetal brain	J. T. Kemshead (unpublished)
UJ127:11	Human foetal brain	Kemshead *et al.* (1983a)
UJ181:4	Human foetal brain	Kemshead *et al.* (1983b)
UJ223:8	Human foetal brain	Kemshead *et al.* (1983b)
UJ167:11	Human foetal brain	Kemshead *et al.* (1983b)
A2B5	Chick retina	Eisenbarth *et al.* (1979)
Anti-Thy-1	Purified antigen	Crowhurst *et al.* (1985)
2D 1	Human mononuclear cells	Pizzolo *et al.* (1980)
Anti-human Ig	Commercial	
J5	Acute lymphoblastic leukaemia cells	Ritz *et al.* (1980)
OKM	Human mononuclear cells	Breard *et al.* (1980)
OKT3	Peripheral blood cells	Kung *et al.* (1979)
FD19	Low-grade astrocytoma	J. T. Kemshead (unpublished)
LE61	Marsupial kidney cell line	Lane, 1982
HMFG 1	Milk fat globule membranes	Taylor-Papadimitriou *et al.* (1981)

conjugated anti-mouse immunoglobulin (Ig). Frozen sections are obligatory for these studies as many of the antigens recognised by the anti-neuroblastoma antibodies are destroyed by formalin fixation and embedding of tissue in paraffin wax.

To establish the reliability of immunohistological diagnosis, samples from 38 known cases of Stage IV neuroblastoma were analysed for binding of monoclonal antibodies (Kemshead *et al.*, 1983b). In all cases antibody reactivity paralleled the clinical diagnosis, although not every anti-neuroblastoma reagent bound to all samples (Malpas *et al.*, 1982) (Table II). To overcome heterogeneity in antigen expression observed in neuroblastoma as well as many other solid tumours, it is necessary to use a panel of monoclonal antibodies, and currently 11 different anti-neural antibodies are employed to assist in the diagnosis of neuroblastoma. None of the anti-lymphoid/myeloid reagents used in this study bound to neuroblastoma tissue/cells: the pan-leucocyte reagent 2D1 (Pizzolo *et al.*, 1980); anti-human Ig; the anti-common acute lymphoblastic leukaemia

TABLE II

PATTERNS OF REACTIVITY OF MONOCLONAL ANTIBODIES TO DIFFERENT BONE MARROW ASPIRATES HEAVILY INFILTRATED WITH NEUROBLASTS (INDIRECT IMMUNOFLUORESCENCE)[a]

Number of samples binding antibody	Number of antibodies bound
21	8/8
7	7/8
5	6/8
2	5/8
3	4/8

[a] Thirty-eight different bone marrow aspirates from different patients, heavily infiltrated with neuroblasts, were analysed for binding of cells to eight different monoclonal antibodies. 5.0×10^5 nucleated cells were incubated with each monoclonal antibody, followed by fluorescein-conjugated goat anti-mouse Ig. Tumour cells were examined for binding with a Zeiss photomicroscope III with epi-illumination optics.

antigen reagent J5 (Ritz *et al.*, 1980); an anti-pan-T cell antibody OKT 3 (Kung *et al.*, 1979); and an anti-myeloid antibody OKM (Breard *et al.*, 1980).

It has proved possible to categorically differentiate between neuro-blastoma and lymphoblastic leukaemia/lymphoma in cases where conventional procedures have proved inadequate (Kemshead *et al.*, 1983b). Immunohistological analysis of these tumours has therefore been of great benefit to the clinician. It is not yet possible to be as certain of the reliability of reagents made to aid the differential diagnosis of rhabdomyosarcoma and Ewing's tumour as panels of antibodies with the required specificities are not yet thoroughly established.

The panel of anti-neuroblastoma antibodies described previously and others produced by Seeger (1982) and Seeger *et al.* (1979, 1981, 1982) and Reynolds and Graham–Smith (1982), have also proved extremely useful in identifying metastatic spread of tumour to bone marrow (Seeger *et al.*, 1982). Neuroblasts infiltrating marrow can be identified to levels of between 1 cell in 1,000 to 10,000 (Reynolds *et al.*, 1984). This is a considerable improvement in the sensitivity achieved by conventional histological and cytological procedures, where it is difficult to detect tumour cells below a level of 1–2% of the total nucleated population. However, it remains questionable if detection of tumour cells in bone marrow aspirates using monoclonal antibodies offers an improvement in efficiency over that achieved analysing trephine bone marrow biopsies by conventional techniques.

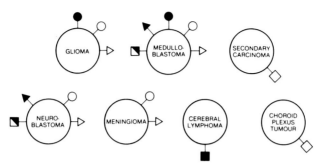

Fig. 1. Antigenic phenotype of seven different cerebral tumours defined by a panel of monoclonal antibodies.

B. Intracranial Malignancies

Over 180 consecutive cranial and spinal tumours have been screened with a large panel of monoclonal antibodies (Coakham *et al.*, 1984b). Analysis of tumours where the diagnosis was established shows that each malignant cell type can be identified according to the particular panel of monoclonal antibodies which bind to the tumour tissue (Fig. 1). For example, all gliomas (26) were found to bind the antibodies UJ13A and A2B5, but only 60% reacted with antibody FD19 [binding to the intracellular antigen glial-fibrillary acidic protein (GFAP)] (Eng *et al.*, 1971). The heterogeneity in antigen expression observed in frozen sections of tumour biopsies is not as marked as that detected amongst malignant cells present in marrow aspirates. This is probably because the sections analysed are 5 μm thick and therefore generally consist of more than one cell layer. The heterogeneity seen in the binding of gliomas with FD19 is expected as, by electron microscopy studies, not all the tumours would appear to contain this antigen. Well-differentiated astrocytomas (Grade 1) contain high amounts of GFAP compared with the undifferentiated glioblastoma multiforme (Grade 4). Secondary deposits of carcinoma in the brain can be identified using the monoclonal antibody LE61 and lymphoid tumours (primary or secondary deposits) by antibody 2D1 (Table I). These reagents were found not to bind to any tumours of neuroectodermal origin.

Based on the characteristic pattern of monoclonal antibody binding to intracranial tumours, it is again possible to use the reagents to establish a diagnosis in cases where conventional histological and cytological techniques fail. Immunohistological analysis of tumours has been found to be of most benefit where (1) the biopsy material is scanty or me-

chanically deformed; and (2) the tumours are composed of either anaplastic or small round cells.

In a similar way to that described above, immunohistological analysis
of tumour cells in the cerebrospinal fluid has proved to be of value
(Coakham et al., 1984a). In 16 of 17 cases studied, malignant cells were
classified as carcinoma (5 of 6 cases), lymphoma (3 of 3 cases) or of neuroectodermal origin (8 of 8 cases). Fourteen of these biopsies were examined by routine cytology and malignant cells reported in 10 cases,
with accurate characterisation of tumour type in only 3 aspirates.

III. RADIOIMMUNOLOCALISATION OF TUMOURS

A. Neuroblastoma

In contrast to the majority of childhood neoplasms, the prognosis of
children with metastatic neuroblastoma has not significantly improved
over the last 20 yr (Jaffe, 1976). Combinations of chemotherapy and radiation therapy used in conjunction with surgery have enabled children
to often reach a state of complete remission (Green et al., 1976; Pritchard
et al., 1982). However, patients frequently relapse, suggesting that contemporary imaging techniques are inadequate at identifying residual
disease in these individuals. The use of radiolabelled monoclonal antibody and the γ camera has been investigated to determine if this technique offers a more sensitive approach to the detection of metastatic
spread of neuroblastoma (Pressman and Keighley, 1948; Goldman et al.,
1984).

Pre-clinical studies showed uptake of radiolabelled antibody UJ13A
(Table I) into human neuroblastoma xenografts established in nude mice
(Table III). No antibody uptake was detected when the experiments werre
repeated with an antibody known not to bind to human neuroblastoma
FD44 (Table III). The level of the radiolabelled antibody conjugate found
in mouse blood and organs fell more rapidly than that in tumours. This
indicated that for clinical studies, ^{131}I (half-life 8.05 days) may be a more
suitable isotope for radioimmunolocalisation (RIL) than ^{123}I (half-life 13.3
hr). This is despite the energy of emissions from the latter isotope being
more suitable for γ-camera scanning.

In the first series, nine children were injected with between 0.9 and
2.8 mCi of^{131}I conjugated to approximately 200 μg of monoclonal antibody
UJ13A (Goldman et al., 1984). Primary tumours were successfully visualised in all six patients with a known primary site at the time of scan-

TABLE III

DISTRIBUTION OF ^{125}I-RADIOLABELLED ANTIBODIES IN NUDE MICE BEARING HUMAN NEUROBLASTOMA XENOGRAFTS

Monoclonal antibody	Antibody uptake[a]		
	Tumor	Other organs[b]	Brain
UJ13A	4–23	0.1–1.0	<0.05
FD44	0.1–1.0	0.1–1.0	<0.05

[a] Nude mice were injected with either radiolabelled UJ13A or FD44 monoclonal antibodies (15 μCi ^{125}I/1.0 μg protein). Five days later blood and major organs were removed from the animals, weighed and radioisotope levels determined using a counter. Uptake of radioisotope per gram of tissue was estimated and the results expressed as a ratio of organ to blood level.

[b] Organs examined liver, kidney, spleen, lung, adrenal, muscle, skin and brain.

ning. Of the three patients in whom no primary site was demonstrated, two patients were, by other imaging modalities, in complete remission after surgery or chemotherapy. In the third patient no primary tumour was ever located. Ten other sites of metastatic spread were identified in this group. Seven of these correlated with known sites of tumour spread. A positive UJ13A scan occurred in three sites where disease was not thought to be present. Two of these represented previously undiscovered sites of tumour and were subsequently shown to be involved either at laparotomy or by ^{99m}Tc-MDP bone scan. One of these three UJ13A sites was proven to be a false positive and two negative UJ13A scans were reported at sites expected to be involved with tumour. All of the sites at which tumour was visualised were evident by 24 hr although clarity of images improved by 3 days as the blood pool levels of isotope decreased.

The sensitivity of tumour detection using this approach still needs to be accurately determined. The smallest tumour identified in the study was present in a lymph node 1.5 cm in diameter. Work is continuing in the laboratory to investigate the use of panels of antibodies to maximise tumour cell detection in children with neuroblastoma (Malpas et al., 1982). It is unfortunate that no other RIL studies in children with this malignancy have been reported. The efficiency of the technique can therefore only be judged by comparison of results in adults with other tumours, using different radiolabelled antibodies (Mach et al., 1980; Epenetos et al., 1982). By these criteria, it would seem that the results of RIL in children (obtained without computer enhancement) are as good as those achieved in adults, where sophisticated computer subtraction techniques are often employed.

The compound meta-iodobenzylguanidine (MIBG) (Vetter *et al.*, 1983) (An analogue of a precursor of epinephrine and norepinephrine) radiolabelled with isotopes of iodine has also been used to attempt RIL of neuroblastoma (Treuner *et al.*, 1984). The reports on the success of the technique are very preliminary and conflicting and therefore it is not possible to compare this procedure with radiolabelled antibody scans. In theory one might not expect this to be as efficient as the antibody approach, as not all neuroblastomas synthesise either epinephrine or norepinephrine (Voorhess, 1968) and not all will therefore anabolise the compound.

Despite the wide distribution of the UJ13A antigen (Allan *et al.*, 1983) on all neuroectodermally derived tissues apart from melanoma, the scans of patients with neuroblastoma showed no antibody uptake in either the brain or the retina. This is because the reagent is kept from these sites by the blood–brain (Vick and Bigner, 1972) and blood–retinal barriers (Tso and Shih, 1976). The operational specificity of the antibody is therefore far more important in this field than the actual true distribution of antigen. Uptake of the antibody to the peripheral nervous system was only detected in one site. In three of the nine patients in the study, the adrenal glands were visualised, suggesting that their size may represent the lower limit of sensitivity of the technique. Whilst the RIL of tumours still offers great potential as a diagnostic tool, problems have been encountered using radiolabelled mouse monoclonal antibodies in children. Variable uptake of the conjugates by the reticuloendothelial system have been observed and there is a relatively low percentage of the total injected dose taken up by the tumour. This has been found to vary from approximately 0.01% to 7% (J.T. Kemshead, unpublished observation). The reasons underlying these major problems and attempts at circumventing them are currently under investigation.

B. Intracranial Malignancies

Intracranial tumours have also not featured widely in RIL studies. Mahaley (1967) was one of the first workers to describe the use of heteroantisera radiolabelled with ^{125}I to image gliomas. More recently, Phillips *et al.*, (1982) demonstrated localisation of a human monoclonal antibody in one patient with a recurrent glioma. It is pertinent to question why so little attention has been paid to RIL of intracranial malignancies in comparison to other tumours (Smedley *et al.*, 1983; Begent *et al.*, 1980). This may be because of the reluctance to use antibodies which cross react with normal neural tissue and/or the uncertainty as to whether the blood–brain barrier will allow access of the antibody to the tumour. As indicated above, radiolabelled antibody UJ13A (of the IgG_1 isotype) does not cross the blood–brain barrier. This has to be broken, therefore, for antibody to gain access to any tumour. Blood–brain barrier disruption has been reported to occur to varying degrees in either the same or different tumour types (Vick and Bigner, 1972). Patients should therefore receive a ^{99m}Tc scan as a prerequisite for attempting RIL of intracranial tumours. If this shows breakdown, it is possible to question if a tumour can be identified specifically with radiolabelled monoclonal antibody.

Despite the non-selective binding of antibody UJ13A to normal and malignant intracranial tissues, the antibody was chosen to visualise tumours because of the experience gained in its use for RIL of neuroblastoma (Goldman *et al.*, 1984). In the first study, four patients were scanned—three with gliomas and one with a meningioma. All patients had received ^{99m}Tc scans and both informed consent and ethical committee approval was obtained for the study (Coakham *et al.*, 1984b; Richardson *et al.*, 1985a). Patients received, by intravenous injection, 1.5–2.0 mCi of ^{131}I conjugated to approximately 250 µg of UJ13A. Immediately after injection and 4 hr later, no uptake of the conjugate into the tumour could be detected in any patient. However, in all cases clear images of tumour could be identified at 24 hr, without computer enhancement, and these were still detectable 16 days after injection of the conjugate (Fig. 2) (Kemshead *et al.*, 1984a).

The kinetics of radiolabelled UJ13A association and disassociation from the tumour are therefore grossly different from that of ^{99m}Tc (tumours can be imaged within 4 hr).

The binding of radiolabelled antibody is restricted to the tumour and possibly normal brain juxtaposing the malignant area. As might be expected from the data obtained by ^{99}Tc scans, tumours do not cause generalised disruption of the blood–brain barrier. The 'operational' specificity of UJ13A is therefore maintained as the reagent cannot reach areas of normal tissue where binding could otherwise occur. Computer analysis of the amount of $UJ13A/^{131}$I conjugate in the tumour against that present in blood of normal brain indicates a ratio of at least 3 : 1, 6 days following the initial injection. This ratio increases with respect to time as the radiolabelled protein is lost from the blood at a faster rate than from the tumour (half-life in blood approximately 24 hr as compared to 72 hr in the tumour). Direct counting of isotope in the tumour and normal brain at the time of operation approximately parallels the data obtained by computer analysis of γ-camera images, and indicates that the ratio of conjugate in tumour to normal brain can be as high as 16 : 1, 16 days after injection of radiolabelled antibody (Richardson *et al.*, 1985b).

Whilst the images obtained in this study suggest antibodies can play

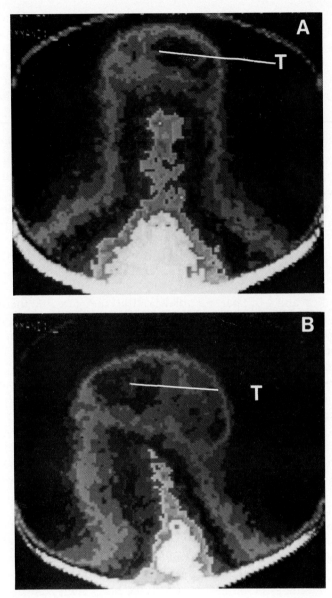

Fig. 2. Radioimmunolocalisation of radiolabelled UJ13A to a meningioma in the frontal lobe of the brain. A 55-year-old patient was injected with 1.9 mCi of ^{131}I conjugated to 200 μg of UJ13A. Images of the tumour were obtained at 24 hr after administration of the conjugate. Uptake of free iodine into the thyroid gland was blocked by Lugol's iodine given 3 days before and during the scanning period. (A) Anterior–posterior image; (B) lateral image. T, tumour deposits. (From Treleaven *et al.*, 1984.)

a role in the *in vivo* diagnosis of intracranial malignancies, the above data do not prove that uptake into the tumour is due directly to antibody binding to antigen. This is particularly relevant in brain tumours as prior to the use of ^{99m}Tc radiolabelled albumen was used as an 'imaging' agent in nuclear medicine. The simplest approach to demonstrate that tumour uptake is specific to antigen is to undertake two scans on an individual, one with UJ13A and one with an alternative antibody known not to bind to the malignant cells. Images obtained from the latter scans should show no uptake into the tumour site. However, whilst this is ideal, it presents ethical problems both in terms of the doses of isotope given to the patient and unwarranted delays in treatment. It is proposed to attempt this study using ^{123}I conjugated to the monoclonal antibodies. With a much shorter isotope half-life it is possible to compact the two procedures and reduce the total dose of radiation to the patient. Other technical problems may limit the feasibility of this, however, such as irreproducibility of radio-labelling protein with ^{123}I.

Two patients with malignant glioma hae been injected with radio-labelled antibody known not to bind tumour cells [UJ181.4 (Table I) and HMFG 1 (Taylor-Papadimitriou *et al.*, 1981)]. The kinetics of association and disassociation from the tumour parallel those for the conjugate in the blood. This is exactly the result one would expect from non-specific entry of the ^{131}I conjugate into tumour sites because of blood–brain barrier breakdown and the opposite of that expected in patients where an antibody known to bind to the tumour is used. Unfortunately, because of the need for surgery, only ^{99m}Tc scans were undertaken on these patients and therefore it was not possible to complete the study with UJ13A/131 conjugates.

Thus, whilst there is no direct proof that the UJ13A monoclonal antibody conjugate binds to antigen in tumours, all data currently obtained suggest this is the case. Further investigations are planned on a series of patients to prove this point.

IV. TUMOUR CELL REMOVAL FROM BONE MARROW HARVESTED FOR AUTOLOGOUS TRANSPLANTATION

Neuroblastoma is a tumour that, in general, responds well to chemotherapy. However, remissions are not prolonged and once relapse occurs it is difficult to find further effective therapy (Finkelstein, 1982). In the absence of new single agents that have been shown to be cytotoxic to neuroblastoma, the only option for improving therapy is to attempt to use new combinations of drugs and/or radiation therapy (Seeger *et al.*, 1984; August *et al.*, 1984). The doses of drugs that can be given to an individual are limited by toxicity to normal tissues. Bone marrow is the organ often most susceptible to drug and radiation therapy (McElwain *et al.*, 1979). To overcome this difficulty, high-dose therapy is applied to the patient after a proportion of marrow is removed. This is then rein- fused to rescue the haemopoietic system after the levels of cytotoxic agents in the patient have fallen to below those known to ablate bone marrow progenitors cells. One of the problems with this type of therapy is that, where metastatic spread of tumour occurs, malignant cells may be harvested along with the bone marrow, and thus not be exposed to the supralethal therapy applied to the patient.

Several techniques have been developed to remove/ablate tumour cells from bone marrow harvested for autologous transplantation. These in- clude treatment of bone marrow with drugs e.g., 4-hydroperoxycyclo- phosphamide (Kaiser *et al.*, 1981) and 4-hydroxydopamine (Joussen and Sachs; 1975; Reynolds *et al.*, 1980) or physical procedures relying on dif- ferential centrifugation (Dicke *et al.*, 1979; Figdor *et al.*, 1984). Immu- nological methods for depleting tumour cells from bone marrow include simply coating malignant cells with antibody for opsonisation (Prentice *et al.*, 1982), treating bone marrow with antibody and complement (Bast *et al.*, 1982; Granger *et al.*, 1982), or with antibodies to which either drugs (Rowland *et al.*, 1981, 1982) or toxins (Krolick and Vitetta, 1982; Thorpe *et al.*, 1982) (e.g., a toxin isolated from the castor bean plant *Ricinus com- munis*) have been attached.

The use of the fluorescence-activated cell sorter for cleansing tumour cells from bone marrow has been explored in experimental systems (Herzenberg and Herzenberg, 1978). Whilst giving extremely good re- sults, the speed of sorting needed to achieve maximal separation (2000– 3000 cells/sec) is too slow to remove malignant cells from approximately 5×10^9 nucleated cells.

An alternative approach to fluorescent sorting is to use a magnetic separation procedure. The concept of separating cells on the basis of their iron content is not new, but has been restricted to cells which either contain or will endocytose particles of iron, e.g., red blood cells and macrophages. Recently it has become possible to target colloidal particles of magnetic material (e.g., cobalt) (Poynton *et al.*, 1983) or microspheres (Ugelstad *et al.*, 1980) containing magnetite to any cell type using mon- oclonal antibodies (Treleaven *et al.*, 1984). Figure 3 shows a scanning electron micrograph of monodisperse polystyrene beads containing

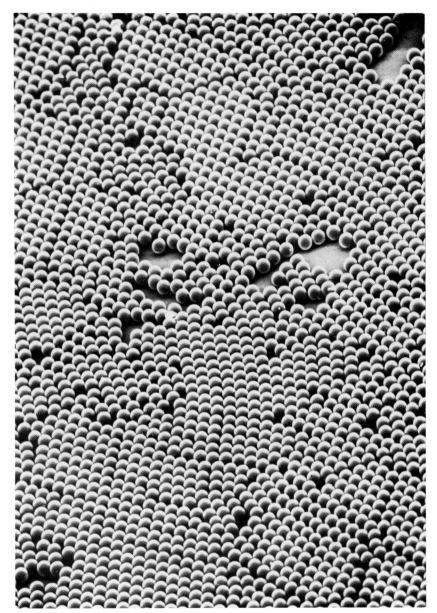

Fig. 3. Scanning electron micrograph of 3-µm polystyrene microspheres illustrating the monodispersity and uniformity of the preparation. (From Treleaven *et al.*, 1984.)

19.4% magnetite (produced by Prof. J. Ugelsted, Department of Polymer Chemistry, University of Trondheim, Norway). These are made by the polymerisation of styrene divinylbenzene and modified to render them hydrophilic (Ugelstad *et al.*, 1983). The beads have a pitted surface of large surface area (100–150 m^2/g). Under appropriate conditions, proteins can be adsorbed onto the surface of the beads and used to target them to any cell type.

An indirect system was chosen to target microspheres to tumour cells. A panel of six anti-neuroblastoma antibodies are used in the procedure to maximise binding to tumour cells and to attempt to overcome the problem of antigenic heterogeneity (Malpas *et al.*, 1982). These reagents are individually purified using protein A affinity chromatography and concentrated to 1.0 mg/ml. Sufficient amount of each antibody is added to a buffy coat fraction of bone marrow to saturate binding to a 5% infiltrate of tumour. Following incubation for 30 min at 4°C, the marrow is washed once with phosphate-buffered saline and 5% purified protein fraction (PPF) to remove unbound antibody. Approximately 85% of the nucleated cells in the buffy coat fraction are recovered.

Microspheres initially sterilised by washing in alcohol are incubated with sheep anti-mouse Ig in 0.1 M phosphate-buffered saline (PBS), pH 7.7, for 18 hr at 4°C (10-mg beads at 1.0 mg/ml). The microspheres are washed free of unbound antibody before use. Trace label studies indicate that approximately 70% of the protein binds to the spheres. These are added to the bone marrow in excess (a minimum of 400 beads : 1 tumour cell) and incubated for 1 hr at 4°C (Fig. 4).

The magnetic separation device used to remove 'magnetic' tumour cells from bone marrow is a completely enclosed system consisting of a series of polycarbonate chambers linked by silicone rubber tubing. Cells coated with microspheres are removed from the marrow using relatively high-field strength samarium cobalt permanent magnets. These are situated in grooves cut into the base of the main chamber so that they are separated from the interior by 2 mm of polycarbonate. To ensure maximum efficiency of separation, a second smaller chamber is linked to the first and has two samarium magnets in its base (Fig. 5). Finally, a third chamber is situated between the poles of a water cooled electromagnet (field strength 1.0 Tesla). Any free microspheres or tumour cells that escape the first two chambers are removed by this magnet. The system is assembled under sterile conditions and primed with PBS and 20% PPF. The treated bone marrow is pumped through the system at a rate of 1.5 ml/min. The apparatus is flushed free of bone marrow cells using PBS, 5% PPF. Approximately 5 × 10^9 bone marrow cells can be purged of at least 99.9% of tumour in 3 hr.

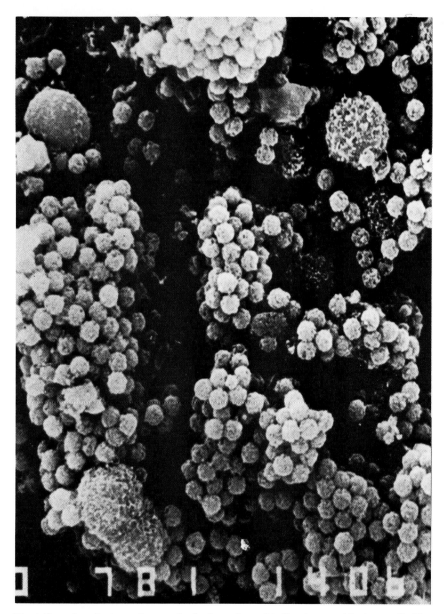

Fig. 4. Scanning electron micrograph of microspheres binding to neuroblastoma cells. The human neuroblastoma cell line CHP100 was incubated with a panel of monoclonal antibodies and anti-mouse Ig-coated microspheres. After concentration of cells using a magnet, the preparation was prepared for scanning electron microscopy.

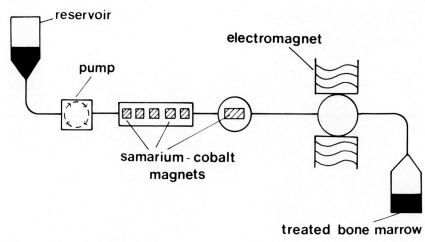

Fig. 5. Diagramatic representation of the apparatus devised for the removal of tumour cells from bone marrow. (Modified from Treleaven *et al.*, 1984.)

Estimates of the number of tumour cells removed from bone marrow are relatively imprecise as it is not possible to identify these at a frequency of more than 1 in 10,000. Experiments can be designed to increase this sensitivity but these are not analogous to the methods needed for large-scale handling of bone marrow containing tumour cells. The only way to accurately assess the effectiveness of this type of procedure is on long-term follow-up studies on patients known to have tumour cells in their bone marrow. To date, four children with overt tumour cell involvement in their marrow (1–5%) have been treated by very high-dose chemo-therapy and haemopoietic rescue via autologous cleaned marrow. The therapy given to each individual has varied slightly in this multi-centre study, but each instance has involved the use of total body irradiation (900–1200 rads fractionated or non-fractionated) and high-dose melphalan (140–180 mg/m^2) (McElwain *et al.*, 1979). In one centre, vincristine has been added to this regime, given over a 5-day period (day 1, 1.5 mg/m^2; days 2–5, 0.5 mg/m^2). All patients that have received this therapy remain well, but the maximum time from treatment is only 10 months; follow-up studies are necessary to ascertain if this is a useful approach to treating either relapsing patients with neuroblastoma or using it as a first line therapy.

To date, 29 patients with either Stage III or Stage IV neuroblastoma have been treated with these ablative protocols and magnetic micro-spheres to purge tumour cells from bone marrow. In addition, by chang-ing the antibodies, bone marrows from 2 children with B cell lymphoma and 1 with acute lymphoblastic leukaemia have been purged of tumour

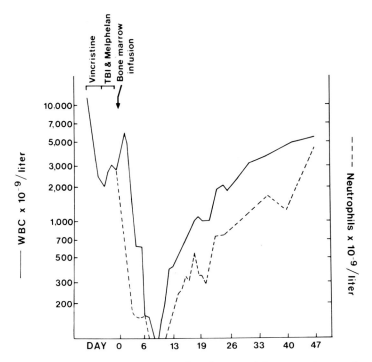

Fig. 6. Recovery of peripheral blood white cell and neutrophil counts after autologous grafting with purged bone marrow. After bone marrow harvest, the patient was treated with vincristine 1.5 mg/m² on day 1, followed by vincristine 0.5 mg/m by infusion on the next 4 days. On days 6–8 she received a total of 1200 rads given in two daily fractions. Finally on day 7, she received 90 mg of melphalan (180 mg/m²). The total nucleated cells returned to the patient was 1.2 × 10⁸/g body weight. (From Treleaven *et al.*, 1984.)

cells. In most cases haemopoietic recovery has been very rapid (time to 500 neutrophils in the blood 12–21 days, and 50,000 platelets 26–36 days) (Fig. 6). The only exceptions to this are patients that have received prolonged and extensive therapy prior to this regime. In these children, the time to 500 neutrophils in the blood has been up to 60 days, and particularly prolonged when individuals have received high doses of alkalating agents.

V. MONOCLONAL ANTIBODIES USED TO TARGET THERAPEUTIC AGENTS *IN VIVO*

Selective targeting of therapeutic agents into tumours, to reduce toxicity to normal tissues, has been attempted for many years. Monoclonal antibodies against iodiotypic determinants on Ig molecules have been shown to be of therapeutic benefit in patients with B cell lymphoma (Miller *et al.*, 1982; Foon, 1982). This approach, however, is extremely specialised due to the interaction of anti-idiotype and Ig, and cannot be applied to other malignancies. Experiments using conjugates of either drugs [e.g., vindesine (Rowland *et al.*, 1981)] or toxins (Thorpe and Ross, 1982) and monoclonal antibodies have not reached the point where they can be applied to the *in vivo* treatment of tumours. A variety of heteroantisera to ferritin, conjugated with ^{131}I, have been used as therapeutic agents in patients with hepatocellular carcinoma and Hodgkin's disease (Order *et al.*, 1983; Lenhard *et al.*, 1983). B irradiation from the ^{131}I with a penetration of 2 mm in human tissues is responsible for the cytotoxic effects of the conjugates.

Human neuroblastoma xenografts in nude mice can be ablated using a monoclonal antibody conjugated with [131]I. Tumours of approximately 1.0 cm diameter were successfully treated by administration of three injections of 150 μc of ^{131}I conjugated to 150μg of UJ13A, given over a 23-week period. This effect was only found when ^{131}I was targeted to tumour sites, and antibody injected alone did not have any tumouricidal effect.

Mice cannot be used to estimate the toxicity of a UJ13A radiolabelled conjugate to normal tissues as the antibody does not bind to normal murine neural tissue. Furthermore, a mouse monoclonal antibody injected into a mouse will be recognised and processed by the reticuloendothelial system in a different way than if it were injected into a primate. High doses of UJ13A/^{131}I conjugates have therefore been injected into marmosets (4 × 2.0 mCi of ^{131}I coupled to 2.0 mg of UJ13A) over a period of 12 months. Animals given this conjugate and others given control injections of either ^{131}I alone or antibody alone suffered no gross physiological disturbance. As was predicted from biodistribution studies of small doses of conjugate in patients with Stage IV neuroblastoma, no ^{131}I was detected intracranially in the marmoset, although uptake into the reticuloendothelial system (liver, spleen and bone marrow) was noted. Thus, whilst certain tissues (brain and retina) are protected from the high doses of isotope/antibody conjugate by blood–tissue barriers, others may suffer damage from the targeted agent.

A Phase 1 study in children relapsing with Stage IV neuroblastoma has begun to investigate toxicity of this type of targeted therapy. Doses of approximately 50 mCi of ^{131}I conjugated to 20 mg of UJ13A were found to cause bone marrow aplasia in two children (J. T. Kemshead, unpublished observation).

This was found to be variable, and may be due to either the degree of prior therapy given, and/or the differential non-specific uptake of the conjugate by the reticuloendothelial system. Preliminary data indicate that one of the children in the initial study received therapeutic benefit from the procedure. After administration of 55 mCi of conjugated ^{131}I, bone marrow remained free of tumour for 8 months and bone scans showed healing of lytic sites in the pelvis and tibia (Kemshead *et al.*, 1984b). Major problems have, however, been encountered in this study. The total dose of conjugate reaching the tumour is small (and variable) in comparison to the total material injected. Much work remains to reduce the uptake of the conjugates by the reticuloendothelial system. The method of targeting therapy, however, looks promising, particularly when only small tumour masses remain. It is hoped that targeted radiation therapy may one day replace total body irradiation in children, and reduce the considerable side effects of this type of therapy.

ACKNOWLEDGEMENTS

This work was supported by the Bristol Brain Tumour Fund and the Imperial Cancer Research Fund. We wish to thank Mrs. J. Farley, Mrs. D. Jones Goulton and Ms. F. Gibson for their excellent technical assistance, and Mrs. S. Watts for typing this manuscript.

REFERENCES

Allan, P. M., Garson, J. A., Harper, E. I., Asser, U., Coakham, H. B., Brownell, B., and Kemshead, J. T. (1983). *Int. J. Cancer* **31**, 591–598.
Ashall, F., Bramwell, M. E., and Harris, H. A. (1982). *Lancet* **1**, 1–6.
August, C. S., Elkins, W., Burkey, E., D'Angio, G. D., and Evans, A. (1984). Submitted for publication.
Bast, R. C., Jr., Ritz, J., Feeney, M., Lipton, J., Sallen, S., Nathen, E., and Schlossman, S. I. (1982). *Am. Soc. Clin. Oncol.* Abstr. 1043.
Begent, R. H. J., Stanway, G., Jones, B. E., Bagshawe, K. D., Searle, F., Jeunes, R. F., and Vernon, P. (1980). *J. R. Soc. Med.* **73**, 629–630.
Breard, J., Reinherz, E. L., Kung, P. C., Goldstein, G., and Schlossman, S. I. (1980). *J. Immunol.* **124**, 1943–1948.
Coakham, H. B., Garson, J. A., Brownell, B., Allan, P. M., Harper, E. I., Lane, E. B., and Kemshead, J. T. (1984a). *Lancet* **1**, 1095–1097.
Coakham, H. B., Garson, J. A., Brownell, B., Allan, P. M., Harper, E. I., Kemshead, J. T. (1984b). *S. Afr. J. Surg.* **22**, 13–22.
Crowhurst, S., Cotmore, S. F., and Waterfield, M. D. (1985). In preparation.
Dicke, K. A., Spitzer, G., Zander, A. R., Lanzotti, V. J., Verma, D. S., Petus, C. P., Val-

divieso, M., Lotzova, E., and McCredie, K. B. (1979). *Transplant. Proc.* **11**, 212–214.
Eisenbarth, G. S., Walsh, F. S., and Nirenberg, M. (1979). *Proc. Natl. Acad. Sci. U.S.A.* **76**, 4913–4917.
Eng, L. F., van der Haeghen, J. J., Bignami, A., and Gerstl, B. (1971). *Brain Res.* **28**, 351–358.
Epenetos, A. A., Britton, K. E., Mather, S., Shepherd, J., Granowska, M., Taylor-Papadimitriou, J., Nimmon, C. C., Durbin, H., Hawkin, L. R., Malpas, J. S., and Bodmer, W. F. (1982). *Lancet* **1**, 999–1004.
Figdor, C., Voute, P. A., de Kraker, J., Bont, W., and Vernie, L. (1984). *In* "Advances in Neuroblastoma Research" (A. E. Evans, G. J. D'Angio, and R. L. Seeger, eds.), Vol. 3, pp. 459–470. Alan R. Liss, Inc., New York.
Finklestein, J. Z. (1982). *In* "Diagnostic and Biological Markers for Neuroblastoma Clinical and Biological Manifestations" (C. Pochedly, ed.), pp. 281–291. Am. Elsevier, New York.
Foon, K. A. (1982). *N. Engl. J. Med.* **307**, 686–687.
Goldman, A., Vivian, G., Gordon, I., Pritchard, J., and Kemshead, J. T. (1984). *J. Pediatr. (St. Louis)* **105**, 252–256.
Granger, S. M., Janossy, G., Francis, G., Blacklock, H., Poulter, L. W., and Hoffbrand, A. V. (1982). *Br. J. Haematol.* **50**, 367–374.
Green, A. A., Hustu, H. O., Palmer, R., and Pinkel, D. (1976). *Cancer (Amsterdam)* **38**, 2250–2257.
Herzenberg, L. A., and Herzenberg, L. A. (1978). *In* "Handbook of Experimental Immunology" (D. M. Weir, ed.), 3rd ed., Vol. 3, p. 1. Blackwell, Oxford.
Jaffe, N. (1976). *Cancer Treat. Rev.* **3**, 61–82.
Jousson, G., and Sachs, C. (1975). *J. Neurochem.* **25**, 509–516.
Kaiser, H., Stewart, R. K., Colvin, M., Korhling, M., Wharam, M. D., and Santos, G. W. (1981). *Exp. Haematol.* **9**, Suppl. 9, 190.
Kemshead, J. T., and Black, J. (1980). *Dev. Med. Child Neurol.* **22**, 816–829.
Kemshead, J. T., and Coakham, H. B. (1983). *J. Pathol.* **141**, 249–257.
Kemshead, J. T., Fritschy, J., Garson, J. A., Allan, P., Coakham, H., Brown, S., and Asser, U. (1983a). *Int. J. Cancer* **31**, 187–195.
Kemshead, J. T., Goldman, A., Fritschy, J., Malpas, J. S., and Pritchard, J. (1983b). *Lancet* **1**, 12–15.
Kemshead, J. T., Jones, D. H., Goldman, A., Richardson, R. B., and Coakham, H. B. (1984a). *J. R. Soc. Med.* **77**, 847–854.
Kemshead, J. T., Goldman, A., Jones, D., Pritchard, J., Malpas, J. S., Gordon, I., Malone, J. F., Hurley, J. D., Breatnach, F. (1984b). *In* "Advances in Neuroblastoma Research" (A. E. Evans, G. J. D'Angio, and R. L. Seeger, eds.), Vol. 3, pp. 533–544. Alan R. Liss, New York.
Krolick, K. A., and Vitetta, E. S. (1982). *Nature (London)* **295**, 604–605.
Kung, P. C., Goldstein, G., Reinherz, E. L., and Schlossman, S. F. (1979). *Science* **206**, 347–349.
Lane, E. B. (1982). *J. Cell Biol.* **92**, 665–673.
Lenhard, R. E., Order, S. E., Spunberg, J. J., Ettinger, D. S., Askell, S. O., and Leibel, S. A. (1983). *Am. Soc. Clin. Oncol.*, Abstr. 825, p. 211.
McElwain, T., Hedley, D. W., Burton, G., Clink, H. M., Gordon, M. Y., Jarman, M., Jutter, C. A., Miller, J. L., Milstead, R. A. V., Prentice, G., Smith, I. E., Spence, D., and Woods, M. (1979). *Br. J. Cancer* **40**, 72–80.
Mach, J. P., Carrel, S., and Forni, M. (1980). *N. Engl. J. Med.* **303**, 5–10.
Mach, J. P., Bucheggar, F., Forni, M., Ritschard, J., Berche, C., Lambroso, J. D., Schreyer, M., Giradet, C., Accolla, R. S., and Carrell, S. (1981). *Immunol. Today* **2**, 238–249.

Mahaley, M. S. (1967). *Clin. Neurosurg.* **15,** 175–189.

Malpas, J. S., Kemshead, J. T., Pritchard, J., and Greaves, M. F. (1982). *In* "Proceedings of the 13th Meeting of the International Society of Pediatric Oncology" (C., Raybaud, R. Clement, G. Lebreuil, and J. L. Bernard, eds.), pp. 90–95. Excerpta Medica, Amsterdam.

Miller, R. A., Maloney, D. G., Warnke, R., and Levy, R. (1982). *N. Engl. J. Med.* **306,** 517–523.

Order, S. E., Ettinger, D. S., Leibel, S. A., Klein, J. L., and Leichner, P. K. (1983). *Am. Soc. Clin. Oncol.,* Abstr. 464, p. 119.

Pallensen, G., Jepsen, F. L., Hastrup, J., Ipsen, A., and Nvidberg, N. (1983). *Lancet* **1,** 1326.

Phillips, J., Sikora, K., and Watson, J. V. (1982). *Lancet,* **1,** 1214–1215.

Pizzolo, G., Sloane, J., Beverley, P., Thomas, J. A., Bradstock, K. F., Mattingley, S., and Janossy, G. (1980). *Cancer (Amsterdam)* **46,** 2640–2647.

Poynton, C. H., Dicke, K. A., Culbert, S., Frankel, L. S., Jagannath, S., and Reading, C. L. (1983). *Lancet* **1,** 524.

Prentice, H. G., Blacklock, H. A., Janossy G., Bradstock, K. F., Skeggs, D., Goldstein, G., and Hoffbrand, A. V. (1982). *Lancet* **1,** 700–703.

Pressman, D., and Keighley, G. (1948). *J. Immunol.* **59,** 141–146.

Pritchard, J., McElwain, T. J., and Graham-Pole, J. (1982). *Br. J. Cancer* **45,** 86–94.

Raney, R. B., Lyon, G. M., and Porter, F. S. (1976). *J. Pediatr. (St. Louis)* **89,** 433–435.

Raschke, W. C. (1982). *In* "Monoclonal Antibodies to Human Tumour Antigens in Human Cancer Markers" (S. Sell and B. Wahren, eds.), pp.1–32. Humana Press, Clifton, New Jersey.

Reynolds, C. P., Reynolds, D. A., Frenkel, E. P., and Smith, R. G. (1980). *Am. Soc. Clin. Oncol.* **21,** 392 (Abstr. 290).

Reynolds, C. P., Smith, R. G., and Frenkel, E. P. (1981). *Cancer (Amsterdam),* **48,** 2088–2092.

Reynolds, C. P., and Graham-Smith, R. (1982). *In* "Diagnostic and Biologic Markers for Neuroblastoma Clinical and Biological Manifestations" (C. Pochedly, ed.), pp. 131–167. Am. Elsevier, New York.

Reynolds, C. P., Moss, T. J., Seeger, R. C., Black, A. T., and Woody, J. N. (1984). *In* "Advances in Neuroblastoma Research" (A. E. Evans, G. J. D'Angio, and R. L. Seeger, eds.), Vol. 3. pp. 425–441. Alan R. Liss, Inc., New York.

Richardson, R., Davies, G., Bourne, S. P., Staddon, G. E., Kemshead, J. T., and Coakham, H. B. (1985a). *J. Neuro oncology* (in press).

Richardson, R., Davies, G., Bourne, S. P., Jones, D., Kemshead, J. T., and Coakham, H. B. (1985b) *J. Neurosurg.* (in press).

Ritz, J., Pesando, J. M., Notis-McConarty, J., Lazarus, H., and Schlossman, S. F. (1980). *Nature (London)* **283,** 583–585.

Rowland, G. F., Simmonds, R. G., Corvalan, J. R. F., Marsden, C. H., Johnson, J. R., Woodhouse, C. S., Ford, C. H. J., and Newman, C. E. (1981). *Protides Biol. Fluids* **29,** 921–926.

Rowland, G. F., Simmonds, R. G., Corvalan, J. R. F., Baldwin, R. W., Brown, J. P., Embelton, M. J., Ford, C. H. J., Hellström, K. E., Hellström, I., Kemshead, J. T., Newman, C. E., and Woodhouse, C. S. (1982). *Protides Biol. Fluids* **30,** 375–379.

Schnegg, J. F., Diserens, A. C., Carrel, S., Accolla, R. S., and de Tribolet, N. (1981). *Cancer Res.* **41,** 1029–1035.

Schulz, G., Bumol, T. F., and Reisfeld, R. A. (1983). *Proc. Natl. Acad. Sci. U.S.A.* **80,** 5407–5412.

Seeger, R. C., (1982). *In* "Diagnostic and Biologic Markers for Neuroblastoma in Neuroblastoma Clinical and Biological Manifestations" (C. Pochedly, ed.)., pp. 169–182. Am. Elsevier, New York.

Seeger, R. C., Zeltzer, P. M., and Rayner, S. A. (1979). *J. Immunol.* **122,** 1548–1555.

Seeger, R. C., Rosenblatt, H. M., and Imai, K. (1981). *Cancer Res.* **41,** 2714–2717.

Seeger, R. C., Danon, Y. L., and Rayner, S. A. (1982). *J. Immunol.* **128,** 983–989.

Seeger, R. C., Lenarsky, C., Moss, T. J., Siegel, S. E., and Wells, J. (1984). *Am. Soc. Pediatr. Res., Abstr.* **18,** 248A.

Smedley, H. M., Finan, P., Lennox, E. S., Ritson, A., Takei, F., Wraight, P., and Sikora, K. (1983). *Br. J. Cancer* **47,** 253–259.

Sweet, E. M. (1983). *In* "Assessment by Radiological Techniques in Paediatric Oncology" (W. Duncan, ed.), pp. 26–36. Springer-Verlag, Berlin and New York.

Taylor-Papadimitriou, J., Peterson, J. A., Arklie, J., Burchell, J., Ceriani, R. C., and Bodmer, W. F. (1981). *Int. J. Cancer* **28,** 17–21.

Thorpe, P. E., and Ross, W. C. J. (1982). *Immunol. Rev.* **62,** 119–158.

Thorpe, P. E., Mason, D. W., Brown, A. N. F., Simmonds, S. J., Ross, W. C. J., Curnber, A. J., and Forrester, J. A. (1982). *Nature (London)* **297,** 594–596.

Treleaven, J. G., Gibson, F. M., Ugelstad, J., Rembaum, A., Philip, T., Caine, G. D., and Kemshead, J. T. (1984). *Lancet* **1,** 70–73.

Treuner, J., Feine, U., Niethammer, D., Muller-Schaunberg, W., Meinke, J., Eibach, E., Dopfer, R., Klingebiel, T., and Grumbach, S. (1984). *Lancet* **1,** 333–334.

Tso, M. O. M., and Shih, C. Y. (1976). *Exp. Eye Res.* **23,** 209–216.

Ugelstad, J., Mork, P. C., Kaggerud, K. H., Ellingsen, T., and Berge, A. (1980). *Adv. Colloid. Interface Sci.* **13,** 101–140.

Ugelstad, J., Soderberg, L., Berge, A., and Bergstrom, J. (1983). *Nature (London)* **303,** 96–98.

Vetter, H., Fischer, M., Muller-Rensing, R., Velter, W., and Winterberg, B. (1983). *Lancet* **1,** 107–108.

Vick, N. A., and Bigner, D. D. (1972). *J. Neurol. Sci.* **17,** 29–39.

Voorhess, M. L. (1968). *J. Pediatr. Surg.* **3,** 147–151.

CHAPTER 15

Analysis, Results, and Future Prospective of the Therapeutic Use of Radiolabeled Antibody in Cancer Therapy

Stanley E. Order

Radiation Oncology
The Johns Hopkins Hospital Oncology Center
Baltimore, Maryland, U.S.A.

The complexity of research efforts concerning the use of radiolabeled antibody in cancer therapy is due to the need for the integration of immunology, physics, and radiation oncology as well as new unexpected variables that have been uncovered as further study has progressed (Order *et al.*, 1979). To allow the reader to integrate these disciplines and the new findings, each area of interest is discussed individually, later integrated, and then new prospectives offering further possible progress are discussed.

MONOCLONAL ANTIBODIES FOR CANCER
DETECTION AND THERAPY

I. THE TUMOR TARGET

The initial impression that tumor-specific and only tumor-specific antigens would be appropriate targets for radiolabeled antibodies placed the requirement of unique tumor specificity on investigators that sought to utilize radiolabeled antibodies for cancer therapy. Often antigens might be considered relatively unique, but if persistent investigation was carried out the specificity could be demonstrated in other tissues and/or tumors. Among the early antigens identified and targeted with ^{131}I antibodies were fibrin (Spar *et al.*, 1967), human chorionic gonadotropin (Bagshawe *et al.*, 1980), carcinoembryonic antigen (CEA) (Goldenberg *et al.*, 1978), and ferritin (Order *et al.*, 1975). In considering the nature of the problem of radiolabeled antibodies targeting cancer, antigens were chosen that were in high concentration and presented a significant target allowing the delineation of tumors diagnostically by comparing the concentration in the tumor over time to the background, i.e., the so called tumor : normal tissue ratio. Even while this research was ongoing, it had long been realized that surface antigens, such as the TL^+ thymic–leukemic antigen (Old *et al.*, 1968), represented a more restricted antigen normally not found outside the thymus gland except if T cell leukemia occurred.

How then, based on these diverse observations, are we to construct a view of solid tumors as antigenic targets? Is unique specificity a requirement? In our laboratory we have demonstrated a phenomenon called the "biologic window" (Fig. 1). This window accounts for the selective binding of ^{131}I anti-ferritin in hepatoma compared to the normal tissues (many which contain ferritin) (Rostock *et al.*, 1983). This selectivity at the tumor target also exists for other antigens. The "biologic window" to date consists of the neovasculature of tumors, tumor cell ferritin synthesis and secretion, and slower blood flow. These are the physiologic and metabolic characteristics of the window which allow selective targeting (Rostock *et al.*, 1984). The data clearly demonstrate that any high-concentration antigenic component in tumors may act as a suitable target for radiolabeled antibodies.

More recently it has been shown that smaller tumors have an ideal ratio of blood vessels to tumor and a high ferritin secretion rate which makes them excellent targets for radiolabeled antibodies (Fig. 1). However, based on dosimetric considerations, a modest size tumor will have a significant radiolabeled antibody concentration ($\mu Ci/g$) and an increased tumor dose due to the overall concentration in a somewhat larger mass.

Antigens should probably be segregated into at least two classes, those

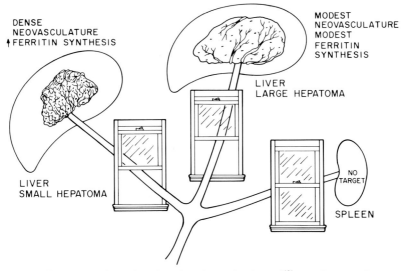

DENSE
NEOVASCULATURE
↑FERRITIN SYNTHESIS

MODEST
NEOVASCULATURE
MODEST
FERRITIN
SYNTHESIS

LIVER
LARGE HEPATOMA

LIVER
SMALL HEPATOMA

NO
TARGET

SPLEEN

Fig. 1. The "biologic window" describes the selective binding of ^{131}I anti-ferritin in hepatoma (or other ferritin-bearing tumors) over normal tissue. Characteristics which seem to influence the targeting are tumor neovasculature, ferritin synthesis, and a slower blood flow; all relate to tumor size. The smaller tumors have the greatest efficiency for uptake. The spleen does not take up more anti-ferritin then would normal IgG.

that are secreted from tumor cells into the circulation, and those that remain in close association with the tumor cell surface or other cell surfaces within tumors but are not represented in the circulation. In addition (Fig. 2), the neovasculature, stroma, and tumor cells all represent a reasonable series of targets because, dependent on the linear energy of the isotope, regional targeting may be cytotoxic to tumor cells.

The solid tumor itself must be considered an integrated mass with variable proportions of diverse antigenic moieties, which may allow amplification of radiolabeled antibody deposition by considering the most effective antigenic sites for targeting (Fig. 3).

If consideration is given to human cell surface non-secreted antigens analogous to the TL^+ antigen, then antigenic modulations that have been found to occur in both systems (Old et al., 1968) must be considered; i.e., the antigen under antibody attack may be modulated by the tumor cell. In contrast, antigens that are secreted by the tumor cell (ferritin), if exposed to high-affinity antibodies, may bind the antigen in the circulation and inhibit tumor targeting. Thus it is necessary to consider, in selection of radiolabeled antibodies for *in vivo* tumor targeting, antibody affinity, antigenic modulation, and the isotope's linear radiation energy so that the proper distance within the cancer may be irradiated.

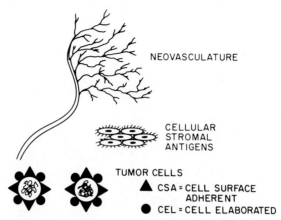

Fig. 2. Solid tumors have both cell surface and cell elaborated antigens as well as potential antigens in the stroma and neovasculature. The complete knowledge of antigenicity and potential targets will be needed to optimize radiolabeled antibody applications.

Finally, tumors in the peritoneal cavity or in the circulation offer different targeting situations and associated cellular interaction. In the peripheral circulation, monoclonal antibodies once adherent to leukemic cells will be cleared rapidly in the spleen and liver (Miller and Levy, 1981). In the peritoneal cavity, antibody may be exposed to tumor cells directly, and experimentally macrophage activation and cytotoxicity has led to tumor cure in a C_3Heb/Fej ovarian cancer (Order et al., 1974).

It is expected, therefore, that as investigators study diverse tumors, the antigenic moieties which offer greatest advantage for tumor targeting will be enumerated based on the dosimetry and therapeutic effectiveness of counterpart radiolabeled antibodies. Thus, antigenic profiles will be developed which characterize cancers and will be the preliminary analysis required prior to therapeutic intervention.

II. THE ANTIBODY MOLECULE

The IgG molecule initially became the carrier for isotope, and the diagnostic localization in tumors was demonstrable in a variety of cancers (Pressman et al., 1957; Goldenberg et al., 1978; Mach et al., 1980; Order et al., 1975, 1980). However, interest grew particularly in the use of Fab fragments for the reversal of digoxin intoxication (Smith et al., 1977) where it was successful. Fab fragments from the immunospecific anti-digoxin cleared the digoxin more rapidly then the intact IgG molecule. Our own

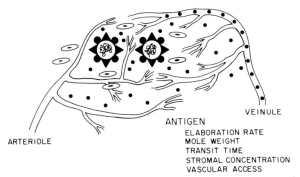

Fig. 3. The cancer cell elaborated antigens pose a kinetic problem as well. In the dynamic state of a viable tumor, antigenic representation and distribution will play a significant role in tumor targeting. Example: AFP was a poor antigenic target for therapy with a low molecular weight, high elaboration rate, and rapid transit time and vascular access.

laboratory investigated Fab or Fab^2 from the viewpoint of radiolabeled antibody and found that (1) nonlabeled Fab was not curative in our ovarian cancer model, whereas heat inactivated antiserum with IgG was (Wright *et al.*, 1979); (2) radiolabeled Fab or Fab^2 led to rapid clearance but poor tumor dose deposition. (Diagnostic scanning requires maximal differences between foreground and background, whereas therapy requires maximal deposition over time.) This, in addition to other data, led to the conclusion that Fab^2 represents an ideal scanning agent with rapid background clearance and a less effective therapeutic agent carrying less isotope and clearing more rapidly from the tumor as well as normal tissue.

The advent of monoclonal technology (Kohler and Milstein, 1975) led to a variety of laboratories seeking high-affinity monoclonal antibodies with the ability to examine subclasses of IgG, of which to date IgG$_{2a}$ has been a superior and more stable subclass of antibody. It remains to be determined what other antibodies and antibody subclasses might be of value other than IgG.

III. THE RADIOLABELING PROCESS

Initially, chloramine T (Pressman *et al.*, 1957) and more recently lactoperoxidase (Marchalonis, 1969) have been used to iodinate the isotopes ^{131}I or ^{125}I to antibody. ^{131}I has the advantage of both irradiation for visualization and β irradiation for treatment (Leichner *et al.*, 1981). The disadvantages of ^{131}I are that in therapeutic doses above 30 mCi, hospital-ization is required for patient isolation due to radiation emanating from the patient; the present dose rates available from maximal labeling indices (8-10mCi/mg) are less than ideal. The use of ^{125}I, although at first glance appealing, would require a longer sustenance at the tumor target than can be achieved; therefore, the dose rate and total tumor dose would be reduced. More recently in our laboratory, Dr. Jerry L. Klein attempted labeling by the Bolton Hunter method but it still held no advantage over previous labeling methods for ^{131}I.

The advent of monoclonal antibody brought a renewed interest in chelation methods of labeling ^{111}In for diagnostic purposes (Halpern *et al.*, 1983). In therapeutic attempts, the finding of dehalogenation of monoclonal murine-derived antibodies has given further stimulus to seek new methods of radiolabeling (Order, 1982), and chelation of other iso-topes is presently under study.

In the therapeutic application of radiolabeled antibodies, a variety of α and β emitters remain attractive. The dangers of release of free isotope, extreme toxicity, and a variety of manufacturing problems have inhibited progress to date. However, it is to be expected that these technical matters will be overcome and will allow outpatient treatment with higher tumor dose rates and total doses of radiation to be achieved.

Of the areas of immediate concern, new isotopic radiolabels remain perhaps the most relevant—the solution of this problem would signif-icantly enlarge the scope of therapeutic applications for radiolabeled an-tibodies.

IV. SPECIES OF DERIVATON OF ANTIBODIES

In a desire to treat patients with multiple courses of radiolabeled an-tibodies, the rather straightforward approach of immunization of a num-ber of species led us to the unanticipated finding that species of origin significantly altered the tumor-effective half-life. Tumor-effective half-life is the resultant of the biological and physical half-lives of the ra-diolabeled antibodies. It, along with the concentration in millicuries per gram, determines the tumor dose. In our experience, rabbit, pig, and monkey antibodies had tumor-effective half-lives of 3–4 days and were associated with tumor remission. Sheep, goat, chicken, and turkey an-tibodies had tumor-effective half-lives of 2 days or less and therefore were not associated with remissions. Our conclusion has been that tumor-effective half-life was most effected by species of origin, whereas tumor concentration was related to specificity.

These observations have particular impact on the development of therapeutic monoclonal antibody since to date most monoclonal antibodies have been murine derived and will be associated with reduced tumor-effective half-lives. Of course, human monoclonal antibodies would not have such restrictions as it would be expected that a longer tumor-effective half-life would be achieved and the antibody could be recycled due to reduced immunogenicity. What is the reason for the association of species of origin and tumor-effective half-life? The biodegradability of the varied immunoglobulin molecules in this xenogeneic application seems to be the factor of importance. It is interesting to note that monkey antibody has had the longest tumor-effective half-life, sometimes up to 5 days. Along these lines we are now investigating bovine and baboon antibodies.

A model for pre-screening foreign species has been developed by Dr. Jerry Klein where he evaluates the whole body-effective half-life of normal IgG from the species of interest in a rodent system. The relationship between tumor-effective half-life and whole body-effective half-life has uniformly shown little difference. The difference in the tumor is the radiolabeled antibody concentration and therefore tumor dose (hepatoma 4.8×1 normal tissue). This pre-screening model has been advantageous in the further development of cyclic radiolabeled antibody therapy.

V. DOSIMETRY OF RADIOLABELED ANTIBODY

In diagnostic applications, the description normally used has been tumor : normal tissue ratios. With any effective antibody this should increase as tumor-bound antibody is retained and background diminishes. Fab fragments, because of their rapid clearance, are particularly useful in this regard. However, it is concentration of radiolabeled antibody in millicuries per gram over time that determines tumor dose. The regulation of radioactivity at the target therefore depends on the biologic half-life and physical half-life of the isotope, the composite result being the tumor-effective half-life. Examples of dosimetric problems include:

1. ^{131}I anti-α-fetoprotein (AFP) deposited in hepatoma 2.7 μCi/g and was not effective, whereas ^{131}I anti-ferritin at 7.3 μCi/g was effective. In this example *specificity dominates efficacy* since species of origin was the same (rabbit) and tumor-effective half-life was the same.

2. ^{131}I anti-CEA led to 1–2 μCi/g in colorectal metastasis to the liver and was not effective, whereas in intrahepatic biliary cancer it was 4.7 μCi/g and was effective. In this example, some *characteristic* concerning the *"tumor target"* yet unknown to us allows more efficient tumor targeting in biliary cancer than in colorectal cancer. Here specificity and tumor-effective half-lives were the same and the tumor target varied.

3. When a given patient's tumor remitted with ^{131}I anti-ferritin, it did so in response to rabbit antibody but it progressed when given ^{131}I anti-ferritin sheep-derived antibody. In this example, the specificity and tumor concentration were equal but the *tumor-effective half-life varied* due to *species* of antibody origin; a reduced dose of radiation on the second cycle allowed tumor progression.

In the administration of radiolabeled antibodies, the dosimetry in *concentration* (millicuries per gram) and *tumor-effective* half-life are the guidelines for intercomparison of antibodies of varying characteristics, isotopic combinations, and future development. Our physics team headed by Dr. Peter Leichner and in cooperation with Hirsch-Chemie is developing an automated system for the integration and display of tumor dose with radiolabeled antibodies. A thorough review of the manual methods required for such computations has been reported (Leichner *et al.*, 1983). Those investigators interested in therapeutic applications of radiolabeled antibodies should require reports to be evaluated (in millicuries per gram) and tumor-effective-half-life in order to determine the dose in Gray (rad). The use of ratios is not meaningful except for diagnostic purposes. The evaluation of potential toxicities as well as tumor effectiveness requires an understanding of tumor dose.

VI. RADIOBIOLOGY OF RADIOLABELED ANTIBODY

The present ^{131}I anti-ferritin antibodies used in the hepatoma program deliver 1000–1200 rad at 5 rad/hr initially (Leichner *et al.*, 1983). In addition, attempts at recycling indicated that sensitization occurred but the time sequence for sensitization had not been established. Based on low-dose rate irradiation results, tumor inhibition should occur (Shipley *et al.*, 1979) but the delay of 2 months between cycles allowed rapidly dividing tumors an opportunity for regrowth. In hepatoma specifically, there was an additional advantage with the use of adriamycin which potentiates low-dose rate radiation effects (Sherman *et al.*, 1982) and 5FU, which has been an additive to irradiation in gastrointestinal tumors

(Moertel *et al.*, 1969). Both agents were also active in hepatoma although the doses used for enhancing the effect of radioimmunoglobulin were far below the normal therapeutic levels. The doses with immunoglobulin were adriamycin 15 mg and 5FU 500 mg, compared to standard therapeutic doses of adriamycin 60 mg/m^2 and 5FU 500 mg/m^2.

In Hodgkin's disease, no other agent than ^{131}I anti-ferritin was used and a 40% partial remission was recorded in 21 patients with 73% remission of B symptoms in patients that had failed MOPP nd ABVD (Lenhard *et al.*, 1983).

VII. METHODS OF ANALYSIS FOR TUMOR REMISSION

The standard techniques of measuring lesions directly or by scans (CT or nuclear) and determining planar dimensions of resolution have been adequate in the past. One of the necessities for the dosimetry of radiolabeled antibody was determination of tumor volume. The method required that CT scans taken every 1 cm throughout the tumor-bearing region be reconstructed into three-dimensional volumes. Plots of the total liver volume and tumor volume have allowed us to determine more accurately the remission of cancer by this means in comparison to the physical examination. An example of tumor targeting and a plot of tumor remission are shown in Figs. 4 and 5.

VIII. RESULTS IN THERAPEUTIC TRIALS WITH RADIOLABELED ANTIBODIES

Our experience to date has indicated lack of efficacy of:

1. Monoclonal anti-ferritin due to dehalogenation regardless of subclass of IgG prepared for iodination. This experience has occurred in other laboratories that have looked at the therapeutic aspects of radiolabeled monoclonal antibody.

2. ^{131}I anti-AFP due to poor tumor target concentration (2.7 μCi/g in contrast to 7.3 μCi/g) for ^{131}I anti-ferritin in the same tumor.

3. ^{131}I anti-CEA in colorectal metastasis to the liver in comparison to intrahepatic biliary cancer with the same specificity but different ra-

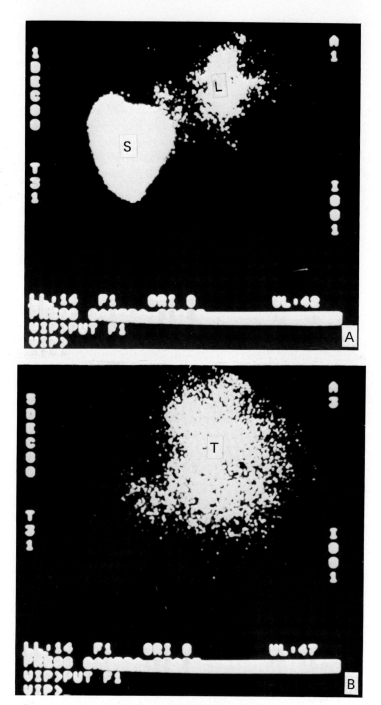

Fig. 4. A pair of emission computerized tomographic nuclear scans showing technetium in the normal liver (minimal) and normal spleen (A) and the ^{131}I anti-ferritin scan with maximal uptake in the tumor (area of defect in ^{99m}Tc) (B). S, Spleen; L, liver; T, tumor.

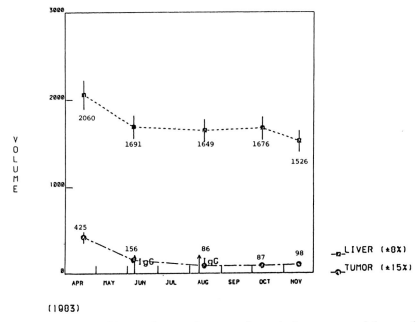

(1983)

Fig. 5. A plot of total liver volume and tumor volume during a course of therapy for primary hepatic malignancy. IgG represents time of ^{131}I anti-ferritin-radiolabeled antibody administration.

diolabeled antibody concentrations in the tumors between 1 and 2 μCi/ g colorectal cancer and 4.7 μCi/g in intrahepatic biliary cancer.

In contrast, Table I demonstrates the affirmative results to date. These trials are being carried out through the efforts of the research laboratory at Johns Hopkins and the Radiation Therapy Oncology Group (RTOG); specifically, the University of California at San Francisco (Dr. Steve Leibel) and Albert Einstein Medical Center in Philadelphia (Dr. Sucha Asbell and Dr. Jerome Spunberg). This demonstration consortium has shown that the biologic effectiveness was reproducible as was the physical science related to radiolabeled antibody; that shipment across the country was feasible; and that community hospitals were able to participate in the administration and care of patients receiving radiolabeled antibody.

It must be emphasized that basic research in experimental models, physics, and dosimetry as well as a scientific clinical team has pioneered this effort which is still in its beginning. However, tumor saturation doses, tumor-effective half-life, and cyclic treatment by alteration of species

TABLE I

^{131}I-RADIOLABELED ANTIBODY AND ASSOCIATED TUMOR REMISSION

Antibody and labeling	Tumor type	Patient number	Remission rate (%)	Method evaluated
^{131}I Anti-ferritin (8–10 mCi/mg IgG)	Hepatoma[a]	81	50	Tumor volumetrics, clinical
^{131}I Anti-ferritin (8–10 mCi/mg IgG)	Hodgkin's, failed MOPP–ABVD[b]	21	40	Direct measurement, chest film, gallium scans, clinical
^{131}I Anti-CEA (8–10 mCi/mg)	Intrahepatic biliary[c]	14	50	Tumor volumetrics, clinical

[a] Order *et al.* (1984).
[b] Lenhard *et al.* (1983).
[c] Order and Leibel (1984).

were but a few of the new innovations in this treatment modality which have proved to be of value in guiding a therapeutic program.

IX. FUTURE PROSPECTIVES

A wide range of needs are basic to the new developments and include (1) automation of dosimetry; (2) better radiolabeling of monoclonal antibodies for therapeutic purposes; (3) radiolabels that will allow outpatient therapy; (4) examination of human monoclonal antibodies; (5) evaluation of multiple antigenic targets within tumors for dose rate and total dose amplification; and (6) integration of radiolabeled antibodies into standard prospective therapy trials.

Based on our present clinical experience there has been no acute toxicity. Toxicity to date has been limited to thrombocytopenia (Ettinger *et al.*, 1982). Tumor remission has been achieved and cyclic therapy has been feasible.

Basic research is also needed to further characterize the "biologic window" and the rules for radiolabeled antibody tumor targeting. Examination of host interaction during this form of radiation and more radiobiologic information will aid future clinical trials. Radiolabeled antibody is not simply a promise for the future, but already is a clinical reality with demonstrable tumor remissions. Let the science and collected clinical data speak for itself.

ACKNOWLEDGEMENTS

This work was supported by American Cancer Society PDT-227, Radiation Therapy Oncology Group NIH-NCI CA29536-03, and NIH-NCI CA06973-18.

REFERENCES

Bagshawe, K. D., Searle, F., Lewis, J., Brown, P., and Keep, P. (1980). *Cancer Res.* **40,** 3016–3017.

Ettinger, D. S., Order, S. E., Wharam, M. D., Parker, M. K., Klein, J. L., and Leichner, P. K. (1982). *Cancer Treat. Rep.* **66,** 289–297.

Goldenberg, D. M., DeLand, F., Kim, E., Bennett, S., Primus, F. J., van Nagell, J. R., Jr., Estes, N., DeSimone, P., and Rayburn, P. (1978). *N. Engl. J. Med.* **298,** 1384–1388.

Halpern, S. E., Hogan, P. L., Graves, P. R., Kiztol, J. A., Chen, A. W. N., Frincke, J. M., Bartholomew, R. M., David, G. S., and Adams, T. H. (1983). *Cancer Res.* **43,** 5347–5355.

Kohler, G., and Milstein, C. (1975). *Nature (London)* **256,** 495–497.

Leichner, P. K., Klein, J. L., Garrison, J. B., Jenkins, R. E., Nickoloff, E. L., Ettinger, D. S., and Order, S. E. (1981). *Int. J. Radiat. Oncol. Biol.* **7,** 323–333.

Leichner, P. K., Klein, J. L., Siegelman, S. S., Ettinger, D. S., and Order, S. E. (1983). *Cancer Treat. Rep.* **67,** 647–657.

Lenhard, R. E., Order, S. E., Spunberg, J. J., Ettinger, D. S., Asbell, S. O., and Leibel, S. A. (1983). *Proc. Am. Soc. Clin. Oncol.* **2,** 211.

Mach, J. P., Forni, M., Ritschard, J., Buchegger, F., Carrel, S., Widgren, S., Donath, A., and Alberton, P. (1980). *Onc. Biol. Med.* **1,** 49–69.

Marchalonis, J. J. (1969). *Biochem. J.* **113,** 299–305.

Miller, R. A., and Levy, R. (1981). *Lancet* **2,** 226–229.

Moertel, C. G., Childs, D. S., Reitemeier, R. J., Colby, M. Y., and Holbrook, M. A. (1969). *Lancet* **2,** 865–867.

Old, L. J., Stockert, E., Boyse, E. A., and Kim, J. H. (1968). *J. Exp. Med.* **127,** 523–539.

Order, S. E. (1982). *Int. J. Radiat. Oncol. Biol. Phys.* **8,** 1193–1201.

Order, S. E., and Leibel, S. A. (1984). *Appl. Radiol.* **13,** 67–73.

Order, S. E., Kirkman, R., and Knapp, R. (1974). *Cancer (Amsterdam)* **34,** 175–183.

Order, S. E., Bloomer, W. D., Jones, A. G., Kaplan, W. D., Davis, M., Adelstein, S. J., and Hellman, S. (1975). *Cancer (Amsterdam)* **35,** 1487–1492.

Order, S. E., Goldenberg, D., Hoffer, P., Rubin, D., and Weissman, I. (1979). *Int. J. Radiat. Oncol. Biol. Phys.* **5,** 729–743.

Order, S. E., Klein, J. L., Ettinger, D. S., Alderson, P., Siegelman, S., and Leichner, P. K. (1980). *Int. J. Radiat. Oncol. Biol. Phys.* **6,** 703–710.

Order, S. E., Klein, J. L., Leichner, P. K., Self, S., Leibel, S., and Ettinger, D. (1984). *Proc. Am. Soc. Clin. Oncol.* **3,** 138.

Pressman, D., Day, E. D., and Blau, M. (1957). *Cancer Res.* **17,** 845–850.

Rostock, R. A., Klein, J. L., Leichner, P. K., Kopher, K. A., and Order, S. E. (1983). *Int. J. Radiat. Oncol. Biol. Phys.* **9,** 1345–1350.

Rostock, R. A., Klein, J. L., Kopher, K. A., and Order, S. E. (1984). *Am. J. Clin. Oncol.* **6,** 9–18.

Sherman, D. M., Carabell, S. C., Belli, J. A., and Hellman, S. (1982). *Int. J. Radiat. Oncol. Biol. Phys.* **8,** 45–51.

Shipley, W. U., Ling, C. C., Gerweck, L., and Jennings, W. (1979). *In* "Population Survival Effects and Interaction in Cell Killing by Conventional Radiation and Chemotherapeutic Aspects." 6th Int. Cong. Rad. Res., Tokyo.

Smith, T. W., Butler, V. P., and Haber, E. (1977). *In* "Antibodies in Human Diagnosis and Therapy" (E. Haber and M. Krouse, eds.), pp. 365–389. Raven Press, New York.

Spar, I. L., Bale, W. F., Marrick, D., Dwey, W. C., McCardle, R. J., and Harper, P. V. (1967). *Cancer (Amsterdam)* **20,** 865–870.

Wright, T., Sinanan, M., Harrington, D., Klein, J., and Order, S. E. (1979). *Appl. Radiol.* 120–124.

CHAPTER 16

Antibody Targeting of Anti-cancer Agents

M. J. Embleton and M. C. Garnett

Cancer Research Campaign Laboratories
University of Nottingham
Nottingham, United Kingdom

I. INTRODUCTION

The concept of drug targeting by antibody molecules is long-standing and has received renewed interest in recent years owing to the intro-

317

duction of methods for producing somatic cell hybrids secreting defined monoclonal antibodies. By means of appropriate immunisation and screening methods, it is theoretically possible to obtain monoclonal antibodies with specificity for a desired epitope, or for a particular cell type within a mixed population. In the field of oncology, the most useful antibodies would be those which bind avidly to tumour cells, but not at all to normal differentiated cells or stem cells. In practical terms this ideal is difficult to attain, and most anti-tumour monoclonal antibodies probably recognise antigens which are expressed quantitatively at a greater level on malignant cells, but may be present at a low level also on certain normal cells or within the extracellular matrix. However, so long as antigen expression on normal cells is very low or the cell population involved is not vital to the continued survival of the host, such 'quantitative specificity' is perhaps sufficient to qualify a monoclonal antibody as a potential vector for targeting chemically coupled therapeutic agents.

The choice of therapeutic agent involves opposing considerations. On one hand, it may be desirable to choose highly toxic substances which can kill cells following entry of only a few molecules, such as plant toxins or their A chains (Eiklid *et al.*, 1980; Yamaizumi *et al.*, 1978). In this case the antibody vector should ideally be absolutely specific for the tumour target cell if the conjugate is to be administered systemically, or the consequences of delivery to inappropriate sites could be disastrous.

A more cautious alternative is to target conventional cytotoxic drugs which are already in clinical use, in which case any side effects produced by drug activity on 'innocent' cells are judged to be clinically acceptable. In fact, the need to deliver relatively large amounts of a cytotoxic drug to achieve cell killing tends to reduce the possibility of toxicity to normal cells binding small amounts of a 'quantitatively specific' antibody vector, so cytotoxic drugs might offer a therapeutic advantage over toxins in this respect. A possible problem with this approach is the more questionable ability of the antibody vector to deliver therapeutic quantities of the drug to the target cell. It is, therefore, anticipated that the antibody should recognise a particularly abundant cell surface structure, and that high molar ratios of drug substitution be achieved without undue loss of antibody-binding activity. These objectives are not impracticable, and this chapter reviews some of our experiences in drug targeting using a monoclonal antibody designated 791T/36, which was raised against a cultured human osteogenic sarcoma cell line.

II. DESIGN OF CONJUGATES

A. Choice of Antibody

1. Biochemical Considerations

While the specificity of the antibody is of paramount importance for the success of antibody-targeted therapy, the biochemical properties of a particular monoclonal antibody are also important. Early work on drug targeting used polyclonal antibodies which appeared from the literature to be quite robust to the effect of substitution by haptens without apparent loss of binding activity. This may have been partly due to the heterogeneity of such antibodies.

It has been our experience with monoclonal antibodies, however, that individual monoclonal antibodies vary in their ruggedness towards substitution. Some antibodies will totally lose antibody-binding activity with even such mild procedures as fluorescein or iodine labelling, while others will permit a relatively high substitution with no loss of binding activity. This can be seen by comparing the published results from different groups using different monoclonal antibodies, in particular that of Rowland et al. (1982) in which vindesine was coupled by the same procedure to four different monoclonal antibodies of three different subclasses. Retention of antibody binding varied from 2% with a molar substitution ratio (moles drug/mole antibody) of 4, to 64% with a molar substitution ratio of 10.

It has also been our experience that this sensitivity is not only dependent on the antibody, but that a particular antibody will be inactivated to varying degrees by different haptens introduced by an equally mild chemical reaction, e.g., 1 mole of 791T/36 can be substituted by 6 moles of vindesine or 8 moles of 14-bromodaunomycin with little loss of binding activity but substitution with 3 moles of methotrexate (MTX) permits only 30% retention of binding activity. The degree of retention of binding activity decreases with increasing substitution for any one hapten. Chemical manipulations may also have an effect on binding activity, e.g., 791T/36 precipitates and loses binding activity in an irreversible manner in borate buffers, yet is stable in citrate, phosphate, tris and carbonate buffers over the pH range 3.5–9.5.

It will therefore be necessary to choose an antibody which will permit the necessary chemical manipulations and which allows an adequate degree of substitution for a particular hapten without an unacceptable loss of antibody-binding activity.

The retention of antibody-binding activity is measured differently by different groups. For our conjugates, we have measured the retention of antibody-binding activity by competition against unmodified antibody using a fluorescence-activated cell sorter (see below for details). We believe that this is a very sensitive and accurate indicator of loss of binding activity, because antibody which competes poorly against unmodified antibody is often still capable of binding to cells bearing the relevant antigen, but presumably with a reduced avidity. While we consider retention of a minimum of 30% of binding activity in our assay desirable, this is a purely arbitrary decision.

2. Monoclonal Antibody 791T/36

Hybridomas were formed by fusing spleen cells from a BALB/c mouse immunised with cells of osteogenic sarcoma Hs791T (abbreviated to 791T) with mouse myeloma line P3-NS1-Ag-4. Following initial screening and cloning, monoclonal antibody produced by one hybridoma (791T/36) was found to react with 7/14 osteogenic sarcoma cell lines in a radioimmunoassay but did not react with normal fibroblast cultures. Several of these fibroblast cultures were derived from donors of positive tumours, including the donor of 791T. The antibody reacted against some unrelated tumour cell lines, notably colorectal carcinomas (3 of 5 positive), although with most tumour types reactivity was restricted to isolated examples or not detected at all (Embleton et al., 1981).

The 791T/36 antibody is of IgG_{2b} isotype and has proved to be stable to labelling with tracers such as radioiodine or fluorescein isothiocyanate (Pimm et al., 1982) and has been estimated to bind to at least 10^6 sites on the surface of 791T cells. The epitope has been identified as a glycoprotein of apparent molecular weight 72,000 (Price et al., 1983). Radioiodinated 791T/36 localised specifically in subcutaneous xenografts of 791T and other antigenically positive tumour lines in immune-deprived mice when administered intraperitoneally (Pimm et al., 1982), and has also been used successfully in the radioimmunodetection of osteogenic sarcoma and colorectal carcinomas in human patients (Farrands et al., 1982, 1983). These properties suggested its suitability as a reagent for drug-targeting studies. It fulfilled the basic requirements for a high number of binding sites on appropriate target cells and adequate resistance to inactivation by chemical substitution, and the availability of tumour targets with known binding activity both in vivo and in vitro

TABLE I

CYTOTOXICITY BY VARIOUS DRUGS AGAINST HUMAN OSTEOGENIC SARCOMA CELL LINE 791T

Drug	$IC_{50}{}^a$ against 791T target cells:	
	ng/ml	Approximate molarity
Methotrexate	5	10^{-8}
Vindesine	10	10^{-8}
Adriamycin	10	2×10^{-8}
Daunomycin	30	5×10^{-8}
cis-Platinum	100	3×10^{-7}
5-Fluorouracil	800	5×10^{-7}
5-Fluorodeoxyuridine	1,400	5×10^{-7}
Melphalan	400	10^{-6}
Retinoic acid	15,000	2×10^{-5}
Interferon	IC_{50} not reached at 10^5 units/ml	

^{a}Drug concentration inhibiting ^{75}Se-met incorporation by 50%.

ensured the provision of adequate systems to test the biological activity of drug–791T/36 conjugates.

B. Choice of Cytotoxic Agents

1. *In Vitro* Cytotoxicity

A wide range of drugs are currently used as anti-neoplastic agents in conventional therapy but few of these are suitable for use in targeted drug delivery systems. The two major factors governing the choice of drug for targeting are that it should be highly cytotoxic to the target cell to be studied and that it has the potential for chemical conjugation to protein. The susceptibility of target cells to drugs is easily determined empirically. For studies with antibody 791T/36, the osteogenic sarcoma cell line 791T was of prime interest, and the sensitivity of this line to various cytotoxic or cytostatic agents was evaluated in a cytotoxicity assay using ^{75}Se-selenomethionine (^{75}Se-met) incorporation as an indication of cell survival (Table I). Target cells were incubated in microtitre plates with various concentrations of each drug for appropriate time periods, then labelled with ^{75}Se-met over an 8- to 16-hr time period (Embleton *et al.*, 1983). Retinoic acid and interferon treatments were continued for 3 and 6 days, respectively, and the cells were exposed to the other drugs for 24 hr before ^{75}Se-met labelling. The most active drugs tested were

MTX and vindesine, and the anthracyclines adriamycin and daunomycin (Table I).

2. Chemical Considerations

To be able to conjugate drugs to immunoglobulins or any other carrier, a free, chemically reactive functional group is required, e.g., carboxyl, amino, hydroxyl or sulphydryl. Of the examples given the first two, carboxyl and amino groups, are likely to be the most useful for immediate research because there is already information in the literature on peptide linkages using these functional groups and their susceptibility to lysosomal cleavage (Masquelier *et al.*, 1980; Trouet *et al.*, 1982; Duncan *et al.*, 1980, 1981; Monsigny *et al.*, 1980; Shen and Ryser, 1981).

While it should be possible to derivatise any drug to give a useful functional group which can be linked in such a way as to give release of free drug intracellularly, this is likely to require more basic chemical research and biological testing before a useful conjugate can be developed. It should also be noted that if the functional group to be used for coupling is required for drug activity, e.g., the sugar amino group of daunomycin/adriamycin (Zunino *et al.*, 1972; Levin and Sela, 1979), it is essential that unmodified drug is released intracellularly. If, however, the functional group to be used for coupling is not essential for drug activity then it may be possible to use a linkage where a modified drug is released intracellularly. For example, MTX coupled to high molecular weight biopolymers via the α-carboxyl group can still bind to dihydrofolate reductase, the target enzyme, but at a reduced level (Whiteley, 1971), so minor modifications of this functional group may be relatively unimportant.

The mode of action of the drug also needs to be taken into account for this mode of therapy as well. Alkylating agents (which probably include *cis*-platinum compounds) are intrinsically unsuitable for targeting using proteins because of their chemical properties. It has been shown by Ross (1974) that alkylating agents alkylate ε-amino groups of proteins causing inter- and intramolecular cross-linking at temperatures above 5°C. This property of alkylating agents would therefore make them unsuitable for this type of work.

If initial work on the targeting of chemotherapeutic agents proves encouraging, it is hoped that a new range of drug derivatives would be produced which were specifically tailored to the needs of this mode of therapy, pre-empting the use of cytotoxic drugs which have been developed using different pharmacological criteria.

C. Advantages and Disadvantages of Carriers

The requirement for delivering a large number of drug molecules to a cell to kill it using the limited antigenic sites available suggests that for antibody-targeted drugs to be effective it will be necessary to achieve a high molar substitution ratio. The two possible approaches would appear to be either to find a particularly robust antibody or to use a drug carrier which is then attached to the antibody. In view of the difficulties encountered in obtaining monoclonal antibodies with the desired specificity, consistent with biochemical stability, the latter alternative offered greater promise.

The use of a carrier has several advantages over that of linking drug directly to antibody. First, the molar substitution ratio using a carrier is limited only by the number of functional groups available for conjugation and the stability of the substituted carrier at physiological pH. This will depend on both the drug and the carrier, but a molar substitution ratio of 20–40 should be feasible for many drug–carrier combinations, compared to a range of 1–10 for direct linkage to monoclonal antibody. Second, because the carrier is only being used as an 'inert' framework to attach the drug to and there is no biological activity to retain, it is possible to use relatively harsh coupling methods, if necessary, to achieve substitution with a particular drug. The major objections to the use of carriers are likely to be seen only *in vivo* and relate to the stability of the carrier–antibody linkage and the molecular weight of the conjugate. Both of these problems will also be found in targeting toxins and immunomodulating agents as well.

The choice of which carrier to use has not yet been investigated thoroughly, but a wide variety of different carriers have been reported in either targeted or non-targeted drug delivery. These carriers have been either natural proteins, e.g., albumins (Chu and Whitely, 1977), fibrinogen and α-globulins (Szekerke *et al.*, 1972a,b), melanotropin (Varga *et al.*, 1977), wheat germ agglutinin (Monsigny *et al.*, 1980) chymotrypsinogen (Chu and Whiteley, 1980), concanavalin A (Kitao and Hattori, 1977) or synthetic polymers, e.g., dextrans (Bernstein *et al.*, Rowland, 1977), polyamino acids, polyglutamate (Rowland *et al.*, 1975), polylysine (Ryser and Shen, 1980), polyaspartate (Zunino *et al.*, 1982), carboxymethyl cellulose (Hurwitz *et al.*, 1980), and N-(2 hydroxypropyl) methacrylamide copolymers (Duncan *et al.*, 1980, 1981). The factors affecting choice between these molecules are likely to include molecular size, numbers of functional groups available for subsitution, homogeneity, ease of handling, ease of coupling, stability and possibly molecular shape (whether globular or random, or straight chain). For our studies we chose human serum albumin (HSA) which seemed to have many desirable properties relating to the above criteria.

There have been two types of drug–carrier–antibody conjugates reported in the literature: first, the type in which drug is attached to carrier by one method followed by coupling to antibody by another method (Rowland, 1977; Rowland et al., 1975; Garnett et al., 1983), and second, where the carrier has been used as a multifunctional agent to link the drug to the antibody (Hurwitz et al., 1978). This second type of conjugate has been termed by the authors a drug–bridge–antibody conjugate. In our experience the first type of conjugate, the drug–carrier–antibody conjugate, is preferable as it allows greater chemical control of the ratio of drug to carrier, and carrier to antibody, and the degree of polymerisation of the final product. Polymerised products are not only undesirable in vivo but also they result in reduced retention of antibody-binding activity. The use of a two-step procedure also permits the selection of different types of linkage between the drug and carrier and between the carrier and antibody. It is anticipated that this latter point will be a significant factor in the development of targeted drug conjugates.

D. Preparation of Conjugates

1. MTX Linked Directly to 791T/36

These conjugates were prepared by an activated ester method. The N-hydroxysuccinimide ester of MTX was prepared by the method of Kulkarni et al. (1981) by incubating equimolar quantities of methotrexate, N-hydroxysuccinimide and dicyclohexylcarbodiimide in a small volume of dimethylformamide for several hours and the precipitate was removed by centrifugation. The substituted antibody was then prepared by reacting small volumes of the unpurified ester as above with solutions of antibody (2–8 mg/ml) in phosphate-buffered saline (PBS) for about 1 hr. Unreacted ester and unwanted small molecular weight products were removed by gel filtration on Sephadex G-25 columns.

Using this method, antibody preparations substituted with varying amounts of methotrexate attached were produced which were assayed for antibody-binding activity. It was determined from these experiments that an average molar substitution ratio in the range 2.0–3.0 was optimal for the MTX–791T/36 drug–antibody combination. This is a very mild chemical reaction which takes place at room temperature involving just small amounts of organic solvent. As the reaction does not involve a cross-linking agent, no polymeric protein material is produced.

2. MTX–HSA–791T/36 Conjugates

These conjugates were made by a three-stage procedure involving first the preparation of MTX-substituted HSA, and second the preparation of an iodoacetyl-substituted antibody and finally the reaction of these two components.

Briefly, HSA-MTX was synthesised by reacting an excess of methotrexate and ethylcarbodiimide [1-ethyl-3-(3-dimethylaminopropyl)carbodiimide] with HSA (20 mg/ml) overnight in PBS. This reaction produced some polymerised HSA-MTX which was removed by size exclusion chromatography. Iodoacetyl-substituted antibody was produced by reacting a three- to fourfold molar excess of N-hydroxysuccinimidyl iodoacetate with antibody in PBS for 1 hr followed by desalting on a G-25 column.

HSA-MTX contains a free sulphydryl group which is in an oxidised unreactive form. This sulphydryl group was freshly reduced using 50 mM dithiothreitol and, after desalting, the freshly reduced HSA-MTX was reacted overnight at room temperature with iodoacetyl-substituted antibody. The reagents and reaction products were then separated by further size exclusion chromatography. For further details of the method see Garnett *et al.* (1983).

III. *IN VITRO* PROPERTIES OF CONJUGATES

A. Retention of Antibody-binding Activity

For this assay we compared the effectiveness of modified antibody to compete for a limited number of antigenic sites against fluorescein-labelled antibody. Target cells (10^5 cells in 750 μl) were incubated for 30 min with 1 μg of fluorescein-labelled antibody and 1 μg of conjugate or modified antibody. The fluorescence of the cells was measured on a flow cytofluorimeter, the mean fluorescence intensity being calculated as the mean channel number of excitation profiles. For each test a standard curve was plotted of fluorescence intensity arising from the competition of known amounts of unmodified antibody (in the range 5–0.1 μg) with

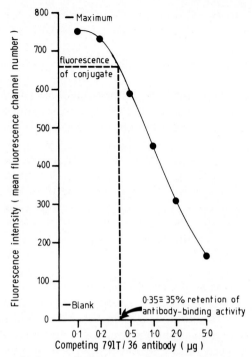

Fig. 1. A typical standard curve showing mean fluorescence intensity of 791T cells treated with 1 μg of fluorescein isothiocyanate-labelled 791T/36/10^5 cells competing against varying amounts of unlabelled 791T/36 antibody. The fluorescence, when antibody of unknown activity is competing in this system, can be read off in terms of equivalent quantities of free antibody as shown.

1 μg of FITC-labelled antibody. The retention of antibody-binding activity was then read directly off the standard curve in terms of the equivalent amount of unmodified antibody giving the same fluorescence intensity expressed as a percentage of competing material (1 μg). This is illustrated in Fig. 1.

This assay is simple and quick to perform and gives very accurate and reproducible results. The major inaccuracy is the determination of the amount of antibody in the conjugate which can be difficult to measure due to the presence of both drug and other protein in the conjugate.

B. *In Vitro* Cytotoxicity

1. Short-term Assays

When testing the cytotoxic potential of materials of unknown activity, it is desirable to test at the highest concentration available and to titrate downwards. Hence, assays that employ small volumes of reagent are preferable to those that require large volumes. In addition, during the development of conjugates it is often desirable to know the results of subtle modifications in conjugation procedures as quickly as possible, so that short-term assays offer an advantage over assays involving long-term culture. Cytotoxicity of MTX–antibody conjugates was tested initially by incubating various dilutions of conjugate for 24 hr with adherent target cells in microtitre plates, followed by labelling with ^{75}Se-met. This assay (termed 24-hr exposure assay) produced reproducible results with free drugs (Table I), and being economical on time and material, was ideally suited to the routine screening of new conjugates. In the event of conjugates proving cytotoxic to relevant target cells in this assay, they were subjected to a modified assay designed to test selectivity for certain target cells. In this case, target cells were pretreated with conjugate for 15 min at ambient temperature, then washed free of unbound conjugate before incubation for 24 hr in microtitre plates and labelling with ^{75}Se-met. Only conjugates binding strongly to target cells (or taken up within 15 min) are cytotoxic in this modified assay (termed pre-treatment assay). In both tests, target cells with both high and low antibody-binding activity were employed.

Direct MTX–791T/36 conjugates were tested against osteogenic sarcoma 791T which expresses 10^6 791T/36 binding sites per cell, and bladder carcinoma line T24 which expresses only 10^4 binding sites. In most cases the direct conjugates were much less toxic than free MTX for both cell lines in the chronic exposure assay, and there was no discrimination between the effects on 791T and T24. In the pre-treatment assay, the direct conjugates showed no activity, even against the 791T line. Results for two representative direct conjugates are shown in Table II. The assumption from such findings was that direct MTX–791T/36 conjugates were unable to deliver sufficient quantities of MTX to the target cells to effect useful levels of cytotoxicity.

Indirect conjugates employing an HSA carrier, however, were much more successful. Table III indicates the relative performance of free MTX, MTX conjugated to HSA (MTX–HSA) and the full drug–carrier–antibody conjugate (MTX–HSA–791T/36) in both forms of the ^{75}Se-met incorporation assay on 791T and T24 cells. The MTX–HSA conjugate was much less toxic to target cells than MTX (see also Garnett et al., 1983). However, the complete MTX–HSA–791T/36 conjugate was highly cytotoxic for 791T cells. In terms of MTX concentration, most MTX–HSA–791T/36 conjugates were almost as active as the free drug and the best preparations have been twice as active. The effect on T24 cells, however, showed on average an IC_{50} approximately two orders of magnitude higher than observed for 791T cells.

TABLE II

CYTOTOXICITY BY DIRECTLY LINKED MTX–791T/36 CONJUGATES

Assay	Reagent	$IC_{50}{}^{a}$ for target cells:	
		791T	T24
(a) Chronic	MTX–791T/36 conjugate		
24-hr exposure	MDC 27	180 ng/ml	100 ng/ml
	MTX–791T/36 conjugate		
	MDC 30	180 ng/ml	180 ng/ml
	MTX	5 ng/ml	2 ng/ml
(b) Pre-treatment	MTX–791T/36 conjugate		
assay	MDC 27	Non-toxic[b]	Non-toxic
		at 40 µg/ml	at 40 µg/ml
	MTX–791T/36 conjugate		
	MDC 30	Non-toxic	Non-toxic
		at 40 µg/ml	at 40 µg/ml
	MTX	9 µg/ml	8 µg/ml

[a]Concentration (in terms of MTX content) inhibiting ^{75}Se-met incorporation by 50%.
[b]No significant difference from growth medium controls.

2. Correlation between Cytotoxicity Tests and Antibody-binding Activity

Although the FACS test for the retention of antibody binding is useful for a rapid assessment of the quality of the conjugation procedure, it does not indicate how much conjugate binds to cells under the conditions of the above cytotoxicity tests. This is important because for drug targeting to be really effective, it is necessary to deliver enough drug to kill the cell before all the relevant antigen sites are saturated by conjugate. While our calculations suggested that the number of conjugate molecules at the cell surface was approximately saturating at the IC_{50} of the 'chronic exposure' assay, we wished to determine this experimentally.

To do this we incubated cells with conjugate under identical conditions to those in the cytotoxicity test, washed the cells once at 4°C and labelled the conjugate with an excess of fluorescein-labelled rabbit anti-HSA antibody also at 4°C where dissociation of 791T/36 from its antigen occurs only slowly. The resulting fluorescence was determined as previously on a flow cytofluorimeter. From this result (Fig. 3) it was apparent that the IC_{50} of the chronic exposure assay occurs at about 20% of conjugate saturation and the IC_{50} for the pre-treatment cytotoxicity test at 300 ng/ml for this conjugate still occurred at just below saturation of antigen sites.

TABLE III

CYTOTOXICITY BY MTX–HSA–791T CONJUGATES

| Assay | Reagent | IC_{50}^{a} for target cells: | |
		791T	T24
(a) Chronic 24-hr exposure	MTX–HSA–791T/36 conjugate MT5	18 ng/ml	250 ng/ml
	MTX–HSA–791T/36 conjugate MT17	2.5 ng/ml	300 ng/ml
	MTX–HSA	900 ng/ml	800 ng/ml
	MTX	5 ng/ml	2 ng/ml
(b) Pre-treatment assay	MTX–HSA–791T/36 conjugate MT5	300 ng/ml	Non-toxic[b] at 40 μg/ml
	MTX–HSA	Non-toxic at 40 μg/ml	Non-toxic at 40 μg/ml
	MTX	9 μg/ml	8 μg/ml

[a]Concentration (in terms of MTX content) inhibiting ^{75}Se-met incorporation by 50%.
[b]No significant difference from growth medium controls.

3. Clonogenic Assays and 'Resistant' Clones

The major disadvantage of ^{75}Se-met incorporation is that is measures the short-term survival of cells capable of protein synthesis, and does not reflect accurately the full cytotoxic potential of the conjugates. At the highest doses, MTX–HSA–791T/36 conjugates rarely achieved more than a plateau of 90% inhibition of ^{75}Se-met uptake over 24 hr, relative to controls. However, once MTX–HSA–791T/36 conjugates had been shown to have proven activity at low concentrations it became feasible to employ clonogenic assays in which the long-term growth potential of target cells was measured. These assays were performed by plating 200 cells in 30-mm culture dishes and incubating for 5–7 days in the continuous presence of conjugates, after which cell colonies were stained and enumerated. An example of such a test, using MTX–HSA–791T/36 conjugate MT5 is shown in Fig. 2. In a clonogenic assay the conjugate was able to inhibit completely colony formation by 791T cells, and the IC_{50} value was 0.3 ng/ml. Comparison with Table II shows that the clonogenic assay was thus more sensitive. T24 target cells were much less susceptible to conjugate than 791T cells, thus confirming the specificity observed in short-term assays. Free MTX, however, was toxic to both cell lines.

Using the colony inhibition assay, it was possible to investigate more

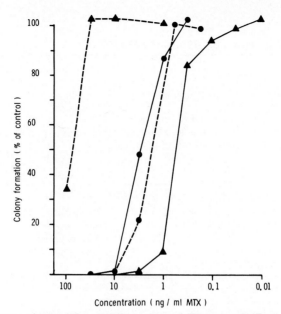

Fig. 2. Cytotoxicity of MTX–HSA–791T/36 conjugate MT5 against 791T osteogenic sarcoma and T24 bladder carcinoma cells as measured by colony inhibition assay. Conjugate concentration is expressed in terms of MTX content and colony formation is expressed as a percentage of the number of colonies formed in growth medium controls. ▲---▲, T24 cells treated with conjugate MT5; ●---●, T24 cells treated with MTX; ▲——▲, 791T cells treated with conjugate MT5; and ●——●, 791T cells treated with MTX.

closely exposure conditions affecting the action of MTX–HSA–791T/36 conjugates. Table IV shows experiments in which 791T cells were treated with conjugate at different concentrations, either continuously or discontinuously with alternating culture in growth medium alone. The concentrations chosen were 0.5 ng/ml which for this batch of conjugate approximated to the IC_{90}, and 10 ng/ml which almost completely inhibited colony growth in continuously exposed cultures.

If exposure to the conjugate was limited to 2 days followed by a further 4 days recovery in growth medium, colony formation was approximately 30% greater than in continuously treated cultures at the IC_{90}, although still substantially suppressed at the higher dose. When cells were allowed to establish small colonies by 2 days culture in growth medium before exposure to MTX–HSA–791T/36, the conjugate did not completely kill them. The high dose (10 ng/ml) inhibited further cell division so that the mean colony size showed minimal change, but the IC_{90} allowed colony growth to continue, albeit at a lower rate and incidence than in controls. These results show that the conjugate is cytostatic rather than

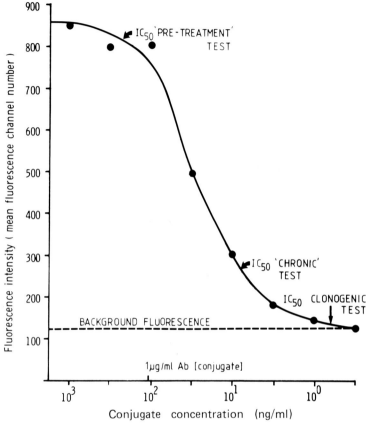

Fig. 3. Quantitation of MTX–HSA–791T/36 binding to cells under cytotoxicity test conditions. Cells were incubated with MTX–HSA–791T/36 conjugate as in the 'chronic exposure' cytoxicity test, washed and treated with FITC-labelled rabbit anti-HSA at 4°C. Mean fluorescence intensity was determined using a flow cytofluorimeter and plotted against MTX concentration of conjugate. The MTX concentration of conjugate at the IC_{50} of the different assays has been indicated on the binding curve.

cytolytic when the target cells are in a logarithmic growth phase. Inhibition is most effective in single cells before division has occurred and it is a relatively slow process in that many cells exposed for 2 days to a partially toxic dose may still recover in fresh growth medium. The slow kinetics of cytotoxicity explains the failure of MTX–HSA–791T/36 to achieve more than about 90% inhibition of ^{75}Se-met uptake over 24 hr at high concentrations. However, when inhibited single cells are forced to remain in the environment of conjugates rather than being allowed to recover, they die within the 5- to 7-day period of the colony inhibition

M. J. Embleton and M. C. Garnett

TABLE IV

EFFECT OF ALTERNATING TREATMENT WITH GROWTH MEDIUM AND MTX–HSA–791T/36 CONJUGATE ON COLONY FORMATION BY 791T CELLS

Treatment		Mean No. colonies±SE	Inhibition of colony formation (%)	Mean colony size (No. of cells±SE)
Days 1–2	Days 3–6			
Growth medium[a]	—	142 ± 4[b]	—	4.8 ± 0.3
Growth medium	Growth medium	215 ± 7	0	61.3 ± 11.0
MT5 0.5 ng/ml[c]	MT5 0.5 ng/ml	20 ± 3	91	
MT5 10 ng/ml	MT5 10 ng/ml	0.7 ± 0.2	99.8	
MT5 0.5 ng/ml	Growth medium	76 ± 2	65	
MT5 10 ng/ml	Growth medium	2 ± 1	99	
Growth medium	MT5 0.5 ng/ml	145 ± 3	33	31.8 ± 8
Growth medium	MT5 10 ng/ml	129 ± 7	40	5.9 ± 0.6

[a]These cells were stained after 2 days.

[b]Cultures contained cell pairs which were not scored as colonies; these would have formed colonies with more prolonged culture.

[c]Expressed as concentration of MTX.

assay, since dishes treated continuously with conjugate contain no single cells at the higher concentrations.

An important question related to cell survival is whether cell clones growing at highly toxic concentrations of conjugate (more than 99% inhibitory) escape because of inherent or acquired properties of low antigenicity or low drug sensitivity. To answer this question, a number of such clones were isolated and propagated in order to expand the populations for antigen and drug susceptibility measurements (Embleton *et al.*, 1984). Of 15 isolated clones, only 4 were capable of indefinite growth, the other 11 dying out after a few cell divisions. This contrasts strongly with the virtually 100% propagation potential of untreated 791T clones. The antigenicity of the four 'escaped' clones was tested, in comparison with normal 791T clones or uncloned stock cultures, by flow cytofluorimetry using fluorescein-labelled 791T/36 antibody, and their sensitivity to MTX was determined by clonogenic assays. The results (Table V) showed that the escaped clones were not deficient in 791T/36-defined antigen and in most cases did not exhibit increased resistance to MTX. The single case of increased resistance to MTX, moreover, was marginal. As might be predicted, the IC_{50} of MTX–HSA–791T/36 conjugate for the 4 clones did not differ significantly from that of stock 791T cells. It thus appeared that cell clones which might have been assumed to be resistant

TABLE V

ANTIGENICITY AND MTX-SENSITIVITY OF 791T CLONES 'ESCAPING' TOXIC CONCENTRATIONS OF MTX–HSA–791T/36 CONJUGATE

A. Selection

Dose of conjugate (ng/ml) MTX	Plating efficiency (%)	No. of colonies isolated / No. of dishes treated	No. of continuous cultures / No. of colonies isolated
0	38.8	—	
50	0.11	11/10 }	4/15
100	0.03	4/13 }	

B. Characteristics

Cell line	Antigenicity (approx. no. antibody-binding sites per cell)	IC_{50} (ng/ml) in free MTX	IC_{50} (ng/ml MTX) in MTX–HSA–791T/36
	B. Characteristics		
Parental 791T	10^6	9	2
Escaped clones:			
791T/MH7R/4	10^6	9	1.5
791T/MH7R/5	2.5×10^6	17	2
791T/MH7R/12	6×10^6	8	2
791T/MH7R/14	10^6	10	3

to the initial dose of conjugate were either incapable of unlimited growth or susceptible to a further exposure to the conjugate. These experiments, together with those in which conjugate and growth medium were alternated, suggest that the best strategy for *in vivo* therapy with MTX–HSA–791T/36 conjugate would be repeated treatment over a prolonged time course in order to maintain an adequate level of targeted drug in the tumour environment.

IV. MODE OF ACTION OF MTX–HSA–791T/36 CONJUGATES

A. General Principles of Cytotoxicity for Targeted Drugs

The ideal on which targeted drug delivery is based is that it will depend entirely on the specificity of the directing agent (usually antibody). While this will be largely true, the drug is likely to have some effect on targeting.

Some drugs, e.g., MTX (Goldman *et al.*, 1968) and some alkylating agents (Byfield and Calabro-Jones, 1981), are taken up selectively by cells, and other drugs, e.g., adriamycin/daunomycin would be expected to have hydrophobic interactions with cell membranes and thus have non-specific interactions with antigen-negative cells. Similarly, some carriers, e.g., poly-L-lysine, are known to facilitate interaction with cells because of their strong positive charge (Shen and Ryser, 1978, 1981) and may also have a significant interaction with antigen-negative cells. For these reasons it is unrealistic to expect absolute specificity of action for targeted drug delivery, but an improvement in the discrimination between tumour and non-tumour cells would be of considerable benefit.

Once the conjugate is within the vicinity of the cell, it has been proposed that the mechanism of action of drugs linked to high molecular weight markers would be as follows. Ingestion of the conjugate into the cell could occur either by phagocytosis for lymphoreticular cells or by pinocytosis for other cell types. If the carrier is a targeted carrier it would be expected to be taken up mainly by membrane phase pinocytosis, but if non-targeted, by fluid-phase pinocytosis, another means of loss of specificity. Once ingested, the conjugate containing vesicles would fuse with primary lysosomes to form secondary lysosomes where hydrolysis of the conjugate would take place into its small molecular weight precursors. The free drug would then be able to diffuse to its target site (De Duve *et al.*, 1974).

While some data are available to support this hypothesis for non-targeted conjugates, there have been no data on the mechanism of action of targeted conjugates. Therefore, we performed a few experiments to determine whether targeted conjugates behaved in a similar manner.

B. Specificity of Action

Chronic exposure and pre-treatment selenomethionine uptake assays and 5-day clonogenic assays (see Table III and Fig. 2, respectively) have all demonstrated specificity of action with the MTX–HSA–791T/36 conjugate, but we wished to demonstrate formally that this specificity was mediated by antibody–antigen interaction. Optimal doses of conjugate (100 ng/ml MTX concentration) were incubated with antigen-positive 788T cells and titrated against increasing doses of competing free antibody in a chronic exposure selenomethionine uptake assay. This showed (Fig. 4) that at low conjugate concentrations the cytotoxic effect could be com-

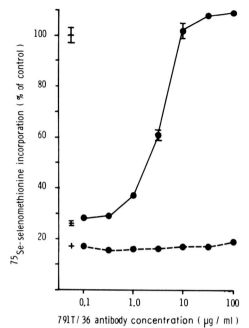

Fig. 4. Inhibition of MTX–HSA–791T/36 cytotoxicity by competing free antibody. 788T (791T/36 antigen positive) cells were incubated with either 100 μg/ml MTX (●----●) or 100 μg/ml conjugated MTX (●——●) and titrated against increasing amounts of unconjugated 791T/36 antibody in a 'chronic exposure' cytotoxicity test, demonstrating the requirement of antibody specificity for conjugate cytotoxicity. Standard error for each point is shown by error bars where it exceeds the plotted point size.

pletely abrogated by competing antibody. This result indicates that almost complete selectivity could be expected by adjusting the dose of conjugate to the appropriate level.

C. Lysosomotropic Action of Conjugate

To ascertain whether lysosomal degradation was taking place, we used two indicators: ammonium chloride and leupeptin.

Ammonium chloride (10 mM) has been reported to raise the lysosomal pH inside lysosomes by almost 2 pH units (Ohkuma and Poole, 1978), causing an inhibition of lysosomal protein degradation (Seglen *et al.*, 1979). If drug–carrier antibody conjugates are degraded in the lysosomes,

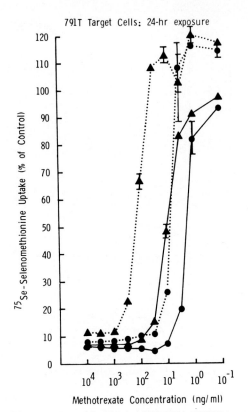

Fig. 5. Effect of 10 m*M* ammonium chloride on MTX–HSA–791T/36 cytotoxicity. 791T cells were treated with either MTX (●) or conjugate (▲) in a 'chronic exposure' assay, with (·····) or without (———) 10 m*M* ammonium chloride. Reduction of cytotoxicity was caused by inhibition of lysosomal enzymes. Standard error for each point is shown by error bars where it exceeds the plotted point size.

this would be expected to reduced conjugate cytotoxicity. In Fig. 5 it can be seen that this was the case: the IC_{50} for the conjugate was raised from 10 ng/ml to 150 ng/ml. Due to the effect of ammonium chloride on the growth of cells, the IC_{50} for MTX was raised from 2 ng/ml to 7 ng/ml; however, this was only a 3.5-fold increase as opposed to a 15-fold increase for the conjugate.

Leupeptin is a potent specific inhibitor of the lysosomal endopeptidases termed cathepsins B, H and L (Seglen *et al.*, 1979). It is apparent from Fig. 6 that when cells were incubated with leupeptin there was no effect on the cytotoxicity of MTX but a 40-fold increase in conjugate cytotoxicity.

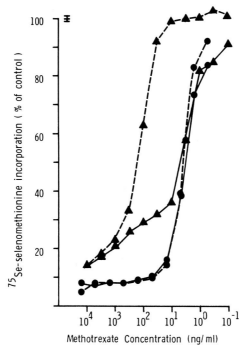

Fig. 6. Effect of leupeptin on MTX–HSA–791T/36 cytotoxicity. 791T cells were treated with MTX (●) or MTX–HSA–791T/36 conjugate (▲) either with (---) or without (———) 100 µ*M* leupeptin in a 'chronic exposure' cytotoxicity test, demonstrating the effect of inhibition of lysosomal enzymes on conjugate cytotoxicity.

D. Intracellular Transport of MTX

Free MTX is taken up into cells by an active transport mechanism transporting folinic acid, but which is separate from the transport mechanism for folic acid. Uptake of free MTX is therefore reduced in the presence of folinic acid (Harrap *et al.*, 1971). This constitutes the basis of leucovorin (folinic acid: N_5-formyl-tetrahydrofolate) rescue after high-dose MTX therapy. It was expected that because of the entry of conjugate into cells via the lysosomes shown above, that folinic acid would have no effect on the cytotoxicity of conjugate, although it does inhibit cytotoxicity to free MTX. The results from this experiment (Fig. 7) showed, however, that the action of the conjugate was inhibited to a greater extent by folinic acid than was MTX and that this was a specific effect because conjugate cytotoxicity was not inhibited by folic acid.

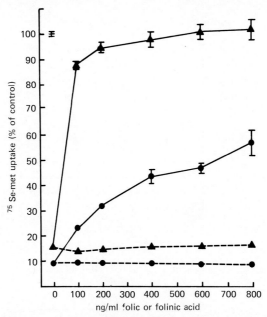

Fig. 7. Effect of folic and folinic acids on MTX–HSA–791T/36 cytotoxicity. 788T (791T/36 antigen positive) cells were treated with 100 μg/ml MTX (●) or 100 μg/ml conjugated MTX (▲) and titrated against either folic (----) or folinic (———) acids, demonstrating the involvement of a specific pathway of MTX transport for both conjugate and MTX. Standard error is shown by error bars where it exceeds the plotted point size.

These results suggested that the conjugate is degraded by the lysosomal hydrolytic enzymes and that the free MTX released in this manner is taken up from the lysosomes into the cytoplasm by a specific transport mechanism. It is unclear and untested as yet what implications these results have for the cytotoxicity of these conjugates on MTX transport-deficient cells.

V. *IN VIVO* ASPECTS OF MTX–HSA–791T/36

A. General Principles

It has been demonstrated that MTX–HSA–791T/36 possesses most of the *in vitro* properties desirable for targeted chemotherapy. While we believe that these *in vitro* assays are good indicators for many of the prerequisite properties for such compounds, there are several parameters which can only be successfully tested by relevant *in vivo* experiments. Some previous investigators in this field have performed either no or only basic *in vitro* assays before testing their conjugates for their ability to prevent the appearance of tumour or extend the life span of animals without reference to problems which may prevent such therapy. We are currently just beginning *in vivo* experiments on our conjugates, so we feel it is worth noting at this stage what problems may arise *in vivo* in order to anticipate what further developments are possible should initial experiments not prove totally successful.

There are probably two important limits of sizes for macromolecules circulating *in vivo*. There is a cut-off point below which molecules are eliminated by the kidney (circa 60,000 Da) and a higher cut-off point (as yet unknown) at which macromolecules are unable to pass out of the vascular system and gain access to all cell surfaces within the body. The higher cut-off point is expected to be between the range of 150,000 and 900,000 Da based on the differing functions of IgG and IgM, respectively. It is apparent, therefore, that any cytotoxic conjugates should be as close as possible to the molecular size of unmodified IgG.

There are two main ways in which conjugates may be eliminated from the circulation: first, the production of antibodies against components of these conjugates (e.g., Borsos *et al.*, 1981) and the resultant precipitation of immune complexes. This problem could be partially resolved by the use of immunosuppressive agents. The second problem is the removal of foreign proteins from circulation by the reticuloendothelial system. This could constitute a problem towards targeted or carrier–drug chemotherapy, but we hope that it will prove no more of a problem than the elimination of free drug in conventional therapy, in that administration of regular small doses of conjugate should result in a sufficiently high circulating level.

In order to target drugs successfully using our conjugate, it is necessary that both the bonds between drug and carrier, and between carrier and antibody, remain intact until the conjugate reaches its target. The peptide linkage between MTX and HSA has been shown previously to be stable (Chu and Whitely, 1972). There is doubt over the stability of the bond linking carrier to antibody although proof of this instability remains to be published. Such a finding would have serious implications for all targeting studies whether using drug carriers, immunomodulating agents or toxins. If this does prove a problem, it is hoped that further research would yield alternative suitable bonding systems.

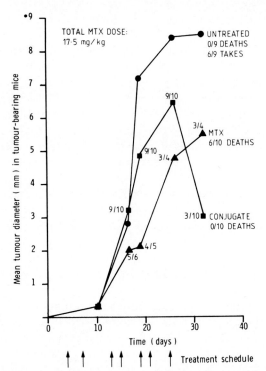

Fig. 8. Therapy of human tumour xenografts with MTX–HSA–791T/36. Thymectomozed, irradiated CBA mice were inoculated with 3–4 × 10⁶ 791T cells at time 0 and treated at the indicated times with either PBS (●), 17.5 mg/kg MTX (▲) or 17.5 mg/kg MTX–HSA–791T/36 (■). The mean tumour diameter of those bearing tumours was plotted for each treatment and the number of animals bearing tumours over the number of animals surviving treatment is given for the relevant point.

B. *In Vivo* Therapeutic Activity of MTX–HSA–791T/36 Conjugates

Following the success of developing the 791T–HSA–MTX conjugate *in vitro*, larger batches of this conjugate and also the optimal direct-linked conjugates were prepared for *in vivo* testing. The results of these preliminary tests are given below.

CBA mice were thymectomised, γ-irradiated and inoculated with 1–3 × 10⁶ osteogenic sarcoma cells and maintained in isolator cabinets. Groups of 7–10 weighed mice were then treated ip at 3- to 4-day intervals with either MTX, conjugate or PBS. Two direct-linked conjugates, total MTX dose 5.5 and 10 mg/kg, showed no effect on the subsequent growth of the xeongrafts.

However, a MTX–HSA–791T/36 conjugate, total dose 17.5 mg/kg, showed a significant therapeutic effect which became manifest after tumours had grown to a measureable size (Fig. 8). This conjugate showed no evidence of host toxicity, compared to a similar dose of free drug which showed considerable toxicity. The toxicity of free MTX for this group of mice was higher than usual—a figure of approximately 20% mortality would have been expected. While it must be stressed that this experiment remains to be substantiated by further such studies, we feel that it offers encouragement for further work.

VI. CONCLUDING REMARKS

The studies outlined in this chapter are based on a model system in which the target cells constitute a relatively homogeneous population in terms of antigen expression and drug sensitivity. This characteristic is unlikely to be shared by primary and metastatic tumours in human patients. On the contrary, neoplastic cells within tumours encountered in clinical practice will undoubtedly differ widely in their expression of an antigen detected by a given monoclonal antibody, and there are also likely to be sub-populations of drug-resistant cells, maintained by a constant mutation rate. To deal with antigenic heterogeneity using monoclonal antibodies, it might be necessary to have available panels of antibodies recognising a range of epitopes associated with the tumour in question. Such an approach has been described in a study in which neuroblastoma cells were removed from bone marrow aspirates *ex vivo*, by means of a panel of anti-neuroblastoma monoclonal antibodies linked to magnetic particles (Treleaven *et al.*, 1984). It would not be impracticable to employ similar panels of monoclonal antibodies in the treatment of patients with disseminated tumours by drug–antibody conjugates, so that antigenic heterogeneity may not be an insurmountable problem clinically. Moreover, if linkages can be devised which result in localised release of a therapuetic agent after binding to target cells has occurred, it may be unnecessary for conjugates to react directly with each target cell.

Drug-resistant sub-populations have been described by a mathematical model (Goldie and Coldman, 1979), from which the use of combinations of drugs with different modes of action was rationalised (Goldie *et al.*, 1982). Such combinations commonly achieve increased therapeutic efficiency over that obtainable using a single drug. A similar approach could be used in the case of drug-antibody conjugates, i.e., conjugates containing different drugs could be administered as part of a standard course of treatment. However, this also may not be necessary in every case. The susceptibility of drug-resistant cells to drug–antibody conjugates has not yet been tested, and it is possible (especially in systems where impaired drug transport is the critical factor) that in some cases the use of an antibody-directed conjugate may overcome the resistance of a given cell clone to the drug in free form.

Potential problems such as the above need to be studied before clinical therapy with drug–antibody conjugates can justifiably be established, and criteria need to be established for the choice of antibody vectors. The main criteria have been considered in this chapter and one of these— specificity—may be checked by careful immunohistological studies using sections of normal and neoplastic tissues (perhaps biopsies from prospective patients), and by observing the ability of radiolabelled antibody to localise at the tumour site. In the meantime, chemical and pharmacological aspects of drug–antibody conjugates relating to their efficiency and specificity of action and their transport *in vivo,* may be adequately studied in model systems such as that described in this chapter. We have shown, for example, that it is possible to link therapeutic quantities of a conventional cytotoxic drug (MTX) to a monoclonal antibody, which then confers upon the drug selectivity of action preferentially against target cells expressing a defined antigen. Similar properties have been demonstrated previously for the anti-mitotic drug vindesine conjugated to antibody 791T/36 (Embleton *et al.,* 1983). This selectivity resulted in a conjugate, which presumably by localising preferentially *in vivo* to tumour xenografts rather than antigenically unrelated tissues (i.e., normal mouse tissues), was less toxic than free drug, while retaining significant anti-tumour properties. This is the aim of targeted therapy, and present progress suggests that the approach taken offers considerable potential for the future.

ACKNOWLEDGMENTS

This work was supported by the Cancer Research Campaign, London, UK.

REFERENCES

Bernstein, A., Hurwitz, E., Maron, R., Arnon, R., Sela, M., and Wilchek, M. (1978). *J. Natl. Cancer Inst. (U.S.)* **60,** 379–384.

Borsos, T., Chapuis, R. M., and Langone, J. J. (1981). *Mol. Immunol.* **18**, 857–862.

Byfield, J. E., and Calabro-Jones, P. M. (1981). *Nature (London)* **294**, 281–283.

Chu, B. C. F., and Whiteley, J. M. (1977). *Mol. Pharmacol.* **13**, 80–88.

Chu, B. C. F., and Whiteley, J. M. (1980). *Mol. Pharmacol.* **17**, 382–387.

DeDuve, C., De Barsy, T., Poole, B., Trouet, A., Tulkens, P., and Van Hoof, F. (1974). *Biochem. Pharmacol.* **23**, 2495–2531.

Duncan, R., Lloyd, J. B., and Kopecek, J. (1980). *Biochem. Biophys Res. Commun.* **94**, 284–290.

Duncan, R., Rejmanova, P., Kopecek, J., and Lloyd, J. B. (1981). *Biochim. Biophys Acta* **678**, 143–150.

Eiklid, K., Olsnes, S., and Pihl, A. (1980). *Exp. Cell Res.* **126**, 321–326.

Embleton, M. J., Gunn, B., Byers, V. S., and Baldwin, R. W. (1981). *Br. J. Cancer* **43**, 582–587.

Embleton, M. J., Rowland, G. F., Simmonds, R. G., Jacobs, E., Marsden, C. H., and Baldwin, R. W. (1983). *Br. J. Cancer* **47**, 43–49.

Embleton, M. J., Garnett, M. C., Jacobs, E., and Baldwin, R. W. (1984). *Br. J. Cancer* **49**, 559–565.

Farrands, P. A., Perkins, A. C., Pimm, M. V., Hardy, J. D., Embleton, M. J., Baldwin, R. W., and Hardcastle, J. D. (1982). *Lancet* **2**, 397–400.

Farrands, P. A., Perkins, A. C., Sully, L., Hopkins, J. S., Pimm, M. V., Baldwin, R. W., and Hardcastle, J. D. (1983). *J. Bone Jt. Surg., Br. Vol.* **65B**, 638–640.

Garnett, M. C., Embleton, M. J., Jacobs, E., and Baldwin, R. W. (1983). *Int. J. Cancer* **31**, 661–670.

Goldie, J. H., and Coldman, A. J. (1979). *Cancer Treat. Rep.* **63**, 1727–1733.

Goldie, J. H., Coldman, A. J., and Gudauskas, G. A. (1982). *Cancer Treat. Rep.* **66**, 439–449.

Goldman, I. D., Lichtenstein, N. S., and Oliverio, U. T. (1968). *J. Biol. Chem.* **243**, 5007–5017.

Harrap, K. R., Hill, B. T., Furness, M. E., and Hart, L. I. (1971). *Ann. N.Y. Acad. Sci.* **186**, 312–324.

Hurwitz, E., Maron, R., Bernstein, A., Wilchek, M., Sela, M., and Arnon, R. (1978). *Int. J. Cancer* **21**, 747–755.

Hurwitz, E., Wilchek, M., and Pitha, J. (1980). *J. Appl. Biochem.* **2**, 25–35.

Levin, Y., and Sela, B. A. (1979). *FEBS Lett.* **93**, 119–122.

Kitao, T., and Hattori, K. (1977). *Nature (London)*, **265**, 81–82.

Kulkarni, P. N., Huntley Blair, A., and Ghose, T. I. (1981). *Cancer Res.* **41**, 2700–2706.

Masquelier, M., Baurain, R., and Trouet, A. (1980). *J. Med. Chem.* **23**, 1166–1170.

Monsigny, M., Kieda, C., Roche, A.-C., and Delmotte, F. (1980). *FEBS Lett.* **119**, 181–186.

Ohkuma, S., and Poole, B. (1978). *Proc. Natl. Acad. Sci. U.S.A.* **75**, 3327–3331.

Pimm, M. V., Embleton, M. J., Perkins, A. C., Price, M. R., Robins, R. A., Robinson, G. R., and Baldwin, R. W. (1982). *Int. J. Cancer* **30**, 75–85.

Price, M. R., Campbell, D. G., Robins, R. A., and Baldwin, R. W. (1983). *Eur. J. Cancer Clin. Oncol.* **19**, 81–90.

Ross, W. C. J. (1974). *Chem.-Biol. Interact.* **8**, 261–267.

Rowland, G. F. (1977). *Eur. J. Cancer* **13**, 593–596.

Rowland, G. F., O'Neill, G. J., and Davies, D. A. L. (1975). *Nature (London)* **255**, 487–488.

Rowland, G. F., Simmonds, R. G., Corvalan, J. R. F., Baldwin, R. W., Brown, J. P., Embleton, M. J., Ford, C. H. J., Hellström, K. E., Hellström, I., Kemshead, J. T., Newman, C. E., and Woodhouse, C. S. (1982). *Protides Biol. Fluids* **30**, 375–379.

Ryser, H. J.-P., and Shen, W. G. (1980). *Cancer (Philadelphia)* **45**, 1207–1211.

Seglen, P. O., Grinde, B., and Solheim, A. E. (1979). *Eur. J. Biochem.* **95**, 215–225.

Shen, W. C., and Ryser, H. J.-P. (1978). *Proc. Natl. Acad. Sci. U.S.A.* **75**, 1872–1876.

Shen, W. C., and Ryser, H. J.-P. (1981). *Biochem. Biophys. Res. Commun.* **102,** 1048–1054.

Szekerke, M., Wade, R., and Whisson, M. E. (1972a). *Neoplasma* **19,** 199–209.

Szekerke, M., Wade, R., and Whisson, M. E. (1972b). *Neoplasma* **19,** 211–215.

Treleaven, J. G., Gibson, F. M., Ugelstad, J., Rembaum, A., Philip, T., Caine, G. D., and Kemshead, J. T. (1984). *Lancet* **1,** 70–73.

Trouet, A., Masquelier, M., Baurain, R., and Deprez de Campeneere, D. (1982). *Proc. Natl. Acad. Sci. U.S.A.* **79,** 626–629.

Varga, J. M., Asato, N., Lande, S., and Lerner, A. B. (1977). *Nature (London)* **267,** 56–58.

Whiteley, J. M. (1971). *Ann. N. Y. Acad. Sci.* **186,** 29–42.

Yamaizumi, M., Mekada, E., Uchida, T., and Okada, Y. (1978). *Cell (Cambridge, Mass.)* **15,** 245–250.

Zunino, F., Gambetta, R., Marco, A. D., and Zaccara, A. (1972). *Biochim. Biophys. Acta* **277,** 489–498.

Zunino, F., Giuliani, F., Savi, G., Dasdia, T., and Gambetta, R. (1982). *Int. J. Cancer* **30,** 465–470.

CHAPTER 17

Effects of Monoclonal Antibody–Drug Conjugates on Human Tumour Cell Cultures and Xenografts

G. F. Rowland[1] and R. G. Simmonds

Lilly Research Centre Ltd.
Eli Lilly and Co.
Windlesham, Surrey, United Kingdom

I. INTRODUCTION AND EARLY STUDIES

The explosive growth of hybridoma technology in recent years has resulted in the production by many laboratories of a large number of monoclonal antibodies whose binding activities suggest they may have selectivity for human tumour-associated antigens. The various applications of such antibodies, both diagnostic and therapeutic, are the subject of this book and have been predicted in numerous reviews and books on monoclonal antibody applications (see, for example, McMichael and

[1]Present address: Department of Biochemistry, University of Stellenbosch, Stellenbosch, South Africa, 7600.

MONOCLONAL ANTIBODIES FOR CANCER DETECTION AND THERAPY

Fabre, 1982). Many reviewers end with a sentence stating "the ultimate prize would be to use monoclonals as carriers of cytotoxic drugs, thus fulfilling Paul Ehrlich's dream of a magic bullet". With perhaps hundreds of laboratories now working in the hybridoma field, it is initially surprising to find that relatively few studies have been published in which drug–monoclonal antibody conjugates have been prepared and used in targeting or cancer therapy experiments, particularly since there was an upsurge of interest in drug–antibody targeting using polyclonal antibodies when monoclonals were first described.

Although there is no convincing evidence that monoclonals can identify truly tumour-specific antigens, the wealth of work in this field has produced many antibodies that show significant selectivity for tumour cells. This selectivity has been quantitated in some cases (Brown *et al.*, 1981; Embleton *et al.*, 1981) and the indications are that some normal antigens, probably differentiation structures, may be present at levels that are several orders of magnitude higher on tumour cells than on normal cells. This theme of selectivity by monoclonals appears in most of the chapters in this book and has been reviewed recently in relation to the potential application of monoclonal antibodies to drug targeting (Rowland, 1983).

An examination of the literature shows that a number of anti-cancer drugs have been used in experimental antibody targeting studies, mainly with polyclonal antibodies. The earliest reports were isolated studies utilizing the anti-metabolite methotrexate (Mathé *et al.*, 1958; DeCarvalho *et al.*, 1964). During the past 10 yr, increasing numbers of reports on studies in experimental animals with other clinically used anti-cancer drugs have appeared. These include studies with adriamycin (Hurwitz *et al.*, 1975), bleomycin (Manabe *et al.*, 1983), chlorambacil (Ghose *et al.*, 1972), melphalan (Everall *et al.*, 1977) and vindesine (Johnson *et al.*, 1981). Methotrexate has also been re-examined more recently (Kulkarni *et al.*, 1981). In addition, other cytotoxic drugs not in current clinical use have been coupled to antibodies as potential targeted warheads. These include neocarzinostatin (Kimura *et al.*, 1980), phenylene diamine mustard (Rowland *et al.*, 1975), triaziquone (Linford *et al.*, 1974) and platinum (Hurwitz *et al.*, 1982).

In these studies drugs were conjugated to antibody by a range of chemical reactions including diazotization, carbodiimide condensation between carboxyl and amino groups, glutaraldehyde coupling between amino groups, periodate oxidation of sugar residues, and active ester formation of carboxyl groups. Drugs have been conjugated directly to amino acid residues on immunoglobulin and indirectly through a range of intermediate carrier molecules such as dextran, polyglutamic acid and albumin. One major reason for coupling drugs through an intermediate carrier was the belief that insufficient numbers of drug molecules would be delivered to target cells by antibodies alone bearing drugs at conjugation ratios of about 10 : 1, the maximum number generally obtainable without loss of antigen-binding function. Effectiveness could theoretically be increased by the greater numbers of drug molecules delivered, as by the use of an intermediate carrier, or by the use of a more potent drug. The vinca alkaloids are in molar terms amongst the most potent anti-cancer drugs in clinical use and thus offer a valuable potential as warheads for direct coupling to antibodies.

Work on vinca antibody conjugates began at the Lilly Research Centre in 1980, the coupling procedure being based initially on that used to prepare a vinca-albumin complex designed as an immunogen to raise anti-vinca antibodies for immunoassay (Conrad *et al.*, 1979). The vinca alkaloid used in the conjugation was desacetyl vinblastine azide, an intermediate in the synthesis of vindesine. Details of the coupling will be described in a later section of this chapter.

The first experiments were based on conjugates of vindesine (VDS) to goat polyclonal antibodies recognising rabbit immunoglobulin. These were prepared using affinity-purified goat anti-rabbit antibody and after characterization in terms of their drug and antibody content were tested *in vitro* in two systems designed to show if the conjugates could produce specific cytotoxic or cytostatic effects. In the first system, mouse EL4 lymphoma cells were exposed to a rabbit anti-EL4 serum at a non-agglutinating level for 30 min. After washing to remove unbound rabbit antibody, the cells were incubated with the VDS–goat–anti-rabbit conjugate at different concentrations for a further 30 min. Removal of unbound conjugate by washing was performed before the cells were placed in tissue culture to observe at daily intervals their growth and survival. One advantage of an indirect system, in which the target antigen is an antibody layer, is that it allows inclusion of a specificity control using the same cells without the first layer of rabbit antibody. Table I shows the results of such an experiment in which a modest but statistically significant reduction in cell numbers was observed using the targeted conjugate.

Similar results were obtained using a human lung carcinoma cell (CALU-6) pre-treated with a rabbit antiserum that had been raised against the cell. As with the mouse EL4 system, a small but significant and selective effect was observed using the vinca conjugate (Rowland *et al.*, 1982).

The experiments described above demonstrated target selective biological action *in vitro* but used a system involving only a brief exposure of the cells to conjugate. In a different series of experiments (Johnson

TABLE I

INDIRECT TARGETING *IN VITRO* USING A VDS–POLYCLONAL ANTIBODY CONJUGATE AND MOUSE LYMPHOMA CELLS

Conc. of VDS in the conjugate[a] used for the second layer pre-treatment[b] (μg/ml)	Viable cells/well ($\times$ 10^{-3}) on day 2[c]	
	Pre-treated[b] with medium as the first layer	Pre-treated with rabbit anti-EL4 serum as the first layer
0	78.4 $\pm$ 7.0	73.1 $\pm$ 8.3
3.4	80.8 $\pm$ 6.6	63.3 $\pm$ 10.3 ($p < 0.01$)[d]
34	74.3 $\pm$ 16.6	58.6 $\pm$ 12.5 ($p < 0.001$)[d]

[a] A conjugate of VDS and affinity-purified goat anti-rabbit Ig antibody (conjugation ratio 3 : 1) was used as second layer.

[b] Pre-treatments were for 30 min.

[c] After the pre-treatments, cells were washed and established in microwell cultures (200 μl) at 20 $\times$ 10^3/well and allowed to grow for 2 days. The results of viable cell counts are expressed as mean $\pm$ SD of 20 replicate cultures.

[d] Based on student's *t* test in comparison with non-conjugate-treated cells.

et al., 1981), vindesine was conjugated to a polyclonal sheep anti-CEA antibody and tested directly with the CALU-6 cells in a system involving 72 hr of exposure. Results from these experiments showed that the cells were killed using conjugated VDS at 1/25th of the dose of unconjugated VDS required. In addition, both sheep anti-CEA alone or a conjugate of VDS coupled to normal sheep immunoglobulin were non-cytotoxic at 50 times the effective level of VDS-sheep anti-CEA.

Encouraging as these *in vitro* results were, it was generally agreed that development of clinically useful conjugates based on polyclonal sheep antisera would be difficult and a major effort was undertaken to produce suitable mouse monoclonal antibodies to CEA that could substitute for the polyclonal sheep preparation.

II. MONOCLONAL ANTIBODIES USED IN VINDESINE CONJUGATION STUDIES

In order to extend the VDS-anti-CEA studies, mouse monoclonal anti-CEA antibodies were produced by the well-established hybridoma technique using purified CEA (Pritchard and Egan, 1978) as the immunogen.

Hybrids secreting anti-CEA antibody were screened using an enzyme-linked immunoassay (Woodhouse *et al.*, 1982). Positive hybrids were maintained in culture and cloned prior to storage in liquid nitrogen. Supernatants from hybrid clones were then examined in more detail for specificity. Tests included an immunoassay for reactivity against non-specific cross-reacting antigen (NCA), and histochemical studies designed to identify monoclonals that would react with CEA-bearing tumours but not with normal tissues. One antibody designated 11.285.14 has undergone extensive testing (Gatter *et al.*, 1982; Corvalan *et al.*, 1984) and emerges as a strong candidate for targeting studies because of its high degree of tumour selectivity. Reactivity was observed with epithelial cells of the normal gastrointestinal tract but there was no binding to normal skin, brain, mammary tissue, lung, liver, bile duct, pancreas, kidney, prostate, testes, thyroid, muscle or lymphoid cells in lymph nodes and tonsil. In other histochemical studies, 11.285.14 has been shown to be free from reactivity with cells in the spleen. Reactivity with myeloid cells in the spleen may be a feature of monoclonal antibodies recognizing NCA (Corvalan *et al.*, 1984) and such reactivity could be responsible for the binding and destruction of granulocytes that has been observed (Dillman *et al.*, 1983). The moderate systemic toxicity observed on administration of granulocyte reactive anti-CEA monoclonals to patients sounds a cautionary note for clinical use of antibodies (Dillman *et al.*, 1984). Antibody 11.285.14 did not bind granulocytes and did not produce the adverse effects described by Dillman *et al.* (1984) when given to a limited number of patients with advanced colorectal carcinoma for imaging studies (Hockey *et al.*, 1983; R. Begent, personal communication). Antibody 11.285.14 has also proved useful in the one-step affinity purification of CEA (Simmonds *et al.*, 1984).

Experiments in which 11.285.14 has been conjugated to VDS and used for drug targeting studies are described in subsequent sections of this chapter. Other monoclonal antibodies that have been conjugated with VDS include antibody 791T/36 (Embleton *et al.*, 1981), obtained by immunising with osteogenic sarcoma cells, anti-melanoma antibody 96.5 (Brown *et al.*, 1981) and the anti-neuroblastoma antibody UJ13A (Kemshead *et al.*, 1982). Discussion of features of these monoclonals will be found in other chapters of this book.

Although antibodies of this nature appear to have selective properties that make them potentially useful for drug targeting, it is important not to forget the problem of antigenic heterogeneity. A study of histochemical reactivity of 11.285.14 with 119 gastric malignancies clearly illustrates this point (Hockey *et al.*, 1984). Although 92% of primary tumours reacted with the antibody, only 61% stained more than one cell in twenty. Similarly 81% of lymph nodes showed metastatic tumour but only 68% contained more than 5% of staining cells in these secondary deposits. A wide range of CEA expression has also been observed using fluorescent-labelled 11.285.14 with cells isolated from fresh surgical biopsy samples of colorectal carcinomas (R. W. Baldwin, personal communication).

In addition to the antibodies described above, which have tumor cell selectivity, VDS conjugates have been prepared and studied using three monoclonals recognising determinants on T lymphocytes. These antibodies designated RFT-1, RFT-2 and RFT-11 (Janossy *et al.*, 1985a) do not bind to non-lymphoid cells and have potential application in the treatment of T cell malignances.

III. PREPARATION AND CHARACTERISATION OF VDS–MONOCLONAL ANTIBODIES

A. Antibody Isolation

Antibodies used for conjugation were of the IgG_1, IgG_{2a} and IgG_{2b} isotypes. In order to achieve a standardised procedure for conjugate preparation, the antibodies were isolated from mouse ascitic fluid using a protein A immunoabsorbent column, applicable to all the antibodies used. The ascites fluid was filtered or centrifuged to remove particulate material and lipid, before adjusting the pH to 8.0 by addition of sodium phosphate buffer. Adsorption onto protein A-Sepharose (Pharmacia Ltd) equilibrated with pH 8.0 buffer was performed at 4°C. Bound immunoglobulin was eluted using 0.1 M citrate/phosphate, pH 3.5 and the eluates adjusted to pH 7.4 by addition of 5 N NaOH. Following dialysis twice against 50 volumes of distilled water, the immunoglobulin was lyophilized.

B. Conjugation Procedures

Two methods have been employed to prepare covalent conjugates of VDS and monoclonal antibodies. The method based on desacetylvinblastine (DAVLB) azide used for the early polyclonal conjugate studies was subsequently replaced by a more efficient process using an active ester of 4-succinoyl-VDS.

1. Azide Conjugation

Lyophilized immunoglobulin was dissolved in 0.34 M borate buffer pH 8.6 at 40 mg/ml. Desacetylvinblastine hydrazide was converted to the azide with hydrochloric acid and sodium nitrite at 4°C, then neutralised and added dropwise to the stirred immunoglobulin solution in the presence of 10% dioxan to give a final concentration of 6 mg/ml. The mixture was adjusted to pH 9.0 and allowed to react at room temperature maintaining the pH at 9.0 ± 0.1 NaOH throughout. After 2 hr, excess azide was destroyed with dilute ammonia and the mixture applied to a Biogel P-6 column equilibrated with PBS. The conjugate was collected in the excluded fraction and characterised for protein and drug concentration by measuring the absorbances of the solution at 270 and 280 nm and relating the values obtained to those for the free drug and unconjugated immunoglobulin at those two wavelengths.

It was observed that the conjugation ratio (CR) achieved using the azide method varied according to the monoclonal antibody used but was reproducible with the same antibody (Rowland *et al.*, 1983). For example, using 11.285.14 (an IgG_1), a CR of 3 : 1 could be obtained without significant loss of solubility or antigen-binding capacity. Losses did however, occur, if attempts were made to increase the CR by increasing the amounts of DAVLB hydrazide in the reaction mixture. By contrast, antibody 96.5, an IgG_{2a} reacting with melanoma antigen p97, could be reacted under conditions giving CR of 10 : 1 with 64% antibody activity retained.

With a limited number of monoclonals examined, it appeared that when using the azide method higher conjugation ratios could be achieved with IgG_{2a} and IgG_{2b} isotypes than with IgG_1 isotypes. The differences could, however, have been fortuitous.

2. Active Ester Conjugation

Batches of 4-succinoyl-VDS N-hydroxysuccinimide ester were prepared by Mr. G. Cullinan of Lilly Research Laboratories, Indianapolis. One volume of the active ester at ca. 10 mg/ml in dimethylformamide was added to six volumes of immunoglobulin at ca. 20 mg/ml in 0.34 M borate buffer pH 8.6. The reaction was stirred at room temperature for 4 hr, then adjusted to pH 7.4 before gel filtration on BioGel P-6 as for the azide method.

Using this method, antibody 11.285.14 was conjugated at a CR of up to 10 : 1 with 60% recovery and 80% antigen-binding activity.

IV. SELECTIVITY OF VDS–MONOCLONAL CONJUGATES
IN VITRO

An extensive series of *in vitro* tests was performed using VDS conjugates with antibody 791T/36 (Embleton *et al.*, 1983) prepared by the azide method. Four osteogenic sarcoma cell lines, able to bind between 5×10^5 and 2×10^6 molecules of antibody per cell, showed cytotoxicity during the 24 hr following brief (15 min) exposure to the VDS–791T/36 conjugate. By contrast, four non-binding cell lines were unaffected over the same dose range. All eight cell lines were susceptible to free VDS, indicating that the selective cytotoxicity was not due to an inherent difference in drug sensitivity. It was also observed that the levels of conjugated VDS required to produce cytotoxicity in the target cell were often higher than when using free VDS. Moreover, the antibody levels were also higher than those expected to saturate cell surface antigen-binding sites. Cytotoxicity probably results from a dynamic process of internalization of surface bound conjugate which can only take place at supersaturating levels in the incubation medium.

The experiments described above assessed cytotoxicity by measuring the incorporation of radioactive selenomethionine into cellular protein. An alternative approach is to determine the effect of conjugate treatment on the ability of the treated cells to form colonies in subsequent culture. This approach was used with VDS–96.5 anti-melanoma conjugates against three cell lines bearing different levels of the target antigen p97 (Rowland *et al.*, 1983). The results showed that VDS–96.5 was able to inhibit colony formation of the two melanoma cell lines with antigen levels of 4×10^5 and 1.3×10^5 per cell but did not affect a lung carcinoma cell line that carried minimal amounts of p97.

In addition to the clonogenic assays previously described, the effect of conjugate treatment was assessed by counting numbers of cells grown in microtitre trays for 7 days after a 30-min exposure to various dilutions of conjugate. An experiment performed by this technique compared the effects of conjugates prepared by the azide and active ester methods on SK Mel-28 melanoma cells that express large amounts of the target antigen p97. Figure 1 shows the dose–response curves with the two preparations. The active ester conjugate was approximately twice as potent as the azide conjugate in this test.

A series of *in vitro* experiments were performed using VDS linked to anti-T cell monoclonals by the active ester method. In order to demonstrate specificity, a control conjugate was prepared using immunoglobulin obtained from the mouse myeloma P3x63Ag8. This IgG$_1$, des-

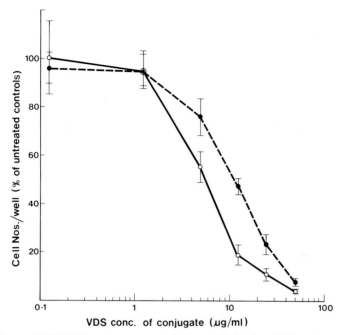

Fig. 1. Effects of VDS–96.5 conjugates on melanoma cells *in vitro*. Cells were pre-treated with various concentrations of conjugate prepared by the azide (●---●) or the active ester method (○—○) and then established in microwell tissue culture. Results are the means (±SD) of three separate experiments in which numbers of treated cells are expressed as a percentage of untreated cells on day 7 of culture.

ignated Ag8, was prepared in ascites by growing the myeloma in BALB/ c mice, and shown to be unreactive with the T cell line (Molt-3) used as the target in these tests. In addition, a B cell line (RAJI) and a pro-mye-locyte line (HL60) were used as antigen-negative cells for control purposes. Cells in log-phase growth were incubated in varying concentrations of conjugate for 2 hr at 37°. After washing in tissue culture medium, the cells were established in culture at 2×10^5/ml and viable counts determined daily. Table II shows results from two separate experiments at day 5 when the cells treated with medium alone had reached maximum concentration, approximately 10 times the starting levels. It can be seen that the antigen-positive Molt-3 cells have been either killed or their growth drastically curtailed by the VDS–(RFT-11) conjugate, whereas the antigen-negative cells were unaffected. Treatment with a much higher concentration of the Ag8 conjugate was without effect on cells, whereas both Molt-3 and RAJI were killed by free VDS. Similar results have been

TABLE II

**DIRECT TARGETING *IN VITRO* USING VDS–MONOCLONAL ANTIBODY
CONJUGATES[a] AND HUMAN CELLS[b]**

Exp. no.	Pre-treatment[c]	VDS conc. (μg/ml)	Viable cells/ml ($\times$ 10[-5]) on day 5	
			Antigen positive[b]	Antigen negative[b]
1	Medium alone	0	23.2	26.2
	VDS–(RFT-11)	30	0	18.4
		15	0	18.2
		7.5	3.9	12.3
2	Medium alone	0	23.8	25.5
	VDS–(RFT-11)	33	2.6	30.3
		16.5	12.2	26.8
	VDS–Ag8	113	22.8	21.8
	RFT-11 alone	—	20.0	25.6
	VDS alone	10	0.4	0

[a] Conjugates of VDS and the anti-T lymphocyte monoclonal RFT-11 were as described in the text.

[b] The human T cell line Molt-3 was used as the antigen-positive cell, HL60 (exp. 1) and RAJI (exp. 2) were the antigen-negative cells.

[c] Pre-treatment was 2 hr at 37°C.

obtained with VDS conjugates of two other anti-T cell monoclonals, RFT-1 and RFT-2. Full details will be reported elsewhere (Janossy *et al.*, 1985b).

V. *IN VIVO* STUDIES USING HUMAN TUMOUR XENOGRAFTS

A major objective in the treatment of cancer is to destroy or prevent the growth of malignant cells whilst minimising such effects on normal cells. A step towards achievement of this objective is to show that the monoclonal antibody–drug conjugates, whose selective action *in vitro* has been demonstrated, can also produce anti-tumour effects *in vivo*.

1. Osteogenic Sarcoma

The first tests of *in vivo* efficacy with VDS–monoclonal conjugates were performed using the 791T/36 system. Immune-deprived CBA mice were given xenografts of the osteogenic sarcoma 791T by inoculation of 10^6 cells. Treatments with VDS–791T/36 conjugates at a dose level, in terms of VDS, of 2.75 mg/kg per injection (seven injections over 15 days) resulted in a partial but significant suppression of growth (Rowland, 1983; Baldwin et al., 1984). No toxicity was seen in the conjugate-treated mice. Mice treated with free VDS at this dose level showed marked tumour suppression although one-third of the treated mice died. Similar results were obtained when commencement of treatment was delayed until day 5, using a dose of conjugate per injection of 5 mg/kg in terms of VDS content (Rowland et al., 1984b). The active ester method was employed to prepare the conjugate in the latter experiment.

2. Melanoma

Similar experiments were performed using VDS–96.5 for treatment of melanoma xenografts. Since the active ester-derived conjugate was somewhat more potent in vitro, this was the method of choice for preparing the VDS–96.5 conjugates. A melanoma xenograft was initiated in athymic nu/nu mice and the mice were treated with seven injections of conjugate at dose levels of 5.1 mg/kg, in terms of VDS, over a 3-week period. Conjugate, but not free antibody, reduced the tumour growth rate during the treatment period. Thereafter the growth rate of the conjugate-treated group, although delayed, paralleled the control group (Rowland et al., 1984b).

3. Colorectal Carcinoma

A colorectal tumour, designated MAWI, was kindly supplied by Drs. F. Searle and J. Lewis (Charing Cross Hospital, London) and maintained as a xenograph in nude mice by serial passage of cell suspensions. The MAWI tumour has been shown to express CEA at levels in the order of 50 µg/g, and to maintain this level of antigen expression through 10 serial xenograft passages (Lewis et al., 1983). This stability of expression by MAWI has been confirmed by an ELISA for CEA using the monoclonal 11.285.14 as the detecting antibody (Simmonds et al., 1984). Levels of CEA extractable from colorectal tumours removed from patients surgically were compared with levels in a batch of tumour xenografts grown in nude mice. Table III shows data from surgical material and from two types of xenograft: the MAWI tumour and tumours obtained by inoculation with a colorectal cell line, designated LoVo, that has been shown to synthesise appreciable levels of CEA in tissue culture (Yang and Drewinko, 1980). The surgical materials show a wide range of CEA levels whereas the xenografts of any one type vary little. The LoVo tumour,

TABLE III

LEVELS OF EXTRACTABLE CEA IN HUMAN COLORECTAL CARCINOMA

Tumours	No. of samples	CEA levels[a] (μg/g wet weight)
Surgical material from patients	8	37 (1–150)
MAWI xenografts	7	105 (83–123)
LoVo xenografts	15	12 (6–18)

[a] Saline extracts of tumours were tested for CEA using an ELISA system based on monoclonal antibody 11.285.14 and determined in relation to an affinity-purified CEA standard. Results are given as the means and range.

however, expresses only 11% of the CEA level found in MAWI when grown in nude mice.

Several experiments have been performed using the MAWI xenograft system and anti-CEA monoclonal antibodies. In the first studies, VDS was conjugated by the azide method to a monoclonal anti-CEA of the IgG_{2a} isotype (designated 14.95.55). Marked suppression of tumour growth was obtained when mice were given conjugate twice weekly for 5 weeks at dose levels of 5 mg/kg (VDS) per injection (Rowland et al., 1984a; b). Monoclonal antibodies of the IG_{2a} isotype recognising human colorectal carcinoma antigens have been shown to suppress tumour xenograft growth by mechanisms involving macrophage arming (Herlyn and Koprowski, 1982). In these studies, no drug or toxin warhead was needed to produce the anti-tumour effects. These effects, however, could not be obtained with monoclonals of other isotypes, despite their ability to recognise colorectal carcinoma antigens. An experiment with 14.95.55 showed that this monoclonal IgG_{2a} anti-CEA can also suppress colorectal tumour xenograft growth (Rowland et al., 1984a,b); the dose levels used, however, were considerably higher than those shown to be effective in the studies by Herlyn and Koprowski (1982).

The anti-CEA monoclonal 11.285.14, which is of the IgG_1 isotype, was used to treat nude mice inoculated with MAWI, both as free antibody and conjugated with VDS by the active ester method. Ten injections of antibody alone over a 5-week period at a dose of 140 mg/kg produced a slight suppression of growth, statistically significant only on termination of the experiment after 63 days. Treatment with VDS conjugated 11.285.14, however, produced an almost complete suppression of tumour growth which was sustained for the 90-day duration of the experiment (Rowland et al., 1984a,b).

In the experiments described above, tumour growth was assessed by weekly estimates of tumour volume determined by measuring three maximum external dimensions (length, width and height) and calculating a value for volume based on one-half of the product of these three dimensions. Confirmation that this calculation gives an accurate estimate of tumour mass has been provided by correlating volume and excised tumour weights over a wide range of tumour sizes (Rowland *et al.*, 1984a). This exercise has been repeated at intervals and the relationship remains firm. It was also of interest to examine directly the weights of tumours excised from nude mice at the termination of xenograft experiments as an indication of the effectiveness of treatment. Table IV shows tumour weights from two separate experiments. Experiment 1 gives the weights of tumours from the mice treated as described above with 11.285.14 alone or VDS conjugated. In this experiment each mouse had been inoculated with less than 20 mg (wet weight) of MAWI cell suspension. By 63 days all the PBS-treated control mice had demonstrated significant tumour growth with some tumours weighing several grams. The conjugate-treated group, when killed on day 90, displayed some small nodules weighing on average little more than the starting inoculum.

In experiment 2, mice were inoculated with a larger tumour load; 45 mg distributed at two sub-cutaneous sites. The dose level of conjugate, in terms of VDS, was increased to 15 mg/kg and the schedule, twice weekly for 5 weeks, was as before. In this experiment, marked but not complete suppression was observed. When the experiment was terminated on day 41, the tumours from conjugate-treated weighed on average 11.5% of that of the controls with only 1 out of the 14 tumours on seven mice showing significant growth.

The same experiment includes three groups of tumour-bearing mice treated with free VDS at three dose levels, 0.33, 1.0 and 3.0 mg/kg per injection. At the lowest dose, no effect on tumour size was obtained. At 1.0 mg/kg, partial reduction in tumour weight was observed (47% on average overall), a result that was just statistically significant. A significant effect was seen at 3.0 mg/kg. At this dose level, however, five out of seven mice died.

VI. LOCALISATION STUDIES

One possible approach to the study of drug targeting is to determine directly the relative drug concentrations in target and non-target tissues at various times following the administration of radioactively labelled conjugate. It could be argued that these studies should precede any at-

TABLE IV

WEIGHTS OF HUMAN TUMOUR XENOGRAFTS EXCISED FROM NUDE MICE FOLLOWING TREATMENT WITH VDS–ANTI-CEA CONJUGATES, ANTIBODY ALONE OR FREE VDS

Exp. no.	Treatment[a]	Dose/injection (mg/kg)		No. of mice	Toxic deaths	Mean tumour wt. (mg ± SEM)	Day of measurement	Significance level[b]
		VDS	IgG					
1	PBS	—	—	11	0	1793 ± 485	63	—
	VDS[11.285.14]	5	140	8	0	22 ± 7	90	$p < 0.001$
	11.285.14 alone	—	140	10	0	527 ± 151	63	$p < 0.05$
2	PBS	—	—	10	0	1351 ± 329	41	—
	VDS[11.285.14]	15	480	7	0	155 ± 76	41	$p < 0.001$
	VDS alone	0.3	—	7	0	1361 ± 116	41	NS
	VDS alone	1.0	—	7	0	721 ± 277	41	$p = 0.05$
	VDS alone	3.0	—	2	5	100 ± 30	41	$p < 0.05$

[a] Mice were injected ip twice weekly for 5 weeks.
[b] Mann-Whitney U test, one-tailed comparisons with PBS control groups.

tempts to demonstrate suppression of tumour growth *in vivo* and be used to pre-determine the parameters for such therapy experiments. We chose, however, to look first for biological effects which could have practical application in cancer therapy and then ask questions regarding localisation and the mechanisms involved. Localisation studies with labelled conjugates may show higher levels of conjugate at the tumour site than in non-tumour tissues, but this does not prove that the tumour-suppressive effects obtained are due to targeting.

1. Labelled Antibody

Localisation studies using conjugates were initially carried out using the techniques employed to show that the antibodies alone can localise. These involved preparing drug–antibody conjugates and subsequently labelling them with ^{131}I or ^{125}I. Results of studies carried out in this way can only demonstrate localisation of the antibody component of the conjugate.

A study of this type using VDS conjugated to polyclonal anti-CEA was carried out in a small group of patients with advanced metastatic carcinoma (Ford *et al.*, 1983). Patients received between 230 and 520 µg of an ^{131}I-labelled conjugate of VDS to a sheep antibody that previously had been shown to localise in human gastrointestinal tumour deposits (Dykes *et al.*, 1980). Localisation was observed using the VDS conjugate, showing that drug conjugation does not impair antibody targeting *in vivo*.

Similar information was obtained in xenograft studies using VDS conjugated to monoclonal antibodies. VDS–791T/36 conjugate was radioiodinated and 10 µg (Ig) was injected into mice bearing 791T xenografts. Tissue distribution of radioactive iodine 4 days later showed that the tumour : blood ratio was at least three times higher than the ratios of other tissues to blood (Rowland *et al.*, 1984b). This result, closely similar to that obtained using iodinated- but not drug-conjugated 791T/36 (Pimm *et al.*, 1982), confirmed that monoclonal antibody localisation is not adversely affected by the drug coupling procedure. It does not, however, show that the drug component of the conjugate can localise.

2. Labelled Drug

A preparation of [^{3}H]VDS-succinate was used to form a radioactive ester-type conjugate of VDS and the anti-CEA monoclonal antibody, 11.285.14. Following the normal purification stages on BioGel P-6, the conjugate was re-chromatographed on Sephadex G-200 in order to re-

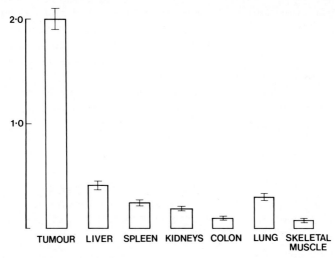

Fig. 2. Tissue : blood ratios of ³H from MAWI tumour-bearing nude mice on day 3 after iv injection of purified [³H]VDS–11.285.14 conjugate. Means ± SE of values from three mice are shown.

move any high molecular weight aggregates and traces of free VDS-suc-cinate. The highly purified ³H-labelled VDS–11.285.14 conjugate was in-jected into MAWI-bearing nude mice at several dose levels. Mice were killed at various times after injection, blood samples taken and tumour and organs collected. Weighed tissue samples were dissolved and ra-dioactivity determined by liquid scintillation counting.

Figure 2 shows the tissue or tumour : plasma ratios of ³H activity per gram wet weight 3 days after an iv injection of 194 µg [³H]VDS–11.285.14 containing 4 µg of VDS. It is apparent that ³H is present in the tumour at twice the plasma level, 5 times the level in liver and more than 25 times the level found in skeletal muscle. Assuming that ³H levels indicate concentrations of VDS, these results clearly demonstrate that drug lo-calisation has occurred in the tumour tissue following iv injection of a drug–monoclonal antibody conjugate. Similar results were obtained when the conjugate was injected ip.

VII. CONCLUSIONS

It has become apparent in recent years that monoclonal antibodies can truly offer a potential means of selective targeting to antigens on cancer cell surfaces. Whether or not this could lead to effective site-specific drug or toxin delivery needed to be tested. Ideally targeting would utilise a monoclonal antibody that bound plentifully to cancer cells alone, through recognition of a ubiquitous fully specific pan-carcinoma antigen. In reality, it is necessary to use a range of monoclonals, recognising cell surface structures present on cancer cells at higher levels than on normal cells. Some monoclonals have wide applicability to many cancer types and some are of a more narrow range.

Experience has now shown that biologically active drug conjugates can be prepared using suitable monoclonals; studies with VDS suggest several points which may also apply to other drugs.

1. Each monoclonal must be examined individually in order to define the optimum conditions for preparing conjugates with the required properties. Despite the theoretical need to produce highly conjugated preparations capable of maximum drug delivery per target cell, over-conjugation can reduce solubility and antibody activity. The optimum conjugation ratio appears to vary from one monoclonal to another (Rowland et al., 1982).

2. The levels of antibody concentration of a drug conjugate needed to saturate cell surface-binding sites are not necessarily adequate to produce cytostatic or cytotoxic effects in vitro. This phenomenon has been observed in all the in vitro test systems examined using VDS–monoclonal antibody conjugates. It appears likely that a biological drug effect requires a high extracellular concentration of conjugate (super-saturating levels) which promotes internalisation of cell surface-bound conjugate through receptor-mediated endocytosis.

3. Using the human tumour xenograft model systems, conjugates can be shown to suppress tumour growth when given by repeated intra-peritoneal injection. The effects vary in their potency depending on the system used and also on the tumour burden at the commencement of treatment but there is no direct evidence that the effects are the result of drug targeting; slow release of drug from a macromolecular conjugate circulating with a long biological half-life could play a part.

4. Localisation of conjugates in tumour xenografts can be demonstrated by the use of radioactively labelled materials. Using a conjugate of monoclonal antibody and tritiated VDS, drug localisation has been demonstrated in tumour xenografts. Since the antibody has itself been shown to localise in tumours of advanced gastrointestinal cancer patients, there is hope that drug localisation would also occur in patients given conjugates.

5. Toxicity of conjugates in experimental animals is considerably less than free drug. The ultimate hope of improving the therapeutic index

of anti-cancer drugs through selective targeting is now closer to fulfill-
ment.

ACKNOWLEDGEMENTS

The authors gratefully acknowledge valuable contributions by the many colleagues and
collaborators whose work is described in this chapter. We thank particularly Dr. J. R. F.
Corvalan and Mr. C. A. Axton, in collaboration with Drs. C. H. J. Ford, C. E. Newman
and C. S. Woodhouse (Surgical Immunology Unit, Birmingham, UK), for studies leading
to the production of anti-CEA hybridomas, and Mrs. C. H. Marsden, Miss V. A. Gore
and Mr. W. Smith for work on production, isolation, characterisation and conjugation of
monoclonal antibodies.

We thank Drs. K. E. Hellström, I. Hellström, and J. P. Brown (Fred Hutchinson Cancer
Research Center, Seattle, Washington) for supplying antibody 96.5 and for testing conjugates
in vitro and *in vivo;* Professor R. W. Baldwin, Drs. M. J. Embleton and M. V. Pimm (Cancer
Research Campaign Laboratories, Nottingham, UK) for supplying antibody 791T/36 and
for carrying out many tests *in vitro* and *in vivo;* Professor G. Janossy and Mrs. E. Rawlings
(Royal Free Hospital, London, UK) for providing the anti-T cell monoclonal antibodies
and for testing conjugates *in vitro;* and Drs. F. Searle, G. T. Rogers and J. Lewis (Charing
Cross Hospital, London, UK) for supplying human material containing CEA and the MAWI
tumour. Finally, we thank Mr. G. Cullinan (Lilly Research Laboratories, Indianapolis, In-
diana) for supply of vinca intermediates for conjugation, and Sue Donovan for typing this
manuscript.

REFERENCES

Baldwin, R. W., Embleton, M. J., Garnett, M. C., Pimm, M. V., Price, M. R., Armitage,
    N. A., Farrands, P. A., Hardcastle, J. D., Perkins, A., and Rowland, G. F. (1984).
    Protides Biol. Fluids **31,** 775–781.
Brown, J. P., Woodbury, R. G., Hart, C. E., Hellström, I., and Hellström, K. E. (1981).
    Proc. Natl. Acad. Sci. U.S.A. **78,** 539–543.
Conrad, R. A., Cullinan, G. J., Gerzon, K., and Poore, G. A. (1979). *J. Med. Chem.* **22,**
    391–400.
Corvalan, J. R. F., Axton, C. A., Brandon, D. R., Smith, W., and Woodhouse, C. (1984).
    Protides Biol. Fluids **31,** 921–924.
DeCarvalho, S., Rand, H. J., and Lewis, A. (1964). *Nature (London)* **202,** 255–258.
Dillman, R. O., Beauregard, J. C., Sobol, R. E., Royston, I., Bartholomew, R. M., Hagen,
    P. S., and Halpern, S. E. (1983). *Proc. Am. Assoc. Cancer Res.* p. 217.
Dillman, R. O., Beauregard, J. C., Sobol, R. E., Royston, I., Bartholomew, R. M., Hagan,
    P. S., and Halpern, S. E. (1984). *Cancer Res.* **44,** 2213–2218.
Dykes, P. W., Hine, K. R., Bradwell, A. R., Blackburn, J. C., Reeder, T. A., Drolc, Z.,
    and Booth, S. N. (1980). *Br. Med. J.* **280,** 220–222.
Embleton, M. J., Gunn, B., Byers, V. S., and Baldwin, R. W. (1981). *Br. J. Cancer* **42,** 582–
    587.

Embleton, M. J., Rowland, G. F., Simmonds, R. G., Jacobs, E., Marsden, C. H., and Baldwin, R. W. (1983). *Br. J. Cancer* **47**, 43–49.

Everall, J. D., Dowd, P., Davies, D. A. L., O'Neill, G. J., and Rowland, G. F. (1977). *Lancet* **1**, 1105.

Ford, C. H. J., Newman, C. E., Johnson, J. R., Woodhouse, C. S., Reeder, T. A., Rowland, G. F., and Simmonds, R. G. (1983). *Br. J. Cancer* **47**, 35–42.

Gatter, K. C., Abdulaziz, Z., Beverley, P., Corvalan, J. R. F., Ford, C., Lane, E. B., Mota, M., Nash, J. R. G., Pulford, K., Stein, H., Taylor-Papadimitriou, J., Woodhouse, C., and Mason, D. Y. (1982). *J. Clin. Pathol.* **35**, 1253–1267.

Ghose, T., Norwell, S., Guclu, A., Cameron, D., Bodurtha, A., and MacDonald, A. S. (1972). *Br. Med. J.* **3**, 495–499.

Herlyn, D., and Koprowski, H. (1982). *Proc. Natl. Acad. Sci. U.S.A.* **79**, 4761–4765.

Hockey, M. S., Ford, C. H. J., Newman, C., Corvalan, J. R. F., Rowland, G. F., Stokes, H. J., Thompson, H., and Fielding, J. W. L. (1983). *Br. J. Surg.* **70**, 300.

Hockey, M. S., Stokes, H. J., Thompson, H., Woodhouse, C. S., MacDonald, F., Fielding, J. W. L., and Ford, C. H. J. (1984). *Br. J. Cancer* **49**, 129–133.

Hurwitz, E., Kashi, R., and Wilchek, M. (1982). *JNCI, J. Natl. Cancer Inst.* **69**, 47–51.

Hurwitz, E., Levy, R., Maron, R., Wilchek, M., Arnon, R., and Sela, M. (1975). *Cancer Res.* **35**, 1175–1181.

Janossy, G., Trejdosiewicz, L., Price-Jones, E., Tidman, N., Prentice, H. G., and Hoffbrand, A. V. (1985a). *Leuk. Res.* (in press).

Janossy, G. *et al.* (1985b). In preparation.

Johnson, J. R., Ford, C. H. J., Newman, C. E., Woodhouse, C. S., Rowland, G. F., and Simmonds, R. G. (1981). *Br. J. Cancer* **44**, 472–475.

Kemshead, J. T., Fritschy, J., Asser, U., Sutherland, R., and Greaves, M. F. (1982). *Hybridoma* **1**, 109–123.

Kimura, I., Ohnoshi, T., Tsubota, T., Sato, Y., Kobayashi, T., and Abe, S. (1980). *Cancer Immunol. Immunother.* **7**, 235–242.

Kulkarni, P. N., Blair, A. H., and Ghose, T. I. (1981). *Cancer Res.* **41**, 2700–2706.

Lewis, J. C. M., Smith, P. A., Keep, P. A., and Boxer, G. M. (1983). *Exp. Pathol.* **24**, 227–235.

Linford, J. H., Froese, G., Berczi, I., and Israels, L. G. (1974). *J. Natl. Cancer Inst. (U.S.)* **52**, 1665–1667.

Manabe, Y., Tsubota, T., Haruto, Y., Okazaki, M., Haisa, S., Nakamura, K., and Kimura, I. (1983). *Biochem Biophys. Res. Commun.* **115**, 1009–1014.

McMichael, A., and Fabre, J., eds. (1982). "Monoclonal Antibodies in Clinical Medicine." Academic Press, New York.

Mathé, G., Loc, T. B., and Bernard, J. (1958). *C. R. Hebd. Seances Acad. Sci.* **246**, 1626–1628.

Pimm, M. V., Embleton, M. J., Perkins, A. C., Price, M. R., Robins, R. A., Robinson, G., and Baldwin, R. W. (1982). *Int. J. Cancer* **30**, 75–85.

Pritchard, D. G., and Egan, M. L. (1978). *Immunochemistry* **15**, 385–387.

Rowland, G. F. (1983). *Clin. Immunol. Allergy* 3(2), 235–257.

Rowland, G. F., O'Neill, G. J., and Davies, D. A. L. (1975). *Nature (London)* **255**, 487–488.

Rowland, G. F., Simmonds, R. G., Corvalan, J. R. F., Marsden, C. H., Johnson, J. R., Woodhouse, C. S., Ford, C. H. J., and Newman, C. E. (1982). *Protides Biol. Fluids* **29**, 921–926.

Rowland, G. F., Simmonds, R. G., Corvalan, J. R. F., Baldwin, R. W., Brown, J. P., Embleton, M. J., Ford, C. H. J., Hellström, K. E., Hellström, I., Kemshead, J. T., Newman, C. E., and Woodhouse, C. S. (1983). *Protides Biol. Fluids* **30**, 375–379.

Rowland, G. F., Corvalan, J. R. F., Axton, C. A., Gore, V. A., Marsden, C. H., Smith, W., and Simmonds, R. G. (1984a). *Protides Biol. Fluids* **31**, 783–786.

Rowland, G. F., Axton, C. A., Baldwin, R. W., Brown, J. P., Corvalan, J. R. F., Embleton, M. J., Gore, V. A., Hellström, I., Hellström, K. E., Jacobs, E., Marsden, C. H., Pimm, M. V., Simmonds, R. G., and Smith, W. (1984b). *Cancer Immunol. Immunother.* **19,** 1–7.

Simmonds, R. G., Smith, W., and Corvalan, J. R. F. (1984). *Protides Biol. Fluids* **31,** 917–920.

Woodhouse, C. S., Ford, C. H. J., and Newman, C. E. (1982). *Protides Biol. Fluids* **29,** 641–644.

Yang, L.-Y., and Drewinko, B. (1980). *JNCI, J. Natl. Cancer Inst.* **65,** 397–403.

CHAPTER 18

Monoclonal Antibodies as Carriers for Immunotargeting of Drugs

Ruth Arnon and Esther Hurwitz

Department of Chemical Immunology
The Weizmann Institute of Science
Rehovot, Israel

Chemotherapy constitutes a major therapeutic approach for the treatment of cancer. Its major drawback is that anti-cancer drugs, although destructive to the tumor cells, are also toxic to normal cells. Therefore, in order to avoid severe damage to normal tissue, doses of drugs which are borderline for killing the cancer cells have to be administered, thus diminishing the effectivity of the treatment. A possible way to overcome this difficulty is by employing affinity chemotherapy, which is based on the biological recognition between a target cell and a site-specific drug counterpart. The target molecule on the cell can be a defined antigen expressed preferentially on the tumor cell or a specific surface receptor; it could constitute an integral membrane component or a compound produced by the cells and only transiently expressed on its membrane.

Therapy by antibodies against tumor-associated antigens, alone or by antibodies and complement, has as a rule not been successful, with the exception of one reported case (Miller *et al.*, 1982) in which a cancer

MONOCLONAL ANTIBODIES FOR CANCER
DETECTION AND THERAPY

patient was cured using monoclonal antibody against its own tumor. The monoclonal antibodies in this case were specific toward the patient's idiotypic protein and their administration led to reduction in tumor load and remission that lasted several years. Similar treatment of several other patients did not lead to the same results. It thus may be assumed that in general, antibodies directed toward tumor cells, though capable of recognizing the cells, are not cytotoxic *in vivo* and hence do not provide an effective means of treatment. The combination of antibody therapy and chemotherapy could be useful, since binding of an anti-cancer drug to a given anti-cancer antibody would combine their cellular and molecular modes of action. Thus, the antibody would selectively deliver the cytotoxic drug to the target cell.

In our studies we attempted to use conjugates, in which drugs were linked chemically to the antibody carrier, for immunotargeting in several experimental tumor systems. We have attached drugs such as daunomycin (Hurwitz *et al.*, 1975, 1976, 1980; Levy *et al.*, 1975; Tsukada *et al.*, 1982a), adriamycin (Hurwitz *et al.*, 1983), cytosine arabinoside (Hurwitz *et al.*, 1984), 5-fluorouridine (Hurwitz *et al.*, 1984), and methotrexate (Arnon and Hurwitz, 1983) to the various anti-tumor directed antibodies, usually *via* a polymeric "bridge" or "handle," consisting mostly of derivatives of dextran. In addition, we have used derivatives in which platinum was directly complexed to the antibodies (Hurwitz *et al.*, 1982), in an attempt to reconstruct *cis*-platinum structure on antibody conjugates. In the preparation of all these conjugates the prerequisite was to acertain the activities of both the antibodies and the drug. In these studies, which are summarized in several recent reviews (Arnon and Hurwitz, 1983; Arnon and Sela, 1982a,b), we showed that it is possible to prepare such drug–antibody conjugates that can penetrate the tumor cells and are considerably less toxic than the corresponding free drugs. As a result, these conjugates were effective both *in vitro* and *in vivo* against the respective tumors.

In order for an antibody to be a suitable drug carrier it has to be highly specific and possess high binding affinity and avidity toward the tumor target cell. When conservative polyclonal antibodies are employed, exhaustive absorption by normal tissue is necessary to ensure the required specificity. The technique of monoclonal antibody preparation (Kohler and Milstein, 1976) by cell fusion has made it possible to obtain monospecific antibodies against tumor cells by direct screening for clones which produce highly reactive and specific antibodies. On the other hand, polyclonal antibodies often show higher avidity to the tumor cells due to their simultaneous reactivity with many antigenic determinants. Their polyclonality also makes them less sensitive to loss of antibody activity during the drug-binding procedures. In our laboratory we have been engaged in drug targeting by antibodies of both polyclonal and monoclonal nature. This chapter compares the results obtained and evaluates the advantages and disadvantages of both types of antibodies.

I. THE PREPARATION OF ANTIBODIES

Polyclonal antibodies against whole cells or against tumor-associated antigens were prepared by immunizing either rabbits, goats, or mice, and subsequent adsorption of the antisera with normal tissues and cells of the relevant mouse strain (Hurwitz *et al.*, 1978, 1979). In most cases the IgG fraction of the antiserum was used, but when possible, the antibodies were affinity purified on immunoadsorbents consisting of fixed tumor cells.

Hybridomas were prepared by fusing spleen cells of immunized mouse or rat cells with NS1 or NSO myeloma cells (Eshhar *et al.*, 1980). For the preparation of antibodies against whole tumor cells, adoptive transfers of immune spleen cells preceded the hybridization; the immune spleen cells were transferred into irradiated recipients which received an additional antigenic challenge (Hadas *et al.*, 1984). Antibodies against purified surface antigens were prepared by direct fusion to the myeloma cells.

The screening for antibody activity was performed by solid phase radioimmunoassay with whole tumor cells (Huang *et al.*, 1975), which were attached to the wells of a soft microtiter plate by drying followed by formaldehyde fixation. The antibody-containing supernatants were then assayed indirectly using ^{125}I-labeled second antibody. For the detection of antibodies against tumor-associated antigens, reverse solid phase radioimmunoassay was used. For that purpose the second antibody was bound to the wells of the microtiter plates, reacted with the antibody-containing supernatant and detected by the use of ^{125}I-labeled antigen. A more detailed analysis following the screening involved direct binding assays with antibodies labeled *in vitro* by the incorporation of $[^{35}S]$- or $[^{75}Se]$methionine.

II. DRUG CONJUGATION PROCEDURES

As mentioned above, conjugates of several drugs were used in our investigations, using the most suitable method for coupling of each drug, as follows: *Daunomycin* was linked to antibodies via dextran-T10 (MW 10,000). The dextran, oxidized by sodium periodate (Hurwitz *et al.*, 1978; Bernstein *et al.*, 1978), was reacted first with daunomycin and then with the antibodies. The coupling, most probably Schiff base formation between the aldehyde groups on the oxidized dextran and the amino groups on the drug and the antibody, was stabilized by partial reduction with sodium borohydride (Arnon and Hurwitz, 1983). *Adriamycin* was bound via a bridge of carboxymethyldextran hydrazide (Hurwitz *et al.*, 1983), utilizing the carbonyl side-chain group on the drug rather than the aminosugar (Hurwitz *et al.*, 1980). The antibody was attached to the dextran hydrazide derivative by cross-linking with glutaraldehyde. Recently we attached adriamycin to monoclonal anti-Thy-1.1 antibodies *via* periodate–oxidate dextran T40 (MW 40,000), similar to the method of coupling of daunomycin. The conjugate was stable at neutral pHs without any reduction process. *Cytosine 1-β-D-arabinofuranoside* (ARA-c) was bound via dextran T10 using a procedure similar to that of the daunomycin bonding, differing only in the reduction step, which was performed by sodium cyanoborohydride in equimolar amount to the periodate (Hurwitz *et al.*, 1984). *Methotrexate* was attached via a copolymer of glutamic acid and lysine (Glu : Lys 4.7 : 1, MW 18,700) by two steps with water-soluble carbodiimide (Arnon and Sela, 1982a). *Platinum* was complexed to the antibodies by direct interaction with the Pt salt K_2PtCl_4 (Hurwitz *et al.*, 1982). In more recent experiments, complexing of Pt to antibodies via polymeric bridges was also attempted.

The extent of drug binding in the different conjugates varied from 25 to 50 mol/mol when antibodies of the IgG class were employed, to 250 to 500 mol/mol for IgM antibodies. Each conjugate was evaluated for its antibody activity as well as for the pharmacological activity of the drug, the latter being determined by inhibition of either RNA or DNA synthesis in various cells ([^{3}H]thymidine, [^{3}H]uridine, or [^{3}H]deoxyuridine incorporation). In most conjugates the drug activity was effectively preserved, and the antibody activity, while diminished to 50 to 70% of its original value, was sufficiently high to enable specific recognition of the relevant tumor cells.

In the following we describe the results achieved in our laboratory with various experimental tumor systems, using drug conjugates of monoclonal antibodies. When available, results obtained with equivalent conjugates of polyclonal antibodies in the same tumor system are described for comparison.

III. THE YAC LYMPHOMA

The Yac lymphoma is a Moloney virus-induced tumor (Klein and Klein, 1964) growing in ascitic or subcutaneous form in A/J mice. In early experiments with this tumor system we used daunomycin conjugates with polyclonal affinity-purified antibodies that were prepared in goats against membrane antigen obtained from the tumor cells by papain digestion. These antibodies were specific towards Yac cells as determined by complement-mediated cytotoxicity, but were nevertheless able to bind to normal splenocytes as well. In therapy studies (10^5 tumor cells transplanted ip and the treatment given 2 days later iv), daunomycin–dextran–anti-Yac at high doses was more effective than either free drug or antibodies alone. A similar effect, however, was sometimes obtained by using the drug conjugated to normal Ig or just to dextran. At lower drug doses, the specific conjugate was more effective than the non-specific conjugate (Fig. 1) but the free drug was also quite effective (preventing the development of the tumor in 60% of the mice).

In view of these results it was envisaged that antibodies with higher specificity might improve the efficacy of the drug–antibody conjugate. Monoclonal antibodies were prepared for this purpose by hybridization of spleen cells from BALB/c $\times$ A/J F_1 mice immunized with whole tumor cells. These antibodies, designated KH_{3-4}, which were of the IgM class, bound to Yac cells 10- to 50-fold better than to normal spleen cells (Fig. 2) and did not react with normal thymocytes or with lymph node cells. The effectivity of the KH_{3-4} dextran–daunomycin conjugate (containing 500 mol of daunomycin per mol antibody) was tested *in vivo* by comparison to the polyclonal goat anti-Yac conjugate described previously. In this experiment (Table I) the tumor was transplanted subcutaneously rather than intraperitoneally. The subcutaneous tumor was quite responsive to daunomycin, and a dose of 12 mg/kg of the free drug led to 60% long-term survival. The drug conjugate with the purified polyclonal goat anti-Yac antibodies was very effective and, when used in the same dose, led to 100% long-term survival. This high effect could be due to the fact that the subcutaneous tumor releases less tumor-associated

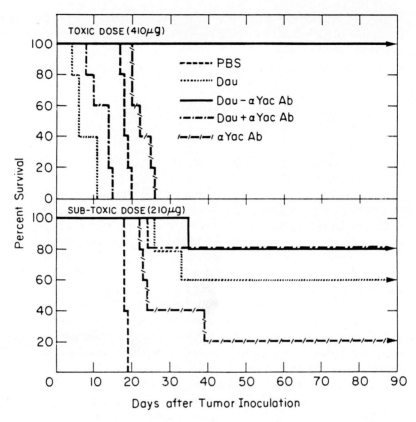

Fig. 1. The therapeutic effect of a daunomycin–anti-Yac conjugate. Yac cells (10^5) were injected ip. Treatment by daunomycin, daunomycin–anti-Yac, a mixture of daunomycin and anti-Yac, anti-Yac, and phosphate-buffered saline (PBS), followed 2 days later by the same route.

antigens into the circulation. However, the daunomycin conjugate of the more specific monoclonal antibody was less effective, and only at a higher drug dose (25 mg/kg), at which a nonspecific Ig–drug conjugate was similarly beneficial. The lower efficacy of this monoclonal antibody as drug carrier could be due to its IgM nature (Kirch and Hammerling, 1981) or to a lower avidity toward the tumor cells. Indeed, experiments of inhibition of binding to cells indicate that the polyclonal antibodies in this case possess higher avidity, which could be the result of their specificity toward many determinants on the tumor cells. The latter argumentation may imply that this could be a general phenomenon unless the monoclonal antibodies are directed toward a particularly abundant antigen on the tumor cells.

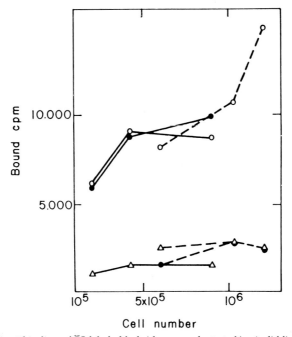

Fig. 2. The direct binding of ^{35}S-labeled hybridoma products to Yac (solid lines) or normal A/J spleen (broken lines) live cells. Specific anti-Yac, KH$_{3-4}$ (●), nonspecific anti-Yac KH$_{2-1}$ (○), and a nonrelevant hybridoma product (△).

IV. THE LEWIS LUNG CARCINOMA

Lewis lung carcinoma (3LL) is originally a spontaneous tumor (Sugiura and Stock, 1955) which is maintained in C57BL mice. It grows at the transplantation site subcutaneously as a local primary tumor and, 2–3 weeks later, develops as visible metastatic foci in the lungs. Enhanced metastasis was obtained by injection of the tumor into the footpad and amputation of the tumoric leg (Gorelik *et al.*, 1978), or by injection of the tumor intravenously. In this system as well, experiments were performed with drug conjugates of both polyclonal (rabbit and syngeneic mice) and monoclonal antibodies. The latter were the product of a rat–mouse hybridoma prepared by fusion of mouse myeloma cells with rat immune splenocytes (Hadas *et al.*, 1984) since, in this tumor system, mouse–mouse hybridizations either with syngeneic (C57BL) or with F$_1$ (C57BL × DBA/2) splenocytes did not lead to the production of specific anti-tumor antibodies.

TABLE I

THE *IN VIVO*[a] EFFECT OF MONOCLONAL ANTI-YAC AS A DRUG CARRIER AND ITS COMPARISON TO DAUNOMYCIN–GOAT ANTI-YAC

Treatment[b]	Drug (mg/kg)	Antibody (mg/kg)	Median (days)	Survival %
PBS	—	—	24	0
Daunomycin	12			60
	17			60
Dau-dex-KH$_{3-4, 10}$[c]	12.5	100	23	20
	20	200		83
Dau-dex-X63[d]	12.5	75	25	20
	22	250		80
Dau + KH$_{3-4, 10}$	12.5	250	28	0
Dau-dex-G anti-Yac(Ab)[e]	12.5	50		100
Dau + G anti-Yac(Ab)	12.5	100		60
G-anti-Yac(Ab)		100	23	20

[a] Yac cells, 10^5 in 0.5 ml PBS were injected subcutaneously into male A/J mice (10 weeks old).

[b] Treatment was given iv on day 3.

[c] KH$_{3-4, 10}$, an anti-Yac IgM obtained from a cloned mouse–mouse hybridoma grown in ascites form and precipitated from the ascitic fluid by ammonium sulfate (40% saturation).

[d] X63, the original IgG produced by the NS1 myeloma.

[e] G-anti-Yac (Ab). The antisera were produced in a goat injected with a soluble papain digest of Yac cells. The antibodies were purified by absorption on and elution from glutaraldehyde-fixed Yac cells.

The polyclonal antibodies prepared against the primary tumor were found to react with the primary and metastatic tumor cells to the same extent and showed almost no reactivity with normal syngeneic cells. Furthermore, their daunomycin conjugates demonstrated prominent *in vitro* efficacy on both types of tumor cells. However, *in vivo* these antibodies showed a relatively low specific distribution factor (less than twofold) in the lungs as compared to other organs (Fig. 3A). The monoclonal antibodies (6B), on the other hand, which reacted *in vitro* almost exclusively with the 3LL cells, showed much more effective homing. As shown in Fig. 3B these antibodies showed strong anti-lung tissue reactivity, but they accumulated in the lungs of normal mice as well. All the same, their specific accumulation factor in the metastatic lungs of tumor-bearing mice was approximately 30, as compared to all other organs.

These monoclonal antibodies served as carriers for attachment of daunomycin, adriamycin, and methotrexate. These drugs are effective inhibitors of the 3LL cells *in vitro* (Table II), but are uneffective against the 3LL tumor or its metastasis *in vivo*. We hoped that in view of the very

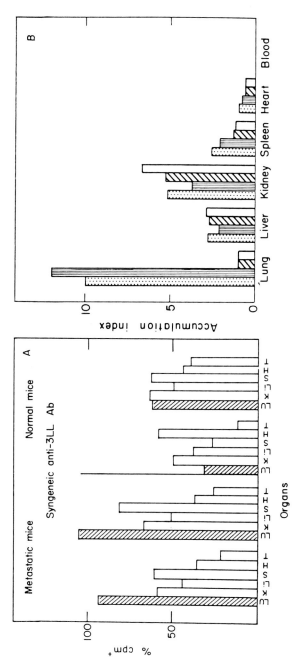

Fig. 3. (A) The *in vivo* distribution of conventional syngeneic antibodies to 3LL cells. Syngeneic anti-3LL, ^{125}I-labeled (obtained by absorption on and elution from formalin-fixed 3LL cells) was injected to normal or metastasis-bearing mice (10 days after the amputation of the local tumor). After 24 hr the mice were killed and the ^{125}I content of various tissues was determined. Lungs (Lu), kidneys (K), liver (Li), spleen (S), heart (H), and thymus (T). The results are presented as percent counts per minute (counts per minute per gram tissue × 100/cpm in 1 ml blood). (B) The *in vivo* distribution of [75Se]methionine-anti-3LL and anti-DNP. The labeled antibodies were injected to the mice as in A. The distribution of the label was determined after 20 hr and presented as the accumulation index (counts per minute per gram tissue/counts per minute per milliliter blood). Columns: Anti-3LL (6B) in metastatic mice (stippled) in normal mice (vertical lines). Anti-DNP in metastatic mice (diagonal lines) in normal mice (clear).

TABLE II

THE DRUG ACTIVITY IN CONJUGATES OF HYBRIDOMA PRODUCTS (ANTI-3LL, 6B, AND ANTI-YAC, KH$_{3-4}$)

Drug dose (µg/ml)	Inhibition of [^{3}H]uridine incorporation (%)				
	Daunomycin	Adriamycin	Dau-dex-KH	Dau-dex-6B	Adr-dex-6B
A. Daunomycin and adriamycin conjugates					
2.5	58				
5	75	84		19	13
10	94			41	48
25			29	61	59
50	98	95	40	80	64
100			50		

Drug dose (µg/ml)	Inhibition of [^{3}H]deoxyuridine incorporation (%)		
	MTX	MTX p(G-L)-KH$_{3-4}$	MTX p(G-L)-6B
B. Methotrexate conjugates			
0.25	39		27
0.5	59	60	74
1.0	70	79	94
2.5	89		93
5	99	91	97

high specific accumulation of the monoclonal antibodies in the lungs, the localization of their drug conjugates at the tumor site may increase their efficacy. However, the conjugates, although inhibitory to the 3LL cells *in vitro*, were not significantly effective *in vivo*. The failure of the conjugates *in vivo* could be due to the ability of the antibody in the conjugate to attach to normal lung cells, as well as to the tumor cells. Another possibility is that this tumor is resistant to these drugs and their delivery to the site did not overcome this resistance. Further studies, with conjugates of tumor-specific monoclonal antibodies and more effective drugs against this tumor, might clarify these points.

V. *IN VITRO* STUDIES WITH HUMAN NEUROBLASTOMA

A mouse hybridoma antibody reactive with a human neuroblastoma cell line LA-N-I was developed by Seeger *et al.* (1982) by immunizing mice with homogenates of first trimester fetal brain. The resulting hy-

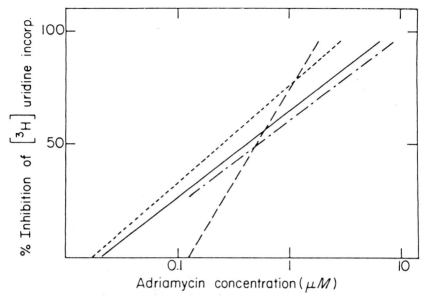

Fig. 4. Inhibition of [³H]uridine incorporation by adriamycin–antibody and Ig conjugates. Adriamycin (------), dextran-hydrazone (dex) (———), adriamycin-dex-Ig X63 (– – –), or adriamycin-dex antineuroblastoma (—·—) was added to neuroblastoma cells, 2 × 10⁴ per well, 20 hr after their plating. Three hours after incubation with the drugs [³H]uridine was added and the plate was reincubated for another 20 hr.

bridoma antibody (390) was characterized as being an anti-Thy-1 antibody. Thy-1, a differentiation antigen, is expressed by many tumors to variable degrees and is scarcely expressed on normal cells, with the exception of fetal and adult brain cells. Thus, it seemed to be a suitable antibody as a drug carrier.

Adriamycin, a drug of choice in the conventional chemotherapy of neuroblastoma, was attached to the anti-Thy-1 antibody via a carboxymethyl–dextran hydrazide bridge (Hurwitz *et al.*, 1980), and the drug activity of the conjugate was tested *in vitro* by the inhibition of labeled nucleic acid incorporation. The results (Fig. 4) showed that the specific conjugate retained the full drug activity, and at low doses it was an even more effective inhibitor for RNA synthesis than the control. The antibody activity in the conjugate, as determined by indirect fluorescence binding in a cell sorter, was also similar to that of the unmodified antibody. As a result, the specific anti-Thy-1 drug conjugates exhibited high specific cytotoxic effect over periods of 5- to 72-hr incubations. Toward the neuroblastoma tumor cells, they were more effective than the nonspecific conjugates, but showed no cytotoxicity to a control myeloid leukemia cell (M-562).

TABLE III

EFFECT OF ADRIAMYCIN AND ADRIAMYCIN CONJUGATED TO 390 MONOCLONAL ANTIBODY ON NEUROBLASTOMA CELL CYCLE[a]

Treatment	Hours in culture	G_1 (%)	S (%)	G_2 (%)
Anti-Thy-1	24	42.1 ± 10.9	42.9 ± 12.6	14.9 ± 2.9
	48	38.4 ± 9.4	46.2 ± 10.8	18.9 ± 7.4
	24	51.1 ± 4	29.7 ± 5	19.2 ± 2
Adriamycin	48	56.1 ± 9.2	12.4 ± 6.6	31.5 ± 8.1
Adriamycin-dex-anti-Thy-1	24	36.1 ± 2	36.4 ± 4.1	27.5 ± 6.8
	48	46.4 ± 6.1	16.9 ± 6.1	37.6 ± 4.1

[a]Neuroblastoma cells, 10^5/well in 100 μl, were incubated with anti-Thy-1, adriamycin, and adriamycin–antibody conjugate. After the appropriate incubation time the cells from three wells for each treatment were removed and subjected to DNA distribution studies.

The method we used for evaluating the activity of the drug–antibody conjugates was to measure their effect on the cell cycle traverse of neuroblastoma cells. The effect of the specific antibody conjugate on the DNA distributions of the LA-N-1 cells was determined in comparison to the perturbations caused by the free drug (Table III). The normal distribution of DNA in neuroblastoma cells after periods of 24 and 48 hr was not altered by the anti-Thy-1 antibody alone; the cells were almost evenly divided between G_1 and S phases and 15–19% were in G_2 + M. Treatment with adriamycin caused some retardation in G_1, a reduction in S phase, and an accumulation of cells in G_2, which probably interferes with subsequent cell mitosis. The adriamycin–anti-Thy-1 treatment of log phase, nonsynchronized cells caused a similar reduction in S phase and mainly an even higher accumulation in G_2 phase than that caused by the free drug. These effects further increased after 48 hr incubation, and might imply that the adriamycin–antibody conjugate is a better cytotoxic agent.

VI. A DRUG CONJUGATE WITH MONOCLONAL ANTIBODIES TO HUMAN-ACTIVATED T CELLS

We tried to employ an antibody–drug conjugate in another tumor system, i.e., a human T cell line (Peer) derived from an acute lymphocytic leukemia patient. A monoclonal antibody toward these cells, denoted V1 (obtained from Drs. Varon and Eshhar) reacted specifically with ac-

TABLE IV

INHIBITIONS OF [³H]-THYMIDINE INCORPORATION INTO PEER CELLS BY ARA-c-V1-10[a]

	Inhibition of [³H]-thymidine incorporation (%)		
μg/ml	ARA-c	ARA-c-dex-V1-10	ARA-c-dex-normal IgM
0.0016	30	23	0
0.0033	51	55	13
0.0165	79	86	49
0.4125	99	99	99

[a]Peer cells 5 × 10⁴/well per 100 μl were plated per well and ARA-c or its antibody derivative were added in 50-μl amounts per well.

tivated T cells and with a few cell lines derived from patients with ALL (Bentwich *et al.*, 1982). To this antibody we have bound the drug 1-β-D-arabinofuranosylcytosine (ARA-c), which is clinically effective in ALL therapy. The conjugate maintained its full original drug activity as assessed by the inhibition of drug [³H]thymidine incorporation (Table IV) and was more effective in this inhibition than a conjugate prepared with a normal mouse Ig. On the other hand, the antibody activity of several preparations of the drug–antibody conjugate, as tested by its binding to Peer cells, was markedly reduced (25–35% of the original binding activity). It is thus apparent that this particular monoclonal antibody is not amenable to modification and drug attachment. Such a phenomenon is one of the drawbacks of monoclonal antibodies and would not occur in polyclonal antibodies with heterogeneous antibody population, which differ from each other not only in the specificity but also in other structural aspects.

VII. ANTI-α-FETOPROTEIN REACTIVE AGAINST RAT HEPATOMA

Rat hepatoma (AH 66) is an α-fetoprotein (AFP)-producing hepatoma maintained in Donryu rats (Isaka *et al.*, 1976). In the case of this tumor system as well, we prepared drug conjugates of both polyclonal and monoclonal antibodies that can be comparatively evaluated. Horse polyclonal antibodies against rat AFP were shown to recognize the tumor cells *in vitro* and to localize on them *in vivo* (Koji *et al.*, 1980). Monoclonal antibodies to rat AFP (312) were prepared by immunizing BALB/c mice

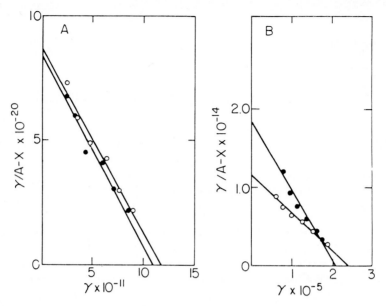

Fig. 5. The association constants of the antibodies to rat AFP. The equilibrium association constants were determined by the binding of the ^{125}I-labeled horse and ^{125}I-labeled monoclonal antibodies to AFP. (A) Experiment done with secreted antigen and the constants were $7.4 \times 10^8 \, M^{-1}$ and $7.1 \times 10^8 \, M^{-1}$ for horse anti-AFP (●) and monoclonal anti-AFP (○), respectively. (B) The antigen was membrane-bound AFP and the constants were $8.1 \times 10^8 M^{-1}$ and $4.7 \times 10^8 M^{-1}$ for horse anti-AFP (●) and monoclonal anti-AFP (○), respectively. The constants were derived from a plot of $\gamma/A - X$ versus γ, in which A is the starting concentration of the antibody, X is the molar concentration of bound antibody, and γ is the number of antibody molecules bond per antigen. (From Tsukada *et al.*, 1982b.)

with rat AFP and hybridizing their spleen cells with mouse myeloma cells. The binding of the monoclonal antibody [the Ig fraction from the ascitic fluid precipitated by 45% saturated $(NH_4)_2SO_4$] to isolated rat AFP or to hepatoma cells was compared with that of the horse anti-AFP. The equilibrium association constants of the two antibodies were determined (Tsukada *et al.*, 1982b) by using ^{125}I-labeled antibodies and studying their binding to AFP attached to paper disks, or by performing reverse-radioimmunoassay and using [^{125}I]AFP. Similar constants were obtained for both types of antibodies with secreted AFP (Fig. 5A) and with whole tumor cells (Fig. 5B).

Daunomycin was linked via oxidized dextran T10 to both the monoclonal and the polyclonal antibodies against AFP. The drug activity in different preparations of the conjugates, as determined by the inhibition

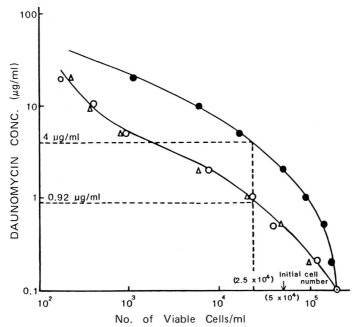

Fig. 6. The specific cytotoxicity of the daunomycin–antibody conjugates. The number of viable cells was determined after 48 hr of incubation of 5×10^4 hepatoma cells (initial cell number shown by arrow) with free daunomycin (●) or its anti-AFP conjugates: daunomycin–dextran–horse anti-AFP (○) and daunomycin–dextran–monoclonal mouse anti-AFP (△). The concentrations needed for 50% killing were compared. (From Tsukada *et al.*, 1982b.)

of [^{3}H]thymidine incorporation, amounted to 60–100% of the free drug activity. The antibody-binding activity was also fully sustained in the conjugates, as determined by their reaction with ^{125}I-labeled antigen.

In their specific cytotoxicity toward the hepatoma cells *in vitro*, the conjugates of daunomycin with the horse anti-AFP and the monoclonal antibodies were also of similar activity, both demonstrating higher efficacy than free daunomycin. Thus, as shown in Fig. 6, when 5×10^4 hepatoma cells were incubated for 4 hr at 37°C with the various drug preparations, the concentration of free daunomycin that caused 50% killing was 4 μg/ml, whereas the same extent of toxicity was obtained with only 0.92 μg/ml of either antibody–daunomycin conjugate.

The most important aspect of this study was to evaluate the chemotherapeutic effectivity of the drug–antibody conjugates on tumor-bearing rats. For that purpose, rats challenged ip with 10^4 AH66 cells were treated with a multiple dose of the specific drug–antibody conjugates and with

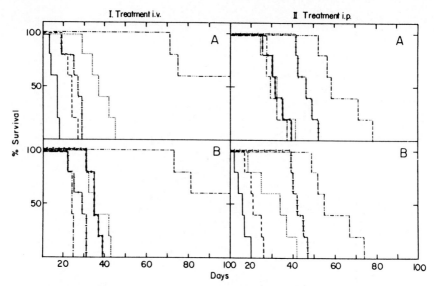

Fig. 7. The therapeutic effectivity of the daunomycin–antibody conjugates. AH66 hepatoma cells were injected into rats at 10^4 cells per rat. Treatments were given 3, 5, 7, 9, and 11 days later, iv (A and B) at a dose of 200 μg of daunomycin and 2 mg of antibody per injection per rat or ip (C and D) at a dose of 40 μg of daunomycin and 400 μg of antibody per injection per rat. (A and C), the specific drug conjugate of horse anti-AFP or this antibody alone; (B and D) the conjugates of hybridoma anti-AFP or this antibody alone. PBS (——); normal horse immunoglobulin (– – – –); anti-rat AFP (• • •); daunomycin (– – – – –); daunomycin–dextran (x-x-x); a mixture of daunomycin and antibodies to rat AFP (⊢—⊢—); daunomycin–anti-rat AFP (–• •– •–). (From Tsukada *et al.*, 1982b.)

the controls which included antibody and drug alone, mixture of the two, as well as a conjugate of drug–dextran and a nonrelevant immunoglobulin. The treatments were given five times, from the third day after the tumor injection, on alternate days, and were administered either iv or ip.

As shown in Fig. 7, the efficacy of the monoclonal anti-AFP and its drug conjugate was similar to that of conventional horse anti-rat AFP and its drug derivative. Both conjugates were more effective than the free drug and antibody, or even than the mixture of daunomycin and antibody, which caused only slight delay in the median survival time by both routes of treatment. An interesting finding is that the ip treatment was the least effective of the two—when so administered the specific conjugate prolonged the survival time but did not prevent death from the tumor. The reason for the lower effectivity of the ip treatment is not clear, particularly in view of the fact that the ip is the more direct route for reaching the ip tumor. A possible explanation is that via this route the free drug is more toxic and consequently can be administered only in lower doses. Hence, the total amount of conjugate that was injected in this experiment, which is five times lower than that given iv, might be insufficient and too low to be effective.

On the other hand, the drug–antibody conjugate injected iv was much more effective and led to remarkable life prolongation as well as to 60% long-term survival. In this case as well, a close similarity was observed between the chemotherapeutic effect of the drug conjugate with the monoclonal antibody and that of the conventional polyclonal antibody. The high efficacy demonstrated by both types of antibody–drug conjugates when injected intravenously may indicate specific homing to the target and confirms a previous observation (Koji *et al.*, 1980) that the horse antibodies to AFP are capable of specifically concentrating at the tumor site. The presumable high abundance of the tumor-specific antigen AFP on the hepatoma cell is probably a decisive parameter which facilitates an efficient immunotargeting in this case.

VIII. SUMMARY AND CONCLUSIONS

In the aforegoing sections we described the results achieved to date in our laboratory by using monoclonal antibodies as carriers of drugs for the purpose of immunotargeting. In tumor systems for which polyclonal antibodies had been previously obtained, and similarly investigated, a comparison between them and the respective monoclonal antibodies was made. Chemotherapeutic drugs such as daunomycin, adriamycin, methotrexate, and cytosine arabinoside were bound to the monoclonal antibodies and the various drug conjugates were evaluated for their efficacy *in vitro* and *in vivo*. All the conjugates retained the full pharmacological activity of the drug and were at least as effective *in vitro* as their corresponding free drugs. As for the antibody activity—with the exception of one, the drug conjugates with the monoclonal antibodies maintained their original antigen-binding capacity. Consequently, for most tumor systems including a rat hepatoma, mouse lung carcinoma (3LL) and a human neuroblastoma line, an *in vitro* specific cytotoxicity toward the tumor the cells to which the antibody was directed was demonstrated.

In the *in vivo* efficacy of the drug conjugates a more extensive variability was observed. For example, in the case of mouse lung carcinoma (3LL), conjugates of the polyclonal and even more so of the monoclonal antibody (directed to lung-associated antigen) exhibited efficient homing to the metastasized lungs. However, the resultant high drug concentration at the tumor site did not overcome the intrinsic ineffectivity of the tested drugs (Daunomycin, adriamycin, or methotrexate) against this tumor *in vivo*. Much more encouraging results were obtained for two other tumor systems. In a mouse T lymphoma (Yac), conjugates of both polyclonal and monoclonal antibodies had a beneficial effect, leading to prolongation of life as well as to long-term survival. However, in this case, the monoclonal antibodies were less effective drug carriers than the polyclonal purified goat antibodies. This could stem from the IgM nature of these particular antibodies, from their low avidity, or from the paucity of the specific antigenic determinants on the surface of the tumor cell. In a rat hepatoma, monoclonal and horse polyclonal antibodies against rat AFP had similar binding affinities for either the immunogen or the whole tumor cell. Both drug–antibody conjugates were effective *in vitro* and *in vivo*, indicating that both types of antibodies worked equally well as drug carriers, leading to very efficient therapeutic effects in tumor-bearing rats. The high efficacy of the monoclonal antibodies in this system could be expected in view of the abundance of AFP on the hepatoma cell surface.

The main conclusions from these studies are that antibodies may indeed serve as carriers for anti-cancer drugs for the purpose of immunotargeting. The monoclonal antibodies have both advantages and disadvantages over the polyclonal ones. They are advantageous since they can be readily obtained by immunization with whole tumor cells, including neoplasms which do not bear a known tumor marker; they can also be prepared from naturally existing antibody-producing peripheral blood lymphocytes by *in vitro* culturing procedures, thus leading to human–human hybridomas; they are uniformly specific and, if directed against an abundant antigen, may show very high efficiency. Their uniformity can be of a disadvantage if they are directed toward a scarce antigen on the tumor cell, or if the drug-binding modification leads to loss of their reactivity. In such cases polyclonal antibodies may be superior. It is thus apparent that both polyclonal and monoclonal antibodies should be considered in future efforts toward immunotargeted chemotherapy.

REFERENCES

Arnon, R., and Hurwitz, E. (1983). *In* "Targeted Drugs" (E. P. Goldberg, ed), pp. 23–55. Wiley, New York.
Arnon, R., and Sela, M. (1982a). *Immunol. Rev.* **62,** 5–27.

Arnon, R., and Sela, M. (1982b). *Cancer Surv.* **1**, 429–449.

Bentwich, Z., Varon, D., Burstein, R., Goldblum, N., and Eshhar, Z. (1982). *Proc. Isr. Immunol. Soc.*, p. 7.

Bernstein, A., Hurwitz, E., Maron, R., Arnon, R., Sela, M., and Wilchek, M. (1978). *J. Natl. Cancer Inst. (U.S.)* **60**, 379–384.

Eshhar, Z., Ofarim, M., and Waks, T. (1980). *J. Immunol.* **124**, 775–780.

Gorelik, E., Segal, S., and Feldman, M. (1978). *Int. J. Cancer* **21**, 617–625.

Hadas, E., Hurwitz, E., and Eshhar, Z. (1984). *Int. J. Cancer* **33**, 369–374.

Huang, J. C.-C., Berczi, I., Froese, G., Tsay, H. M., and Sehon, A. H. (1975). *J. Natl. Cancer Inst. (U.S.)* **55**, 879–886.

Hurwitz, E., Levy, R., Maron, R., Wilchek, M., Arnon, R., and Sela, M. (1975). *Cancer Res.* **35**, 1175–1181.

Hurwitz, E., Maron, R., Arnon, R., and Sela, M. (1976). *Cancer Biochem. Biophys.* **1**, 197–202.

Hurwitz, E., Maron, R., Bernstein, A., Wilchek, M., Sela, M., and Arnon, R. (1978). *Int. J. Cancer* **21**, 747–755.

Hurwitz, E., Schechter, B., Arnon, R., and Sela, M. (1979). *Int. J. Cancer* **24**, 461–470.

Hurwitz, E., Wilchek, M., and Pitha, J. (1980). *J. Appl. Biochem.* **2**, 25–35.

Hurwitz, E., Kashi, R., and Wilchek, M. (1982). *JNCI, J. Natl. Cancer Inst.* **69**, 47–51.

Hurwitz, E., Arnon, R., Sahar, E., and Danon, Y. (1983). *Ann. N. Y. Acad. Sci.* **417**, 125–136.

Hurwitz, E., Kashi, R., Arnon, R., Wilchek, M., and Sela, M. (1985). *J. Med. Chem.* **28**, 137–140.

Isaka, H., Umehara, S., Yoshii, H., Tsukada, Y., and Hirai, H. (1976). *Gann* **67**, 131–135.

Kirch, M. E., and Hammerling, U. (1981). *J. Immunol.* **127**, 805–810.

Klein, E., and Klein, G. (1964). *J. Natl. Cancer Inst. (U.S.)* **32**, 547–568.

Kohler, G., and Milstein, C. (1976). *J. Immunol.* **6**, 511–519.

Koji, T., Ishii, N., Munehisa, T., Kusumoto, Y., Nakamura, S., Tamenishi, A., Hara, A., Kobayashi, K., Tsukada, Y., Nishi, S., and Hirai, H. (1980). *Cancer Res.* **40**, 3013–3015.

Levy, R., Hurwitz, E., Maron, R., Arnon, R., and Sela, M. (1975). *Cancer Res.* **35**, 1182–1186.

Miller, R. A., Moloney, D. G., Warnke, B. S., and Levy, R. (1982). *N. Engl. J. Med.* **306**, 517–522.

Seeger, R. C., Danon, Y. L., Rayner, S. A., and Hoover, F. (1982). *J. Immunol.* **128**, 983–989.

Sugiura, K., and Stock, C. C. (1955). *Cancer Res.* **15**, 38–51.

Tsukada, Y., Bischof, W. K.-D., Hibi, H., Hirai, H., Hurwitz, E., and Sela, M. (1982a). *Proc. Natl. Acad. Sci. U.S.A.* **79**, 621–625.

Tsukada, Y., Hurwitz, E., Kashi, R., Sela, M., Hibi, N., Hara, A., and Hirai, H. (1982b). *Proc. Natl. Acad. Sci. U.S.A.* **79**, 7896–7899.

Index

A

Active ester conjugation, of drugs with antibody, 351

Adenosine triphosphate, cellular content of, immunotoxins and, 275–276

Adrenal glands, radioimmunolocalisation of neuroblastoma and, 288

Adriamycin, 346, 366
  conjugation to antibody, 368
  cytotoxicity of, 321, 322
  potentiation of radiation effects and, 310–311

Affinity, of monoclonal antibodies for breast tissues, 6

Ammonium chloride
  cytotoxicity of immuno-A-chain-toxins and, 228, 232, 235, 245
  potentiation of WT-1-ricin A by, 255–256, 257

Animal studies
  efficacy of immuno-A-chain-toxins *in vivo*, 243–244
  of toxicity of immuno-A-chain-toxins, 241–242

Antibody
  administration regime, influence on tumour levels, 113–115
  alone, tumour therapy and, 34–38
  anti-mouse, development in patients, 36–37, 150, 155
  choice for preparation of conjugates
    biochemical considerations, 319–320
    monoclonal antibody 791T/36, 320–321

combinations of in clinical imaging, 191–192

demonstration of specific localisation with xenografts, 101–104

dose, relationship to localisation in xenografts, 115–116

equilibrium between tumour-localised and blood-borne, 116–117

gastrointestinal diseases and, 131–132
  labelling, 132–133
  purification, 132

to GD3 ganglioside, 26–27

interpretation of immunoscintigraphy and, 91

molecule, in radiolabelled antibody therapy, 306–307

neuroectodermal tumours and, 283

possible disadvantages of, 75

preparation of, 367

quantitative evaluation of localisation in xenografts
  equilibrium between tumour-localised and blood-borne antibody, 116–117
  influence of variations in antibody administration on localisation, 113–116
  influence of variations in tumour site and size on efficiency of localisation, 109–113
  kinetics of localisation of 791T/36 Fab fragments in xenografts, 118–120
  rate and extent of, 106–109

radiolabelled
  dosimetry of, 309–310

385